Low-Cholesterol Cookbook For Dummies®

Cheat Sheet

Smart Shopping Guidelines for Your Grocery List

You can take a big step towards feeding yourself quality foods if you make good choices at the supermarket. Here are some guidelines to set you on the right path:

- Check the ingredient list on labels and avoid products that contain partially hydrogenated oils or lots of added salt.

- Read labels for the saturated fat content of products to ensure that you're not underestimating the amount of fat.

- Buy low-fat and reduced-fat dairy products.

- Favour low-sodium, reduced-fat soups.

- To make sure that you're eating nutrient-rich, fresh produce, bring home only as many fruits and vegetables as you expect to eat within a few days. Shop little and often.

- Opt for organic meats, poultry, and produce when possible.

- Eat liver and kidneys, which are exceptionally high in cholesterol, only occasionally.

- Look for low-fat alternatives to fattier foods, such as reduced-fat sausage and lean mince.

- For the most flavour and nutrients, buy local and seasonal produce. Check out farmer's markets and farm shops, for example.

- If you must have a splurge food, such as rich premium vanilla ice cream, treat yourself to the very best available to fix your craving, and promise yourself you won't indulge again for a long time.

- Stock up on wholegrain breads, cereals, pastas, and antioxidant-rich sweet potatoes – the type of starchy foods that have minimal impact on blood glucose levels.

Fruits and Vegetables with the Most Antioxidant Power

When low-density lipoprotein (LDL) cholesterol (the 'bad' cholesterol) oxidises, it's more likely to lead to hardening and furring up of artery walls. All fruits and vegetables are rich sources of antioxidants and help prevent this. Look for fresh seasonal produce where possible. Here's a list of great foods to shop for, starting with the best:

- Blueberries
- Pomegranates
- Watercress
- Blackberries
- Kale
- Cranberries
- Raspberries
- Strawberries
- Broccoli
- Plums

Great Sources of Soluble Fibre

Soluble fibre helps soak up cholesterol and eliminate it from the body. Here are the ten sources that experts most commonly recommend, listed in alphabetical order. Make sure that you buy and eat these foods regularly:

- Asparagus
- Barley
- Broccoli
- Brussels sprouts
- Green beans
- Green peas
- Kidney beans
- Butter beans
- Oats and oatmeal
- Sweet potatoes

Wiley, the Wiley Publishing logo, For Dummies, the Dummies Man logo, the For Dummies Bestselling Book Series logo and all related trade dress are trademarks or registered trademarks of John Wiley & Sons, Inc., and/or its affiliates. All other trademarks are property of their respective owners.

Copyright © 2008 Wiley Publishing, Ltd. All rights reserved. Item 1401-0.

For more information about John Wiley & Sons, call (+44) 1243 779777.

For Dummies: Bestselling Book Series for Beginners

Low-Cholesterol Cookbook For Dummies®

Cheat Sheet

Foods You May Think You Shouldn't Have But Can

Controlling cholesterol is more about limiting saturated fat than cutting back on total fat intake, and cholesterol-containing foods are fine if you don't exceed your daily quota. So get ready to enjoy the following foods:

- Nuts such as macadamias, almonds, and walnuts, which are sources of heart-friendly oils.
- Wholegrains such as barley, rye, buckwheat, quinoa, brown rice, and wholewheat.
- An omega-3 enriched egg a few times a week and all the egg white you want.
- Cooking oils such as extra-virgin olive oil and grapeseed oil.
- Shellfish such as scallops and clams, which are both low in saturated fat.
- A little (150 millilitres) red wine every day.

Cholesterol Content in Typical Recipe Ingredients

To help you budget your cholesterol quota for the day, refer to this list of cholesterol amounts, in milligrams, in common recipe ingredients. Check with your doctor to determine your ideal daily cholesterol amount, so that you better know how to plan your meals. Most people are advised to keep their dietary cholesterol intake to between 20 milligrams and 300 milligrams per day.

- Almonds, walnuts, and macadamias (most recommended), and all other nuts, any amount: 0 milligrams cholesterol.
- Beef, stewed extra-lean minced, per 100 grams: 75 milligrams cholesterol.
- Broccoli (most recommended) and all vegetables, any amount: 0 milligrams cholesterol.
- Chicken breast, roast, skinless, per 100 grams: 82 milligrams.
- Eggs, large: 213 milligrams cholesterol.
- Milk, semi-skimmed, per 100 millilitres: 6 milligrams cholesterol.
- Parmesan cheese, grated, per 1 tablespoon: 4 milligrams cholesterol.
- Olive oil and other vegetable oils, any amount: 0 milligrams cholesterol.
- Salmon, grilled, per 100 grams: 60 milligrams cholesterol.
- Yogurt, low-fat, per 100 grams: 1 milligram cholesterol.

Saturated Fat Amounts in Common Foods

Limit the amount of saturated fat in your diet and know which items contain it and which don't, starting with this list of common foods. Check with your doctor or dietician to determine your 'acceptable' daily amount of saturated fat intake, and then adjust your menu accordingly. The usual guideline daily amount is no more than 20 grams saturated fat per day for women, and no more than 30 grams saturated fat per day for men.

- Beef, stewed, extra lean, minced, per 100 grams: 3.8 grams saturated fat.
- Butter, per 1 tablespoon: 7.6 grams saturated fat.
- Carrots, per 1 medium: 0 grams saturated fat.
- Chicken breast, roast, skinless, per 100 grams: 0.7 grams saturated fat.
- Chicken, dark meat, roast, skinless, per 100 grams: 2.0 grams saturated fat.
- Kidney beans, boiled, per 100 grams: 0.1 grams saturated fat.
- Milk, semi-skimmed, per 100 millilitres: 1.1 grams saturated fat.
- Milk, whole, per 100 millilitres: 2.5 grams saturated fat.
- Olive oil, per 1 tablespoon: 1.8 grams saturated fat.
- Cheddar cheese, per 100 grams: 22 grams saturated fat.

Low-Cholesterol Cookbook

FOR DUMMIES®

by Dr Sarah Brewer, GP,
and Dr Molly Siple, RD

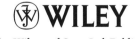

WILEY

A John Wiley and Sons, Ltd, Publication

Reading Borough Council

3412601025576 1

Low-Cholesterol Cookbook For Dummies®

Published by
John Wiley & Sons, Ltd
The Atrium
Southern Gate
Chichester
West Sussex
PO19 8SQ
England

E-mail (for orders and customer service enquires): cs-books@wiley.co.uk

Visit our Home Page on www.wiley.com

Copyright © 2008 John Wiley & Sons, Ltd, Chichester, West Sussex, England

Published by John Wiley & Sons, Ltd, Chichester, West Sussex

All Rights Reserved. No part of this publication may be reproduced, stored in a retrieval system or trans-mitted in any form or by any means, electronic, mechanical, photocopying, recording, scanning or other-wise, except under the terms of the Copyright, Designs and Patents Act 1988 or under the terms of a licence issued by the Copyright Licensing Agency Ltd, Saffron House, 6-10 Kirby Street, London EC1N 8TS, UK, without the permission in writing of the Publisher. Requests to the Publisher for permission should be addressed to the Permissions Department, John Wiley & Sons, Ltd, The Atrium, Southern Gate, Chichester, West Sussex, PO19 8SQ, England, or emailed to permreq@wiley.co.uk, or faxed to (44) 1243 770620.

Trademarks: Wiley, the Wiley Publishing logo, For Dummies, the Dummies Man logo, A Reference for the Rest of Us!, The Dummies Way, Dummies Daily, The Fun and Easy Way, Dummies.com and related trade dress are trademarks or registered trademarks of John Wiley & Sons, Inc. and/or its affiliates in the United States and other countries, and may not be used without written permission. All other trademarks are the property of their respective owners. Wiley Publishing, Inc., is not associated with any product or vendor mentioned in this book.

LIMIT OF LIABILITY/DISCLAIMER OF WARRANTY: THE PUBLISHER, THE AUTHOR, AND ANYONE ELSE INVOLVED IN PREPARING THIS WORK MAKE NO REPRESENTATIONS OR WARRANTIES WITH RESPECT TO THE ACCURACY OR COMPLETENESS OF THE CONTENTS OF THIS WORK AND SPECIFI-CALLY DISCLAIM ALL WARRANTIES, INCLUDING WITHOUT LIMITATION WARRANTIES OF FITNESS FOR A PARTICULAR PURPOSE. NO WARRANTY MAY BE CREATED OR EXTENDED BY SALES OR PRO-MOTIONAL MATERIALS. THE ADVICE AND STRATEGIES CONTAINED HEREIN MAY NOT BE SUITABLE FOR EVERY SITUATION. THIS WORK IS SOLD WITH THE UNDERSTANDING THAT THE PUBLISHER IS NOT ENGAGED IN RENDERING LEGAL, ACCOUNTING, OR OTHER PROFESSIONAL SERVICES. IF PRO-FESSIONAL ASSISTANCE IS REQUIRED, THE SERVICES OF A COMPETENT PROFESSIONAL PERSON SHOULD BE SOUGHT. NEITHER THE PUBLISHER NOR THE AUTHOR SHALL BE LIABLE FOR DAMAGES ARISING HEREFROM. THE FACT THAT AN ORGANIZATION OR WEBSITE IS REFERRED TO IN THIS WORK AS A CITATION AND/OR A POTENTIAL SOURCE OF FURTHER INFORMATION DOES NOT MEAN THAT THE AUTHOR OR THE PUBLISHER ENDORSES THE INFORMATION THE ORGANIZATION OR WEBSITE MAY PROVIDE OR RECOMMENDATIONS IT MAY MAKE. FURTHER, READERS SHOULD BE AWARE THAT INTERNET WEBSITES LISTED IN THIS WORK MAY HAVE CHANGED OR DISAPPEARED BETWEEN WHEN THIS WORK WAS WRITTEN AND WHEN IT IS READ. SOME OF THE EXERCISES AND DIETARY SUGGESTIONS CONTAINED IN THIS WORK MAY NOT BE APPROPRIATE FOR ALL INDIVIDU-ALS, AND READERS SHOULD CONSULT WITH A PHYSICIAN BEFORE COMMENCING ANY EXERCISE OR DIETARY PROGRAM.

For general information on our other products and services, please contact our Customer Care Department within the U.S. at 800-762-2974, outside the U.S. at 317-572-3993, or fax 317-572-4002.

For technical support, please visit www.wiley.com/techsupport.

Wiley also publishes its books in a variety of electronic formats. Some content that appears in print may not be available in electronic books.

British Library Cataloguing in Publication Data: A catalogue record for this book is available from the British Library

ISBN: 978-0-470-71401-0

Printed and bound in Great Britain by Bell & Bain Ltd., Glasgow

10 9 8 7 6 5 4 3 2 1

WILEY

About the Authors

Dr Sarah Brewer, GP, qualified from Cambridge University. Having worked as a GP and as a hospital doctor, she now specialises in nutritional medicine, taking an holistic approach to well-being. She is the author of 50 popular self-help books including the Natural Health Guru series, which you can find out about at www.naturalhealthguru.co.uk.

Dr Molly Siple, RD, is also the author of *Healing Foods For Dummies*. She writes a nutrition column that appears in *Natural Health* magazine and she has taught nutrition at the Southern California School of Culinary Arts in Pasadena, California. She is the coauthor, with Lissa DeAngelis, of *Recipes for Change,* which was a finalist nominee for the International Association of Culinary Professionals' Julia Child Cookbook Awards in the Health and Special Diet category. Ms. Siple also founded a successful catering business in New York City.

Publisher's Acknowledgements

We're proud of this book; please send us your comments through our Dummies online registration form located at www.dummies.com/register/.

Some of the people who helped bring this book to market include the following:

Acquisitions, Editorial, and Media Development

Development Editor: Steve Edwards

Content Editor: Jo Theedom

Commissioning Editor: Nicole Hermitage

Copy Editor: Martin Key

Proofreader: Andy Finch

Technical Editor: Sue Baic

Recipe Tester: Emily Nolan

Nutritional Analyst: Patty Santelli

Publisher: Jason Dunne

Executive Editor: Samantha Spickernell

Executive Project Editor: Daniel Mersey

Cover Photos: © Robert Morris/ GettyImages

Cartoons: Ed McLachlan

Composition Services

Project Coordinator: Lynsey Stanford

Layout and Graphics: Christin Swinford

Proofreader: Susan Moritz

Indexer: Cheryl Duksta

Brand Reviewer: Rev Mengle

READING BOROUGH LIBRARIES	
Askews	
641.5638	£15.99

Contents at a Glance

Recipes at a Glance

Cooking with Poultry, Fish, and Meat

Cooking with Cholesterol-Controlling Vegetables, Beans, and Grains

Serving up Sweet Finishes

Table of Contents

Introduction

*T*he first place to start in controlling cholesterol and lowering your risk of heart disease is with your lifestyle – in particular, by changing and improving what you eat. Sounds hard? Don't despair. The advice in this book is easy to swallow, as we're sure you'll find when you sample the delicious recipes!

Good nutrition is the most important foundation for good health. Nutrients in food work in amazing ways, on both the cellular and molecular level, to restore and maintain normal body function. The vitamins and minerals in the foods you read about in this book help to lower the level of 'bad' cholesterol in your body, while at the same time raising the good kind, and protecting your arteries from damage. And that's just the beginning of a long list of things they do. Of course, you've already taken the right first step by deciding to pick up this cookbook. Getting healthier starts in the kitchen!

The dishes in this book have been specially developed for the needs of someone whose cholesterol level is elevated. You may also need medication to treat your condition, but dietary and lifestyle changes alone often can improve your health enough to avoid the need for medicine. Do discuss your own situation with your doctor, though.

About This Book

The *Low-Cholesterol Cookbook For Dummies* provides a good overview of effective ways to control cholesterol levels, backed up by the experience of nutritionists and the results of scientific studies. Between the covers of this book, you can find the basics about fat and cholesterol in foods and about putting together meals that give you healthy amounts of both. You also discover lots of information on the various nutrients that lower 'bad' LDL (low density lipoprotein) cholesterol or raise the 'good' cholesterol, including soluble fibre which soaks up cholesterol and escorts it out of your body. To ensure that this book is as up-to-date as possible, it also touches on some newly recognised risk factors for heart disease that tie in with managing cholesterol.

As well as all this information, you can find chapters that each cover a category of food, such as vegetables, poultry, or fish, giving you basic tips for cooking these and identifying which ones best suit a cholesterol-lowering diet. Use these recommendations to write your shopping lists. The recipe pages are also packed with useful health advice, and the introductions to the recipes are filled with nutritional information on what you're about to cook.

These recipes are so delicious that you're guaranteed to want to eat them even putting their nutritional benefits aside! Each dish features nutritious, fresh, and natural foods that have beneficial effects on your cholesterol balance. Ingredients and procedures are kept as short and simple as possible, but without sacrificing their all-important flavour.

Conventions Used in This Book

The recipes in this book are complete, but may not spell out every detail of preparing and cooking the food. For example, certain steps and techniques in cooking are standard (such as removing shells from eggs), no matter what you're preparing. Take a quick look at the following list for points that apply to all the recipes:

- Organic foods aren't required but try to buy organic when you can, because they generally contain more antioxidants and nutrients that have a beneficial effect on cholesterol balance. If you use non-organic fruit and vegetables, wash and peel them first because this helps to remove any lingering agricultural chemicals.

- Fruits and vegetables should be washed under cold running water before using.

- Pepper is freshly ground black pepper. Invest in a pepper mill and give it a few cranks when you want pepper bursting with flavour.

- Fresh herbs are specified in many of the recipes for their bright, authentic flavour. But you can still make a recipe if you don't plan to use these by substituting dry herbs, using one-third the amount of fresh.

- Dairy products are low-fat.

- Eggs are large unless otherwise indicated.

- Canned goods are the low-sodium or no-added-salt versions.

- Food products don't contain any partially hydrogenated oils – check the labels.

- Keep pots uncovered unless we tell you to put on the lid.

Keep the following points about the recipes in mind:

- Most of the recipes are for four servings, an easy number to multiply or divide if you're feeding a crowd or you need just two servings for you and a friend. If the recipe makes any more or any fewer servings, we tell you so at the start.

- The nutrient information given at the end of each recipe is the amount of those items in a single serving. If you choose a larger serving size, you need to increase these numbers.

> ✔ If you can't find the exact ingredient that a recipe calls for in a specific amount, don't worry. A little more or less of an item is unlikely to ruin the dish, and – who knows – if you tinker slightly with the ingredients you may invent something that you like even better.

> ✔ The preparation time estimated for each recipe includes cutting veg and assembling ingredients and measuring them. Doing this before you start cooking also makes the whole process more efficient. And you don't discover that you're out of olive oil just at the moment you need to add some.

> ✔ The temperature for all recipes is in degrees Celsius.

Here are some non-recipe conventions to be aware of when reading this book:

> ✔ *Italic* text emphasises and highlights new words or terms that we define.

> ✔ **Boldfaced** text indicates the action part of numbered steps.

> ✔ Monofont highlights any web addresses we refer to.

> ☼ This tasty little tomato indicates a vegetarian recipe. You see it in the 'tabs' at the front of the recipe names in the recipe chapters.

What You're Not to Read

You don't have to read every single word we've written. We do recommend reading the regular paragraphs, however. These sections tell you the basics about controlling your cholesterol. But you don't have to read items marked with the Technical Stuff icon, which although interesting, give you more details and facts than you may want or need.

Sidebars are also optional reading. They provide supporting material on the subject of heart disease but aren't absolutely essential for finding out how to manage your cholesterol balance. And if you're already a pro at cooking, certainly skip over any cooking advice that you find obvious. But don't worry, you won't find instructions on how to boil a kettle.

Foolish Assumptions

We designed these recipes to suit a certain kind of cook:

> ✔ You're fairly handy in the kitchen. You know how to clean mushrooms without someone showing you what to do, and stuffing a chicken is no big deal; but making a *galantine* of chicken (a simmered and boned, stuffed chicken glazed in aspic) is beyond your scope, which is okay, because you won't find many elaborate cooking techniques in this book.

✔ You know how to shop for food. At least, you know your way around a supermarket, but when you wander into a health food store, or an ethnic supermarket, you spot all sorts of ingredients you don't even know exist. You soon will. Some recipes purposely include special ingredients, such as date sugar, Italian Prosciutto, and oil-cured olives in various recipes to lead you into a few delicatessens.

✔ You want dishes with personality and flavours that get your attention, start you salivating, and keep your taste-buds tingling.

✔ Fiddling with recipes is normal for you when you're trying out a dish, and you're comfortable doing so. You're the only person who knows how much garlic or onion you like, for example.

✔ You realise that spending time cooking at least one nutritious meal per day is an important part of taking care of your health and controlling your cholesterol balance. But you're not signing on for hours of fussing in the kitchen. A recipe that lets you get in and out in an hour or less is what you're after, or you at least prefer a dish you can throw together and cook without watching the pot.

How This Book Is Organised

We've organised the chapters in this book around ways of eating and types of food proven to improve cholesterol balance. Each part is divided into chapters that address specific subjects. The following sections describe the main themes in each part.

Part 1: Understanding Cholesterol Basics

These five chapters tell you what to eat and why, presenting a diet that features nutritious wholefoods, cuts back on saturated fat, and balances wholegrain carbohydrates with healthy oils. These pages are also packed with information on the nutritional components of the foods in the recipes and how they affect health in terms of biochemistry – the metabolic reactions occurring inside your cells. Useful shopping lists feature the best foods to eat.

You also get some tips on what to order in restaurants. If you intersperse cooking with eating out, you can refer to Chapter 4 to find out about the healthy foods you can order. And in Chapter 5, we give you some tips on setting up your kitchen and getting ready to cook.

Part II: Mastering the Beneficial Breakfast

Breakfast deserves its own section because it's usually the least nutritious meal of the day, and yet is also the most important. Oats are in the spotlight, of course, as a source of soluble fibre, but you also find information here about other healthy breakfast grains. In Chapter 7 on cooked breakfasts, we steer you in the direction of eating a little protein-rich fish before the sun is high in the sky. You also find out about the health benefits of eggs and how many are fine to eat per week. Chapter 8 tackles the issue of wanting breakfast but having no time to make it, and gives you ways to ensure that you eat something quick, yet healthy, to start your day right.

Part III: Making Your Day with Heart-Healthy Snacks and Starters

This part is especially helpful for beginner cooks, because you really can't go far wrong making soup or salads. These foods are forgiving, and so if you want to add ingredients or experiment with changing amounts, dabble away. These dishes include lots of cholesterol-controlling foods and also provide ways of eating red meat, because a little goes a long way in soups and salads. Chapters 11 and 12 give you a chance to have fun by putting together some tasty party foods – all sorts of healthy starters and nibbles that dress up easily to impress company.

Part IV: Cooking with Poultry, Fish, and Meat

Find out how to include animal protein in your diet without over-dosing on saturated fat and pre-formed cholesterol. It's all about knowing which cuts are the leanest and controlling portion sizes so you eat less over all. You find some good reference materials here that you can use as a guide on these matters, as well as recipes that taste rich and leave you feeling well-fed. If you like fish, with their ever-so-healthy oils, look for the preferred fish shopping list and guidelines on how frequently to eat seafood. Then you can start cooking up some delicious fishes for your dishes.

Part V: Cooking with Cholesterol-Controlling Vegetables, Beans, and Grains

This part enables you to explore many enticing ways to cook plant foods that are naturally low in saturated fat and cholesterol. Read the how-tos on buying, storing, and preparing grains, beans, and vegetables so that you become more confident about cooking these foods and start to eat them more often. You also find a shopping list of the top 10 vegetables that are good for health and cholesterol balance. Look out for the fine details on bean cookery and the useful chart giving recommended cooking times for different grains.

Part VI: Serving Up Sweet Finishes

This part gives you the chance to create some extra-special desserts. As well as great fruit puddings, you find guilt-free recipes for baking using healthy wholefood ingredients. You can even satisfy your sweet tooth with creamy concoctions based on tofu, fromage frais, and yogurt.

Part VII: The Part of Tens

This last part covers two important topics: healthy drinks to enjoy and ways to save money when you're stocking your kitchen with all these quality foods. We present the information in each chapter as a list of ten points.

Icons Used in This Book

Throughout the book, you'll see icons that mark the vital information in low-cholesterol cooking. Here's a listing of what they mean:

The tips in this book offer you useful shortcuts and information for food preparation, cooking, shopping, and more.

This icon alerts you to things you should avoid eating or that need to be handled in a specific way, or possible complications that come up while you're watching your diet or preparing certain foods.

This icon points out general suggestions about shopping, cooking, and eating that are good to keep in mind.

Text marked with a Technical Stuff icon gives you the low-down on nutrient and vitamin details and scientific studies and findings. You don't have to read this information to use the recipes in the book, but you may find it interesting.

Where to Go from Here

The nice thing about using a *For Dummies* book is that you can open it at any chapter and find all you need to know about a certain topic without having to flip to other sections. You may well have picked up this book right now simply because you're hungry and all you want to do is make yourself a salad, in which case just move to Chapter 10. After all, this is a cookbook, and people usually head for the recipes.

However, at some point, perhaps while munching through that healthy green salad, try poking your nose into the first three chapters, especially Chapter 1. This opening chapter gives you a complete overview of the main themes of the book. Also, at least skim over the recommended foods in Chapters 2 and 3. Then you don't just fulfil the role of a reader. You become the expert!

Part I
Understanding Cholesterol Basics

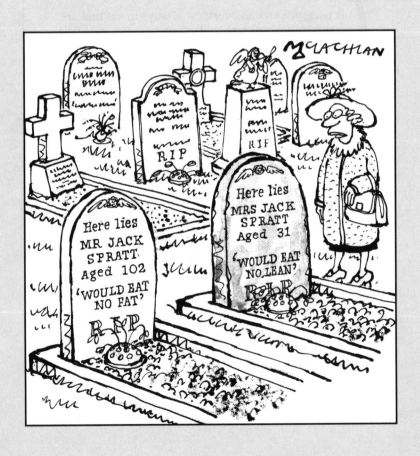

In this part . . .

This part provides an overview of ways to eat that are proven to help control cholesterol balance. We explain how all sorts of delicious foods can lower a raised cholesterol level in specific ways, and why soluble fibre and other ingredients are good for your heart. We also show how you can continue to eat foods such as nuts, red meat, and even certain shellfish, which cholesterol-lowering diets often exclude. In addition, we help you figure out what to order in restaurants. Finally, this part offers advice on how to set up your kitchen to cook in healthy ways, and which basic cholesterol-lowering ingredients to shop for so you can start trying some of the recipes.

If you look at only one chapter in this part, look at Chapter 1, which includes the essence of all the major points in the book.

Chapter 1

Conquering Cholesterol Is Easier Than You Think

. . . .

In This Chapter

▶ Sorting out the different types of cholesterol

▶ Reducing your heart disease risk factors

▶ Developing a way of eating to control cholesterol balance

▶ Linking cholesterol to carbohydrate intake

▶ Having firsts but not seconds

▶ Introducing the recipes

. . . .

*Y*our heart goes about its business, beating over 100,000 times a day, and yet you probably give it little thought, until you have your cholesterol checked and discover it's too high. Then, suddenly, caring for this precious part of your body takes centre stage.

In fact, you need to take care of your heart even if your cholesterol levels are normal. And that's where this cookbook comes in – to give you a tool for controlling your cholesterol balance and keeping your heart healthy with good nutrition.

This chapter starts with a brief description of cholesterol before introducing you to a healthy way of eating, and the types of foods to include in a heart-healthy diet. We describe other risk factors for heart disease and explain how the same foods that lower cholesterol levels can help these conditions, too. Next, we warn you about portion control before moving on to discuss the recipes and the inspiration behind them.

Knowing That Cholesterol Doesn't Grow on Trees

Cholesterol is a wax-like fat. Animal livers produce cholesterol, whether it's your liver or the liver of a chicken or cow. Only animal products, such as eggs, meat, and dairy foods, contain cholesterol. As plants don't have livers, they don't contain any cholesterol, which is one reason why a cholesterol-friendly diet includes eating lots of plant-based foods.

Your liver manufactures cholesterol by joining together 15 two-carbon molecules known as acetates (or vinegars) end to end. Then, after a few other steps, a 27-carbon cholesterol molecule is formed. But here's what's really interesting – those two-carbon acetates can come from several sources, including fatty acids, proteins, sugars, starches, and alcohol.

Normally, your body produces less cholesterol as you consume more *pre-formed* cholesterol (in other words, cholesterol made by the animal you're eating rather than made in your body from saturated fat) in your diet. However, in some people, the opposite is true, and the level of cholesterol in their blood increases as they eat more and more cholesterol in animal-based foods. Individual responses to dietary cholesterol vary widely – depending partly on the genes you inherit, so choose your parents carefully!

Excess cholesterol is potentially dangerous because it can build up in artery walls and reduce the flow of blood to your internal organs, including the heart. This blockage results in a disease called *atherosclerosis*, where the arteries harden and fur up, which is a major cause of heart attacks and strokes.

Cholesterol circulates in your bloodstream in the form of a package called *lipoprotein*, which is made up of cholesterol, protein, and fat assembled in your liver. For more details about cholesterol and the heart, take a look at *Controlling Cholesterol For Dummies* by Carol Ann Rinzler and Martin W. Graf (Wiley).

Lipoprotein comes in many different types, but the two you hear most about are low-density lipoprotein (LDL) and high-density lipoprotein (HDL).

LDL transports cholesterol away from your liver and it's this cholesterol that deposits in arterial walls and starts the formation of *plaques* – the lumpy bits that cause arteries to narrow. Blood flow slows at these narrowings and a blood clot can form that quickly blocks the flow of blood and triggers a heart attack or stroke. That's why people think of LDL as 'bad' cholesterol. In contrast, HDL carries cholesterol back to the liver where it gets converted into bile acids and excretion via your intestinal tract. HDL helps to protect against atherosclerosis, which is how it earns its nickname of the 'good' cholesterol.

So, the purpose of a good cholesterol-friendly diet is not just to lower your total cholesterol, but also to lower LDL and raise HDL. It's all about obtaining the right cholesterol balance.

If you don't know your cholesterol levels and plan to have them checked, you ideally need more than one test because cholesterol levels can fluctuate. If your total cholesterol is more than 5 mmol/L (millimoles per litre), ask your doctor when he or she can repeat the test again. If the results of the two tests are within 0.80 mmol/L of each other, average them (by adding the two figures and dividing by two). If the difference is greater than 0.80 mmol/L, take a third test and average the three (by adding the three results and dividing by three). If the result remains above 5 mmol/L, discuss it further with your doctor.

Doing the numbers

What constitutes a healthy cholesterol level is controversial, even among doctors, and the upper level accepted as normal (by the Joint British Societies – a group of UK expert societies involved in cardiovascular disease) is reducing as doctors develop more ways to reduce the risk of heart disease. The National Institute for Health and Clinical Excellence (NICE) and Department of Health offer these general guidelines to assess cholesterol levels. When you have a cholesterol test, compare the results with these figures. Doctors measure cholesterol levels in millimoles (mmol) of cholesterol per litre (L) of blood.

Category	Level
Total cholesterol	less than 5.0 mmol/L
LDL cholesterol	less than 3.0 mmol/L
HDL cholesterol	greater than 1.2 mmol/l

However, the Joint British Societies recommend lower cholesterol limits for people who have, or are at risk of, coronary heart disease, as follows:

Category	Level
Total cholesterol	less than 4.0 mmol/L
LDL cholesterol	less than 2.0 mmol/L
HDL cholesterol	greater than 1.2 mmol/l

Eating for the Right Cholesterol Balance

The goal of controlling cholesterol balance with diet is not just to keep your total cholesterol within normal range. You also want to choose foods that lower LDL cholesterol and elevate HDL, while avoiding foods that do the opposite.

Lowering your 'bad' LDL levels

One of the most forceful messages about lowering cholesterol that has come through loud and clear over the years is to reduce your intake of saturated fats and dietary cholesterol, because they raise cholesterol levels. However, as research has progressed, this recommendation is altering slightly. Doctors now consider dietary cholesterol to be less of a risk factor in raising cholesterol levels than saturated fat, and another factor is trans fatty acids – the new bad boys on the block.

Restricting saturated fat intake

Saturated fat has a chemical structure that contains as many hydrogen atoms as possible and is usually solid at room temperature. Major dietary sources of saturated fat include full-fat dairy products, fatty meats, and tropical oils (coconut and palm oils).

All the traditional diets for reducing heart disease give high priority to restricting your intake of saturated fat. However, for people of normal weight, with no significant family history of high blood cholesterol levels, and with a good intake of dietary antioxidants from fruit and vegetables, the amount of saturated fat you eat is probably less important than previously thought. Over a third of the saturated fat in milk, butter, and meats doesn't raise cholesterol levels. This is backed by the Framingham Heart Study, which shows no link between high blood cholesterol levels and saturated fat intake. The study showed that, although saturated fat intake increased as a proportion of energy from 16 per cent in 1966 to 17 per cent in 1988, the study population enjoyed significant decreases in total and LDL cholesterol levels.

Hold your horses, though – this result doesn't mean that a high saturated fat intake isn't harmful. Like all fats, saturated fat has a high calorie content and an excess is linked with obesity. If you have a family history of atherosclerosis, coronary heart disease, or high blood cholesterol levels, you've probably inherited genes that mean you process saturated fat less effectively than other people, and you need to follow a diet that is low in saturated fat.

The next question to ask is whether to replace that saturated fat with carbohydrates or other more healthy kinds of fat such as olive oil. We cover this topic in the section 'Controlling your Cholesterol Balance through Diet', later in the chapter.

Watching dietary cholesterol

By *dietary cholesterol*, we mean foods that are high in ready-made cholesterol, such as pig's liver (700 milligrams/100 grams), lamb's kidney (610 milligrams/100 grams), and caviar (588 milligrams/100 grams). Doctors don't consider dietary cholesterol to be as harmful as they previously thought. Research shows that some cholesterol-rich foods, such as egg yolks and shellfish, are also relatively low in saturated fat and have minimal effect on LDL cholesterol levels.

Researchers at Harvard School of Public Health and Brigham and Women's Hospital in Boston examined the association between egg consumption and incidence of cardiovascular disease in a study published in the *Journal of the American Medical Association* in 1999. Data came from a population of over 100,000 male and female health professionals. The study results show that eating up to one egg a day has no significant association with the risk of coronary heart disease or stroke. This is true even for individuals with elevated cholesterol.

The Food Standards Agency and other UK organisations don't recommend a limit on how many eggs you can eat, even though an egg contains about 213 milligrams of cholesterol. They are a good choice for an excellent source of protein and vitamins as part of a healthy, varied, and balanced diet.

When deciding whether to consume a food that contains cholesterol, consider what else you're eating that day so that you keep your intake within sensible limits.

Avoiding trans fatty acids

When certain oils are partially *hydrogenated* to solidify them in the production of cooking fats and margarines, some are converted into an artificial type of fat not normally found in nature known as *trans fats*. Trans fats lurk in breakfast cereals, salad dressings, all sorts of baked goodies such as muffins, pastries, breads, cakes, and biscuits, instant hot chocolate, frozen dinners, and many more foodstuffs. Any time you eat deep-fried foods such as chips or fried chicken, at home or out, you're taking in some trans fats that form in the hot oil.

Research shows a strong link between trans fats and coronary heart disease. People with the highest intake of trans fats are 50 per cent more likely to have a heart attack than those with the lowest intake. A link is also appearing between trans fats and an increased risk of developing type 2 diabetes. (If this affects you, *Diabetes For Dummies* by Alan L. Rubin and Sarah Jarvis (Wiley) gives information and advice to help you live with the condition. *Diabetes Cookbook For Dummies* by Alan L Rubin, Sarah Brewer, Alison Acerra, and Denise Sharf (Wiley) is another good source of information.) Doctors think that this is because trans fats increase the activity of an enzyme CETP (cholesteryl ester transfer protein), which raises levels of LDL cholesterol and lowers levels of beneficial HDL cholesterol. Trans fats also raise *triglycerides*, another type of blood fat associated with increased risk of heart disease. (Chapter 3 gives you an even longer list of the harmful effects of trans fats.)

Check food labels and select products that say they are 'free from trans fats' or which don't list hydrogenated vegetable oil, partially hydrogenated vegetable oil, vegetable shortening, or margarine.

The most effective way to avoid trans fatty acids is to select natural ingredients such as fresh fruits and vegetables rather than processed foods when you're out shopping. Cooking your own meals using unrefined oils also helps keep trans fats off your plate. The recipes in this book let you bake your own muffins, dressings, sauces, and all sorts of main courses free of trans fats.

Choosing ingredients that lower LDL

As you plan your meals and experiment with recipes, include foods that are known to lower LDL cholesterol. Many common ingredients contain components that significantly lower your risk for heart disease. The following information helps you select foods that are good for you:

✔ Some polyunsaturated fats lower LDL cholesterol levels. Sunflower and corn oils contain these fats, but these oils are highly processed, so try to avoid them. A better choice is safflower oil, which you can buy unrefined. (See Chapter 3 for more about why processed oils are less healthy than unrefined oils.)

✔ *Omega-3 fatty acids*, a type of polyunsaturated fat found in oily fish, lower LDL levels and benefit the heart in other ways too, such as reducing the tendency to form unwanted blood clots.

✔ *Monounsaturated fats*, when substituted for saturated fats, can lower LDL cholesterol and stabilise and may even raise HDL cholesterol levels. Almonds are a good source, and macadamia oil, for example, is 81 per cent monounsaturated fat – more than rapeseed oil (60 per cent), avocado oil (62 per cent), and olive oil (73 per cent). In addition, monounsaturated fats don't raise triglyceride levels.

✔ Soluble fibre, to a lesser extent, also lowers cholesterol because it helps to eliminate it from the body. Chapter 2 gives you a list of foods that contain soluble fibre.

✔ Soya beans also have a beneficial effect when substituted for animal protein and may be particularly useful for individuals at high risk of coronary heart disease.

Aiming for more antioxidants

If LDL cholesterol oxidises (which is a chemical change occurring when it gets 'attacked' by oxygen), it's more likely to deposit in your arteries and contribute to the formation of plaque. Fortunately, nature provides a wealth of nutrients that can reverse this process – substances found in fruit and vegetables known as *antioxidants*. The recipes in this book are full of these nutrients and, because foods high in antioxidants are also the most colourful, the dishes look great, too!

Antioxidants mop up and neutralise *free radicals*. Free radicals are molecules that contain an unpaired electron that's missing a mate. This makes it unstable and it therefore darts here and there trying to steal one from another molecule to restore its stability. When a free radical comes in contact with LDL cholesterol, it steals an electron from it, thereby 'oxidising' the cholesterol and changing it. The cholesterol is then more likely to contribute to hardening and furring up of your arteries, a condition known as atherosclerosis. Antioxidants help to reduce atherosclerosis by intercepting and neutralising free radicals, to prevent cholesterol oxidation.

The best known dietary antioxidants are betacarotene, vitamin E, and vitamin C. Several minerals, including selenium, also play a role in preventing oxidation. Numerous plant substances, known as *phytochemicals*, function as antioxidants, too. These compounds, such as *lycopene* – the red pigment in tomatoes – are in the plant to protect it from sun damage, but when you eat the plant, you reap the benefit!

You can best take in antioxidants in their natural form from food. Diet always comes first. An analysis of data from the Health Professionals Follow-up Study and the Nurses' Health Study shows that eating eight or more servings per day of fruits and vegetables rich in the antioxidant, vitamin C, reduces the risk of coronary heart disease by 20 per cent compared with eating less than three servings of these foods a day. An apple a day can keep the doctor away!

Consuming several antioxidants together, as you find them in fruits and vegetables, provides you with a bonus of antioxidant power because antioxidants work together, bolstering each other's activities.

Raising your 'good' HDL levels

Although lowering LDL levels is the main goal in preventing heart disease, raising HDL levels is also an important preventative action. About 30 per cent of people with coronary heart disease have low HDL cholesterol levels while their LDL cholesterol level is normal. In fact, according to some experts on heart attack prevention, increasing HDL is as important as lowering LDL.

Quitting smoking, exercising more, and losing weight all have a beneficial effect on cholesterol balance by raising HDL cholesterol levels. Certain dietary changes can also produce worthwhile results:

- ✔ Replacing saturated fat with monounsaturated fat increases HDL levels. But substituting saturated fat with carbohydrates can lower HDL levels.

- ✔ Eating foods with a lower *glycaemic index* (see the sidebar later in this chapter), an indicator of a food's ability to raise blood sugar levels, is associated with higher levels of HDL. Low glycaemic index foods also reduce triglycerides.

✔ If you drink alcohol at all, consume a moderate amount (no more than one or two units per day). This can also raise your HDL level. All types are beneficial, but red wine is a good choice because of the purple antioxidant pigments it contains. (See Chapter 24 for more on healthy beverages.)

Please don't start drinking alcohol just because red wine is beneficial for your health. Excess alcohol increases blood pressure, can damage your heart and nervous system, as well as your liver, and also makes you gain weight. Always drink alcohol sensibly and in moderation.

Calculating your total cholesterol to HDL ratio

One way to assess your risk of heart disease is to work out the ratio of your total cholesterol to your HDL cholesterol. The *Total:HDL ratio* is consistently reliable in predicting the risk of future heart disease.

Your doctor calculates your Total:HDL ratio from the results of your cholesterol test, and divides your total cholesterol by the amount of HDL present. In round numbers, doctors consider that a ratio of 5:1 or higher is risky and a ratio below 3.5:1 is ideal.

Say that your total cholesterol is 6 mmol/L and your HDL cholesterol is 1.5 mmol/L. Your doctor divides 6 by 1.5 to obtain 4, and so the ratio between total cholesterol and HDL cholesterol is 4:1 – less than the risky level of greater than 5:1, but not as low as the ideal ratio of 3.5:1.

To help tip the ratio in your favour, here's how to eat:

✔ Eat enough of the right kinds of fat, meaning monounsaturated oils and foods that contain omega-3 fatty acids, such as avocados, almonds, macadamias, and fish. Low-fat diets tend to lower HDL levels more than LDL levels, making the ratio between the two even worse.

✔ Add lots of garlic to your recipes, because garlic can raise HDL levels and lower LDL levels. Take one to three cloves of garlic per day in any form – raw, cooked, or as an extract in supplement form. The latter has the advantages of containing a known amount of the garlic active ingredient, *allicin*, and of coming in odour-reduced forms. Raw onion also raises HDL levels.

✔ Beans are beneficial because of their low glycaemic index and their fibre content, increasing HDL levels slowly over time while reducing LDL levels more quickly. (See Chapter 19 for recipes and more information about beans.)

✔ Avoid trans fatty acids because they increase the ratio of LDL to HDL.

✔ Curb foods with a high glycaemic index and avoid simple, refined sugars.

Losing any excess weight is also helpful as is brisk exercise. You don't have to train up to Olympic standard, but exercising for at least 30 minutes per day – ideally more – is a good amount to aim for.

Replacing saturated fat with carbohydrates lowers total cholesterol and LDL cholesterol but also decreases beneficial HDL cholesterol.

Keeping an Eye on Your Risk Factors

Preventing high cholesterol is important for warding off heart disease, but the development of heart disease involves many other risk factors that you also need to pay attention to. The more risk factors a person has, the greater the chance of developing coronary heart disease such as atherosclerosis.

High blood pressure and carrying excess weight raises risk and we address both problems in this cookbook. Chapter 3 gives you some tips on lowering high blood pressure with a diet that contains plenty of fruits and vegetables and wholegrains. And the way of eating that the recipes offer can help you reach a healthy weight. The dishes are made with nutritious ingredients that satisfy hunger so you don't need extra food to feel well-fed.

Being *overweight* (10 per cent above ideal body weight) or *obese* (20 per cent above ideal body weight) increases your risk of heart disease. One way of measuring weight is to use the body mass index (BMI), a figure that takes into account your weight and height. As BMI rises, LDL cholesterol levels and blood pressure also tend to increase. In addition, HDL cholesterol levels decline. To find out your BMI, go to the NHS Direct website at www.nhs direct.nhs.uk/magazine/interactive/bmi/index.aspx.

Two other indicators of the risk of heart disease are also good to know about, namely homocysteine and *C-reactive protein* (CRP). Homocysteine and CRP are probably new to you, but as time goes by you'll hear more about them from your doctor. (You can bring up these topics first, of course.) The medical world, taking a fresh look at the research, is now starting to take both these substances more seriously.

Having your homocysteine or CRP levels measured in the UK isn't easy, because they aren't routinely available on the NHS from your GP. The tests are available privately, however, if you're willing to pay for them, and some specialist NHS consultants may request them.

Having elevated cholesterol and/or a raised homocysteine level and/or a high CRP level increases your risk of having a heart attack several-fold.

Having a peek at homocysteine

Homocysteine is a potentially harmful amino acid, a protein building block, associated with an increased risk of coronary heart disease. Elevated homo-cysteine appears to have a similar damaging effect on artery linings to high levels of the 'bad' LDL cholesterol. Homocysteine promotes the growth of smooth muscle cells in the arteries, making them narrower, as well as inhib-iting the growth of cells that protect against atherosclerosis. Doctors think that the body responds to these changes by depositing cholesterol to mend the damage to the arteries.

Damping down inflammation

Doctors now recognise atherosclerosis as an inflammatory disease like arthritis, because the arterial walls become inflamed. This inflammation isn't like the kind when you cut your finger and it swells and turns red. This is chronic inflammation and produces no obvious symptoms. The main test for inflammation measures the amount of a molecule called *C-reactive protein* (CRP), which makes your blood more sticky. People with high CRP levels tend to go on to develop coronary heart disease and have a heart attack. A study published in the journal *Circulation* in 2003 also concluded that CRP may directly contribute to the formation of unwanted blood clots that can cause heart attacks.

Gaining extra benefits from cholesterol-friendly foods

All these various risk factors, just like elevated cholesterol, are partly con-trollable by diet and often with the very same foods! These multi-tasking ingredients show up in many recipes in this book.

Take a look at Chapter 2 for lists of foods we recommend. You can find a sec-tion on what to eat to help reduce homocysteine. The entire range of homo-cysteine-lowering vitamins is present in green leafy vegetables, citrus fruits, fish, and dairy products.

Another section in Chapter 2 tells you about all the flavoursome foods, such as onions, garlic, ginger, and the spice turmeric, which dampen inflammation.

Lowering Cholesterol for Very High Risk People

Anyone can ask their GP for a blood cholesterol level test, but this is especially important for people at high risk. UK guidelines recommend that doctors screen people if they:

- ✔ Are aged 40 years or over.
- ✔ Have a close family history (for example, in parents or siblings) of raised cholesterol levels.
- ✔ Are overweight or obese.
- ✔ Have high blood pressure.
- ✔ Have diabetes or another medical condition that can increase cholesterol levels, such as kidney or thyroid problems.

As well as offering lifestyle advice to help you with diet, exercise, and stopping smoking, doctors start treatment with a drug known as a *statin*, which reduces production of cholesterol in your liver. The current national targets use LDL cholesterol as the goal and by using statins doctors aim to lower LDL cholesterol to less than 3.0 mmol/L, or to reduce it by 30 per cent from your initial level, whichever figure is the lowest. An alternative approach is to reduce total cholesterol to less than 5.0 mmol/L or by 30 per cent from your initial level (whichever result is lowest). Doctors review the effect of the treatment after 4 to 12 weeks (typically at 8 weeks) to see if you need to increase the dose of statin that you're taking, or add in an additional treatment. A blood test at the same time checks that you're not experiencing liver or muscle side effects from the statin medication.

Statin drugs block formation of a substance called *co-enzyme Q10* (CoQ10) and reduce the amount of cholesterol that your liver makes. Taking a CoQ10 supplement (which you can buy over the counter from high street shops) can help overcome the muscle side effects some people experience as a result of taking a statin drug.

Grapefruit juice interacts with a number of prescribed drugs, including statins. This effect is surprisingly large. For example, taking one particular statin drug (lovastatin) with a glass of grapefruit juice produces the same blood levels of the drug as taking 12 tablets with water! If you take medications, check the drug information sheet provided for grapefruit interactions.

Controlling Your Cholesterol Balance through Diet

The easiest way to change how you eat to control cholesterol is to use the same principles used in the recipes in this book. Cook with *wholefoods* – natural ingredients as nature made them and not refined or processed. Rely on ingredients that provide healthy fats, including monounsaturated fats and polyunsaturated omega-3 fatty acids, as well as soluble fibre, garlic, and other nutrients that maintain heart health. Incorporate plenty of vegetables, fruits, nuts, beans, wholegrains, fish, and poultry in your menus. Remember that lean meats, reduced-fat dairy foods, and eggs are also permissible in a low-cholesterol diet, but in smaller quantities.

The recipes in this book feature carbohydrates that have only a moderate effect on blood sugar levels, such as pearl barley and brown rice. For more on this subject, take a look at *The GL Diet For Dummies* by Nigel Denby and Sue Baic (Wiley). Saturated fat is present only in small amounts, and pre-formed cholesterol content is limited. You can adapt many of your recipes to follow these same heart-healthy cooking guidelines.

The ingredients in this cookbook feature in the traditional diets of Italy, Greece, and other countries bordering the Mediterranean. Heart disease rates are low in this region, and researchers conclude that this way of eating, the now widely publicised Mediterranean Diet, is the prime reason.

A growing body of research supports this dietary approach. Walter C. Willett, MD, and the Harvard School of Public Health co-developed a way of eating based on the results of three very large studies. These are the Nurses' Health Study, with 121,700 participants; the Health Professionals Follow-Up Study, which included 52,000 men; and the Nurses' Health Study II, a survey of 116,000 younger women. In total, researchers tracked the food intake and health of over 250,000 men and women.

Here's what the data reveal:

- Replacing saturated fat with carbohydrates does not significantly lower the risk of coronary heart disease.

- Substituting polyunsaturated or monounsaturated fat for saturated fat is associated with a large reduction in risk of coronary heart disease.

- Substituting carbohydrates for either monounsaturated or polyunsaturated fats increases the risk of coronary heart disease.

- The risk of coronary heart disease increases for individuals who are overweight and sedentary.

✔ Having a high trans fat and low polyunsaturated fat intake triples the risk of heart disease as compared with low trans fat and high polyunsaturated fat intake.

✔ Total fat consumption is not associated with a risk of coronary heart disease.

✔ Higher nut consumption is associated with a lower risk of coronary heart disease.

Switching fats versus lowering fats

The benefits of a diet rich in healthy fats rather than one that is low in fat is clearly shown in the Lyon Diet Heart Study, which began in 1988 and involved more than five years of follow-up. The final results were published in 1999. Researchers assigned 600 people who had experienced a first heart attack to a Mediterranean-style diet or a Western-type diet low in total fat. Those on the Mediterranean diet ate more olive oil, fish, vegetables, and fruit than those on the low fat diet. They also took omega-3 fatty acid supplements to help prevent heart disease and manage cholesterol levels.

Results from the Lyon study show that the Mediterranean-style diet is much more effective at preventing additional heart problems than a low fat diet. Of those consuming the Mediterranean diet, only 14 individuals had a second heart attack or fatal heart problems compared with 44 patients on the low fat diet. In fact, the benefits of the Mediterranean diet were so pronounced that after two and a half years, the trial was stopped early so that those on the low fat plan could benefit from switching to the more healthy Mediterranean way of eating.

The study researchers admit that a diet must be 'gastronomically acceptable' to be truly effective, or people don't stick to it. No problem there! The Mediterranean diet includes the delights of Greek, Italian, and French Provençal cooking. For a sample, try the recipe for Garlicky Butter Beans in Chapter 19, the Grilled Scallops and Herby Vegetables in Chapter 14, and Roast Chicken with Marinated Olives, Rosemary, and Oranges in Chapter 13.

Working out what's best for you

The healthy fats approach to diet offers some leeway, permitting varying amounts of healthy fats. The percentage of fat isn't strictly fixed, and consequently, neither is the percentage of protein or carbohydrates. However, a reasonable division of calories to aim for is 30 to 35 per cent of calories from fat, 50 to 55 per cent of calories from wholegrain carbohydrates, and 15 per cent of calories from protein. You can experiment with more or less protein to see how you feel, while monitoring your weight and checking your cholesterol.

Glycaemic Index

The Glycaemic Index (GI) of a food shows the likely effect it has on blood sugar levels, because the GI rating depends upon how quickly a food is digested and absorbed. Low GI foods (in other words, those that don't have a major impact on blood glucose levels) receive a rating of 55 or less. Intermediate foods are in the range of 56 to 69. And high GI foods are 70 and above. For example, white bread and corn flakes are a high GI food, whereas wholegrain barley and most fruits are low GI foods. The recipes in this cookbook mainly feature ingredients with a low GI rating.

To know the GI of a food before you buy it, a good source of information to check out is www.glycemicindex.com. *The GL Diet For Dummies* by Nigel Denby and Sue Baic (Wiley) can help, too.

 Talk with your doctor about your particular risk factors for heart disease. Diet recommendations and recipes in this book are only a guide to adapt to your individual needs.

Watching what carbs do to cholesterol

Cholesterol problems can originate in a condition known as *metabolic syndrome*. Metabolic syndrome is a group of medical findings linked with abnormally raised levels of both *glucose* (a blood sugar) and *insulin* – the hormone needed to help glucose enter your muscle and fat cells. Together, they increase your risk of coronary heart disease. The condition arises when these cells fail to respond correctly to insulin – a condition known as *insulin resistance*. Your pancreas makes more and more insulin in an attempt to overcome the resistance and, in turn, stimulates your liver to produce higher amounts of very low-density lipoproteins (VLDL) cholesterol. These small, dense particles convert to 'bad' LDL cholesterol and, at the same time, the production of good HDL cholesterol declines. In addition, the level of triglycerides, another potentially harmful type of blood fat, increases. Insulin resistance also causes your blood pressure to go up, and increases the risk of abnormal blood clotting. High levels of insulin and glucose also can damage the lining of the coronary arteries, making the accumulation of plaque more likely. This collection of health problems is together known as metabolic syndrome.

 Doctors link metabolic syndrome with being overweight – in particular with *central obesity*, which is the accumulation of fat around your waist. Before reading any further, find a tape-measure and check the size of your waist in centimetres. If your waist measurement is greater than 80 centimetres and you're female, or if it's larger than 94 centimetres and you're male, you're at risk of metabolic syndrome. The good news is that you can take lots of steps to improve your health, such as taking exercise, eating more healthily, and losing weight. The bad news is that if you ignore the warning signs and carry on with your current diet and lifestyle, you're at increased risk of developing diabetes, a heart attack, or a stroke. In fact, 80 per cent of people with metabolic syndrome develop type 2 diabetes if they don't take steps to avoid it.

Exploring the Recipes in This Book

A diet for controlling cholesterol, as with any diet, begins with preparing food at home, and that's where the recipes in this book come in. After all, this is a cookbook!

We've designed the recipes in this book for everyday cooking when your time and energy are limited. You can easily turn out lots of tasty things even if you're not an expert cook. As long as you know how to do the basics like stirring, chopping, and sticking something in the oven, you'll do just fine. And although using quality cookware helps, you don't need anything as specialised as a pasta maker – though a garlic crusher is always handy.

Relying on wholefoods and traditional cuisines

All sorts of familiar and appetising dishes fit quite naturally into a cholesterol-controlling way of eating. The reason the recipes in this book are so healthy is that they're made with unprocessed and unrefined ingredients that aren't stripped of their important fibre, vitamin, and mineral-bearing parts – in other words, they're *wholefoods*. These wholefoods play an important role in controlling cholesterol and maintaining heart health. A reliance on wholefoods also limits your intake of the trans fatty acids in processed and ready-foods.

Traditional cuisines from around the world are wonderful sources of inspiration for wholefood cooking using local and seasonal foods. The recipes in this book bow to the various Mediterranean cultures, making the circuit from Morocco to Spain, France, Italy, and Greece. Asian flavours show up too with such recipes as the Steak Stir-Fry with Chinese Vegetables in Chapter 15, the Chicken Tandoori with Minted Yogurt Sauce in Chapter 13, and the Red Lentil Dahl with Caramelised Onions in Chapter 19.

Don't worry. You don't have to go hunting for unusual ingredients such as kefir, cuttlefish, or elk. You can find most ingredients right in your usual supermarket.

Adapting recipes to your taste

Don't be afraid to put your own twist on these recipes if it suits you. Few of the specified amounts are written in stone. As you make your way through a recipe (and presumably taste your way through it, too), you'll discover what to add or subtract to suit you. Boost the chilli content if you think a dish is too mild. Skip the coriander leaf if you hate it (but what's there to dislike?) Substitute asparagus for runner beans if that's the vegetable you happen to have on hand. The recipes are meant to set a direction for your cooking, but you're still in charge. Just don't destroy the health benefits of the dish by dumping in more fat, sugar, or salt, or deep-frying a dish that you're meant to bake!

The recipes use various ingredients that start out lower in fat, such as turkey or reduced fat sausage versus pork sausage, or an ingredient that has some of its fat removed, such as semi-skimmed milk.

If your doctor wants you to follow a leaner diet, just lower the fat content of recipes further. For instance, use soya sausage instead of turkey and cook with skimmed milk. You may also want to fiddle with the carbohydrate and protein content. Just ensure that you use healthy ingredients, such as wholegrains and lean meats, to keep the dish heart friendly.

Making your own recipes more heart healthy

After trying out some of the recipes in this book, you can easily adapt some of your own tried-and-tested recipes to your new cholesterol-friendly way of eating. Here's how to start:

- Use vegetables and fruits that provide soluble fibre such as carrots, green beans, strawberries, and apples.

- Make sure that a dish is full of colour by adding red, orange, purple, and yellow fruits and vegetables to give yourself more antioxidants and phytonutrients.

- Prepare a main-course dish with fish instead of meat.

- Garnish with nuts.

- Replace some of or all the refined flour with wholegrain flour. At a minimum, add some vitamin- and mineral-rich wheat germ to white-wheat flour to return what was removed in processing the wheat. (For more info about flour, see Chapter 20.)

- Always cook with unprocessed oils, rather than refined cooking oil and products made with partially hydrogenated oil. Select oils that contain monounsaturated fats and omega-3 fatty acids. (Chapter 3 tells you about these oils.)

- Skip all the white sugar, and if the recipe doesn't work without it, make something else instead.

Chapter 2

Favouring Cholesterol-Friendly Foods

*T*he world is full of foods you can eat while still watching your cholesterol balance. This chapter, and Chapter 3, discuss these types of foods and explain how they keep your heart healthy.

The edibles in this chapter also help your heart in other ways. You find out what foods to cook to reduce high blood pressure and to lose weight. You also discover ingredients that counteract newly identified risk factors as well, such as elevated levels of homocysteine, raised blood levels of inflammatory chemicals that damage artery walls, and insulin resistance, all of which add to the stress placed on your heart, so that controlling your cholesterol becomes even more important.

In the following sections, you find out about high-fibre foods and why you need some soluble fibre in your meals. We introduce you to sources of antioxidants in all their glory, including the amazing and colourful pigments – phytonutrients – a whole new field of study. Then there are the anti-inflammatory foods, the ingredients that lower elevated homocysteine and those friendly, gentle carbohydrates that help keep your insulin levels normal, which as a side effect, also helps to control cholesterol. (See details of the other risk factors for heart disease in Chapter 1.)

All the recipes in this book feature these beneficial ingredients. Read on and start writing your own, special cholesterol-controlling shopping list, which you can use on your very next trip to the supermarket or corner store.

Making Friends with Fibre

Fibre sounds bland and boring, and having to eat more fibre sounds about as appealing as chewing a salad made with hay! But fibre is the great stuff in plant foods that gives them their crunch and texture (although admittedly it contributes little to their flavour). All you need to remember is that by eating more plant foods, and cooking with them more often, your fibre intake takes care of itself.

Because the modern diet is full of processed foods, many people get too little fibre. For instance, grains lose most of their natural fibre (and vitamins and minerals) in the refining process. The average person obtains only about 15 grams of fibre per day, far short of the 25 grams or more that the Department of Health recommends as a guideline daily amount of total fibre.

Guidelines for lowering cholesterol always include having enough fibre, and nutrition research supports this advice. In research published in the *American Journal of Clinical Nutrition*, an analysis of 67 controlled studies found that consuming sufficient fibre lowers both total cholesterol and the 'bad' LDL cholesterol. Although trimming fat and cholesterol produces more dramatic results, eating enough fibre, especially the soluble kind, is part of the picture. As fibre intake increases, your risk of coronary heart disease declines.

Soaking up cholesterol with soluble fibre

Soluble fibre earns its name because it dissolves in water. It acts like a sponge to mop up cholesterol in bile acids, reducing their reabsorption and increasing their loss from the body, and is especially effective in lowering 'bad' LDL cholesterol. Types of soluble fibre include the following:

- **Beta glucans, gums, and methyl cellulose:** These types of soluble fibre, found in oats, seeds and nuts, beans, and pulses bind to bile acids like glue so they're not reabsorbed from your intestines but pass through your body, and travel on towards the loo. They can help reduce both cholesterol and triglycerides (another harmful type of blood fat).

- **Mucilage:** As its name suggests, this is a slimy, viscous substance found in some foods, such as dried beans, brown rice, sesame seeds, and oat bran, which also traps bile acids in your gut.

- **Pectin:** This is the same pectin used to thicken home-made jams and jellies. Pectin forms a gel, slowing the absorption of cholesterol from bile acids in the intestinal tract and meaning that more leaves the body. Eating apples, carrots, beets, bananas, cabbage, oranges, dried peas, and okra regularly increases your pectin intake.

In the small intestine, soluble fibre performs its task by surrounding and trapping bile acids. Bile acids are essential for the digestion of fat and are made out of cholesterol. When the soluble fibre escorts bile out of the body, the liver has to make more bile, using more cholesterol, which it pulls from your blood. Voila! Cholesterol levels decline. You benefit from the law of supply and demand.

Writing a soluble fibre shopping list

Don't go 'ugh' at the slithery texture of foods such as okra. The part that feels slippery is the soluble fibre. You find soluble fibre in many less gelatinous foods as well. Try to eat the following foods regularly:

- **Fruits:** Apples, pears, bananas, strawberries, peaches, apricots, oranges, grapefruit, plums, and prunes.
- **Vegetables:** Carrots, cabbage, potatoes, Brussels sprouts, beets, broccoli, spinach, okra, green beans, tomatoes, sweet potatoes, and aubergines.
- **Legumes:** All beans and pulses including baked beans, soya and soya products, lentils, and peas.
- **Nuts and seeds:** Peanuts, Brazil nuts, sunflower seeds, and sesame seeds.
- **Wholegrains:** Oats and oat bran, barley, and brown rice.

Remember when oats were the new wonder food for preventing heart disease, because of the soluble fibre they contain? Take a look at Table 2-1, and notice that oats aren't the only ones. Of course, we're not suggesting you have a bowl of beans for breakfast instead of porridge, but do try to eat these fibre-rich foods regularly. In the table, the amount of fibre given is for 100 grams of each food.

Table 2-1	Soluble Fibre in Legumes Compared to Oatmeal
Food, 100 grams	*Total Soluble Fibre, in Grams*
Cooked oatmeal	0.7
Kidney beans	1.1
Lima beans	0.4
Black-eyed peas	0.4
Green peas	0.3

Getting a day's worth of soluble fibre

The research study referred to earlier in this chapter shows that consuming 3 grams of soluble fibre per day, the equivalent of three apples or three bowls of oatmeal, reduces total cholesterol by 2 per cent and the risk of coronary heart disease by 4 per cent. To really make an impact on cholesterol levels, you need a daily intake of soluble fibre between 5 and 10 grams. To achieve this, you just need to eat 1 serving of bran flakes; 1 orange; 1 pear; 1 serving each of kidney beans, green beans, and avocado; a potato with the skin; and 1 slice of wholegrain bread. Not so difficult, is it? If you choose the right foods through-out the day, the grams of soluble fibre can really add up.

Counting insoluble fibre, too

The total fibre in food is a sum of both soluble and insoluble fibre. *Insoluble fibre* is mostly the indigestible cellulose that you find in the skin of vegetables and fruit, and in the bran sheath that covers cereal grains. When you eat a stalk of celery, you're chomping on cellulose. And eating a whole pear, including the skin, or wholewheat bread rather than white, also increases your intake of insoluble fibre. Insoluble fibre provides the bulk that promotes bowel regularity, as well as binding with toxins to speed their elimination from the body. All good stuff for intestinal health, although most insoluble fibre – the cellulose – doesn't directly lower cholesterol.

Lignins, however, are a type of woody, insoluble fibre that does lower choles-terol because, like insoluble fibre, they bind with bile acids. Choose vegetables such as carrots, green beans, peas, tomatoes, potatoes, and wholegrains, to increase your intake of lignins. This insoluble fibre is also present in peaches and strawberries, as well as Brazil nuts and flaxseed.

Although most insoluble fibre doesn't directly reduce cholesterol levels, consuming enough total fibre does help to maintain a healthy heart because it prevents problems that go beyond cholesterol. This is true for all age groups, especially older people who are at greater risk of heart attack and stroke. A number of studies published in the *Journal of the American Medical Association* in 2003 found that a good intake of cereal fibre reduces the risk of cardiovascular disease in both men and women aged 65 and older.

Here are some of the benefits of a high-fibre diet:

- ✔ Fibre helps in weight loss because it fills you up without adding calories.

- ✔ Fibre prevents high blood pressure. Several large studies show that fibre in fruit, vegetables, and wholegrains helps to reduce the risk of hypertension in both men and women.

- ✔ High-fibre carbohydrate foods help control cholesterol by slowing the absorption of glucose into the blood and helping to keep insulin levels normal. High levels of insulin in the blood can lead to high cho-lesterol. (See Chapter 3 for more details.) In the Coronary Artery Risk Development in Young Adults (CARDIA) Study, involving nearly 3,000 young adults over 10 years old, the data revealed that fibre intake pre-dicted insulin levels, weight gain, and other heart disease risk factors more accurately than their intake of total or saturated fat.

The fine print on fibre

According to the UK Food Standards Agency, if a label claims that a food product is a 'good source of fibre', it must contain 3 grams of fibre per 100 grams or 100 millilitres, or at least 3 grams in the reasonable expected daily intake of the food. A food 'high in fibre' must provide at least 6 grams per 100 grams or 100 millilitres, or at least 6 grams in the reasonable expected daily intake of the food. To ensure that you eat enough fibre, buy cereals, breads, and crackers with at least 3 grams of fibre per serving.

To give yourself the good minimum of 25 grams of fibre a day, you need to eat 2 apples, 1 pear, a serving of beans, and 3 slices of wholegrain bread – not much, really, in a day's worth of eating. A low-fat vegetarian diet provides even more – as much as 50 to 60 grams of fibre.

When increasing your fibre intake, do so slowly so that your bowel doesn't complain about the increased bulk. Drink plenty of water so all the fibre can work properly. You want it passing through you like a wet sponge, not like a dried up pile of husks!

Arming Yourself with Antioxidants

You have lots of good reasons to cook with ingredients that contain plenty of antioxidants. As you go about your day, these little chaps are busy in the byways of your arteries, preventing problems before they even start. *Antioxidants* are substances that prevent oxidation, a type of chemical reaction that, in some instances, can do harm to body tissues and substances such as cholesterol. In fact, one of the major theories of the way the body ages concerns oxidation. Oxidation occurs when *free radicals* (tiny unstable molecules) go dashing about your insides, reacting with anything they meet and causing damage. But antioxidants come to the rescue. They intercept free radicals and trap them before they can oxidise cholesterol, preventing them from triggering any hardening and furring up of your arteries.

Various studies focusing on the standard dietary antioxidants – vitamin C, vitamin E, and beta carotene – show that taking supplements of antioxidants just isn't enough. The antioxidants in foods are the most effective in protecting the heart. So vegetable haters, it looks like you're stuck. Eating more veg and fruit is the only way out.

Asking for antioxidant-rich foods

To increase your antioxidant intake, add the following foods to your shopping list, with an emphasis on those that provide vitamin C and vitamin E. These provide the most ammunition for fighting heart disease:

- ✔ **Vitamin C:**
  - **Vegetables:** Red peppers, broccoli, Brussels sprouts, cabbage, alfalfa sprouts, and tomatoes.
  - **Fruits:** Papayas, guavas, kiwis, lychees, oranges, grapefruit, mangoes, cantaloupe melons, watermelon, and strawberries.
- ✔ **Vitamin E:**
  - **Grains:** Millet, oats, wholewheat, and sweetcorn.
  - **Nuts:** Almonds, Brazil nuts, hazelnuts, and peanuts.
  - **Seeds:** Sunflower.
  - **Fish:** Prawns, haddock, mackerel, herring, and salmon.
  - **Unrefined cooking oils:** Safflower oil and extra-virgin olive oil.
- ✔ **Betacarotene:**
  - **Vegetables:** Sweet potatoes, carrots, butternut squash, pumpkin, spinach, kale, and red peppers.
  - **Fruit:** Cantaloupe melons, mangoes, apricots, guava, and papayas.

The trace mineral, selenium, enhances the action of vitamin E. A quick way to get more selenium is to eat a couple of Brazil nuts, which are loaded with this mineral. You also find selenium, in lower amounts, in wholegrains, common vegetables such as cabbage and mushrooms, sesame and sunflower seeds, and in fish, poultry, and meats.

Calling all antioxidants

Besides the several vitamins that function as antioxidants, compounds called *phytonutrients* also have antioxidant power. These phytonutrients make up a huge new cast of characters within the world of nutrition. Scientists are still in the process of discovering the many ways these compounds protect against disease.

Antioxidants show up in plant foods because plants also need these clever compounds to protect them from free radical damage. As plants convert sunlight to life-giving energy – the process of *photosynthesis* – this chemical activity generates huge amounts of free radicals. Spotting some of the foods that contain antioxidant phytonutrients is easy because many phytochemicals are also pigments. For instance, carotenoid phytonutrients colour sweet potatoes a golden orange, and another group of phytonutrients, anthocyanins, put the pink in pink grapefruit.

Crowing about carotenoids

Carotenoids are one of the two main classes of plant pigments. They come in various shades of yellow, orange, and red and consist of a group of over 600 compounds, including betacarotene, a form of vitamin A. However, only about 50 are in the foods you eat, and you can absorb only about half of these. That carrots contain carotenoids is probably no surprise, but you also find carotenoids in tomatoes, sweet potatoes, mangoes, cantaloupe melons, pumpkins, apricots, and bananas.

Carotenoids are hiding in green vegetables such as spinach, but are masked by the deep green colour of chlorophyll.

Praising anthocyanins

The other main category of plant pigments, besides carotenoids, is the *anthocyanins*, pronounced with the accent on the 'cy.' Anthocyanins range from reddish-blue crimsons and magentas to violet and purplish blue indigo. Various studies have taken a close look at the antioxidant activity of anthocyanin pigments in such foods as blackcurrants, blueberries, cranberries, and pomegranates. Results suggest that these compounds protect against heart disease in several ways, from preventing the oxidation of the 'bad' LDL cholesterol (check out Chapter 1 for more on LDL), to helping prevent blood clots and breaking down plaque after it has formed.

Rich food sources of anthocyanins include raspberries, red grapes, pomegranates, plums, blueberries, and blackberries. You also find them in red cabbage, red onions, and red beetroots.

Heat damages anthocyanins. To enjoy the maximum benefits, eat at least some of your anthocyanin-rich foods raw. Have a bowlful of the Strawberry and Blueberry Sundae in Chapter 8, made with fresh raw berries and yogurt.

Looking at more antioxidant phytonutrients

Besides these pigments, many other compounds in plant foods supply you with antioxidant power:

- ✔ *Catechins* in dark chocolate are powerful antioxidants. (Yes, chocolate can be a health food in moderation!) Milk chocolate has fewer catechins, and white chocolate has none. Catechins are also present in tea leaves.

- ✔ *Quercetin* in apple skins neutralises a particularly damaging form of free radical. Onions, mangoes, apricots, sour cherries, sweet potatoes, and berries also contain quercetin.

✔ *Hesperetin* in oranges, limes, and lemons revives vitamin C after it has quenched a free radical, so your Cs can quench more free radicals.

✔ *Flavonoids*, a large class of compounds, many of which have antioxidant activity, also prevent blood from clotting. The Zutphen Elderly Study, a 5-year study involving over 800 men conducted in the Netherlands, showed that intake of flavonoids in regularly consumed foods such as tea, onions, and apples lowers the risk of fatal heart disease.

No supplement delivers the range of beneficial nutrients that are present in the average piece of fruit or portion of vegetables.

Testing foods for antioxidant content

So which foods have the most antioxidant punch from all these different compounds? Researchers at Tufts University in Boston worked out a way to measure this and scored various foods in ORAC units. ORAC is short for 'oxygen radical absorbance capacity'. The higher the number, the more antioxidant power a food has. In the following table, dark chocolate has the most ORAC units, but no limit exists to the ORAC units possible. To ensure a good intake of antioxidant nutrients, aim to take in at least 7,000 ORAC units a day in the fruits and vegetables you eat. To put this in perspective, the average person eating two and a half portions of fruit and vegetables per day obtains 5,700 ORAC units. Table 2-2 shows how different fruits and vegetables rate according to a study published in the *Journal of Agriculture and Food Chemistry*.

Your body: An antioxidant factory

The body itself produces several powerful antioxidants, including glutathione and alpha-lipoic acid, both of which are believed to support heart health. Alpha-lipoic acid in turn facilitates the production of glutathione. Alpha-lipoic acid is soluble in both water and in fatty tissues, making it a potentially powerful antioxidant in preventing heart attacks and stroke. Alpha-lipoic acid also helps to prevent wrinkles.

The body makes most of these antioxidants from common components such as amino acids in the food you eat, but as you age – wouldn't you know it? – production of these invaluable antioxidants declines. Fortunately, you can also add to your supply by eating foods that contain them:

✔ Glutathione: Asparagus, avocados, potatoes, spinach, okra, strawberries, grapefruit, peaches, oranges, cantaloupe melons, and watermelon.

✔ Alpha-lipoic acid: Spinach, broccoli, tomatoes, potatoes, peas, and Brussels sprouts.

Table 2-2	Antioxidant Power in Common Foods per 100-Gram Serving		
Foods	*ORAC Units*	*Vegetables and Legumes*	*ORAC Units*
Dark chocolate	103,971	Kidney beans	14,413
Cranberries	9,456	Red lentils	9,766
Blueberries	9,260	Black beans	8,040
Plums (red)	6,237	Red cabbage	3,146
Blackberries	5,348	Beetroot	2,774
Raspberries	4,925	Spinach (raw)	2,640
Strawberries	3,577	Green cabbage	1,359
Cherries	3,361	Broccoli (cooked)	1,259
Avocado	1,933	Onions	1,220
Oranges	1,814	Red bell peppers	901
Red grapes	1,260	Sweetcorn	728

Derived from Wu, X. et al., 2004. Journal of Agriculture and Food Chemistry. 52, 4026–4037.

If you follow a low-carbohydrate diet that involves cutting out fruits and many vegetables from your diet, at least in the early stages, you're denying yourself more than just the sugars in these nutrient-dense foods. You're also denying yourself the many colourful phytonutrients in these foods that support heart health.

Picking Powerful Phytonutrients

Phytonutrients, also sometimes called phytochemicals, are compounds manufactured by plants. They consist of a broad range of compounds, some of which are pigments, whereas others provide flavours and scents and deter insects from eating the plants. Many phytonutrients function as antioxidants. But that's not all these marvellous compounds can do. Some phytonutrients lower cholesterol. No one is recommending that you rely on phytonutrients alone to control cholesterol, but cooking with foods that contain these compounds is a good habit when choosing what to eat. Here are some phytonutrients that lower cholesterol:

✔ **Betasitosterol:** Betasitosterol is very similar, structurally, to cholesterol. This phytonutrient competes with cholesterol for absorption and comes in first! The result is lower levels of cholesterol in the bloodstream. Stanols and sterols that manufacturers add to spreads and mini drinks designed to lower cholesterol act in the same way. Peanut butter contains lots of betasitosterol, and oranges, cherries, bananas, and apples also contain some. Ponder this information as you nibble on the Grilled Chicken with Creamy Peanut Sauce in Chapter 13!

✔ **Inulin:** This is a fibre-like carbohydrate in raisins, garlic, chicory, leek, and Jerusalem artichokes. During digestion, inulin ferments in the intestinal tract, producing short-chain fatty acids that help lower cholesterol.

✔ **D-glucaric acid:** This is a cholesterol-lowering compound present in grapefruit, Granny Smith apples, cherries, apricots, and oranges.

✔ **Sulphur:** Sulphur compounds in onions and many green leafy vegetables are why these vegetables raise 'good' HDL cholesterol – another good reason to eat up your greens! To obtain good amounts of sulphur, eat half an onion a day. Onions also contain flavonoids and people eating just 5 grams of onions per day are significantly less likely to die from coronary heart disease than those eating none. The greatest benefit comes from eating raw onions – try spring onions and sweet red onion rings in salads. Delicious!

✔ **Lycopene:** Lycopene in tomatoes significantly lowers 'bad' LDL cholesterol, and works even better when you eat it in cooked form, such as in tinned tomatoes, tomato ketchup, and tomato sauces such as passatta. Tomato juice is a good source, too.

Minding Your Minerals

Besides antioxidants and an array of phytonutrients, foods also contain minerals that come to your aid in fighting cholesterol. Again, you need to eat plenty of fresh, minimally-processed foods to ensure that you get good amounts of these nutrients. Refined and heavily processed foods, which are stripped of nutrients, are hardly up to the task of controlling your cholesterol. Here are the minerals to watch out for in your diet:

✔ **Copper:** Copper lowers elevated cholesterol and, conversely, lack of copper can lead to high cholesterol. Copper may also help prevent heart rhythm disorders and high blood pressure. Wouldn't you know, copper also functions as an antioxidant. Some of the best food sources of copper are lean meat, tea, coffee, and cocoa, and also wholegrain products, nuts, green leafy vegetables, and legumes, the same foods known to lower cholesterol. Most seafood is also a good source. How about some Sweet and Spicy Mexican Black Beans from Chapter 19 to accompany the Halibut with Coriander and Lime Salsa in Chapter 14?

Taking high dose zinc supplements for longer than a month can deplete your copper reserves.

✔ **Manganese:** When you're lacking in manganese, it can lead to lower levels of 'good' HDL cholesterol. Lack of manganese may also promote the binding of LDL cholesterol to artery walls, increasing the risk of heart disease. Wholegrain cereals, nuts, seeds, fruit, and green vegetables are sources of manganese. However, one of the best places to find manganese is in a cup of tea, which contains 1 milligram of this magic nutrient, on average. Processing of food removes a good portion of its manganese. Do try a bowl of Cherry-Studded Three-Grain Porridge from Chapter 6.

✔ **Chromium:** In combination with niacin (vitamin B3), chromium lowers cholesterol in one out of two people with high cholesterol. Good sources of chromium are lean red meat, but also vegetable sources such as mushrooms, beetroot, wholegrain cereals, nuts, seeds, pulses, and yeast. The Beetroot, Pear, and Chicory Salad in Chapter 10 is waiting for you!

B-ing careful about homocysteine

A bonus from eating all the foods that help control cholesterol is that they also contain certain B vitamins that help to lower homocysteine. *Homocysteine* is an amino acid that your body uses to make protein. High levels seem to have a damaging effect on the lining of the arteries, however, similar to the effect of LDL cholesterol. (See Chapter 1 for more on this compound.)

Homocysteine causes no problems at normal levels, but researchers recognise a close association with elevated blood levels of homocysteine and the likelihood of clogged arteries. Your body needs certain B vitamins – B6, B12, and folate – to convert homocysteine to other things so that it doesn't accumulate and reach high levels. Consuming sufficient amounts of these nutrients can control homocysteine levels and reduce homocysteine when it is elevated.

Here are some foods that provide these important nutrients:

✔ **Folic acid:** Lentils, beans, orange juice, green leafy vegetables, strawberries, asparagus, oatmeal, yeast, and all wholewheat products such as breads and flour.

The UK Food Standards Agency recently recommended adding folic acid to bread to reduce the risk of some developmental disorders occurring in early pregnancy, such as spina bifida. Women who are planning a pregnancy or who are pregnant are also advised to take a folic acid supplement supplying 400 micrograms of folic acid per day.

✔ **Vitamin B6:** Wholegrains such as brown rice, potatoes, beans, nuts, seeds, and green leafy vegetables such as spinach or turnip greens, mangoes, fish, poultry, lean red meat, and milk.

✔ **Vitamin B12:** All animal products are a good source of B12 including meat, fish, poultry, dairy, and eggs. Manufacturers also add B12 to many breakfast cereals in the UK.

Studies show that vegetarians in particular are at risk of deficiency in folic acid and B12 and that they can have higher levels of homocysteine. Supplements that are ethically acceptable to vegetarians are widely available to help prevent nutritional deficiencies.

Intercepting Inflammation

Atherosclerosis is an inflammatory disease, involving chronic low-grade inflammation of the arteries. Plaque developing on artery linings is separated from the blood by a fibrous 'cap.' Inflammation can degrade this protective cap so the plaque ruptures, and a blood clot may form, cutting off the flow of blood to the heart. The combination of inflammation and elevated cholesterol increases the risk of heart attack many times over because elevated cholesterol levels promote the formation of plaque and inflammation makes plaque more dangerous.

Various stresses, including toxins in the environment, and a diet low in antioxidants, can trigger chronic inflammation. But you can take many actions to prevent inflammation:

- ✔ Not all processed foods are bad but try to cut down on heavily processed foods containing a lot of added fat and salt and where valuable nutrients such as fibre, vitamins, and minerals may have been lost.

- ✔ Opt for organic produce and meats if you can.

- ✔ Stay away from food additives and products such as artificially flavoured beverages.

Certain foods can also directly cause inflammation because they contain substances from which inflammatory compounds are made. Arachidonic acid, found in meat and egg yolks, is one such compound. Polyunsaturated oils that contain omega-6 fatty acids (see Chapter 3) also generate the formation of arachidonic acid as well as others that promote inflammation. Eating more omega-3 fish oils helps to counter balance this.

To control inflammation, cut back on red meat, egg yolks, and vegetable oils. Instead, emphasise those foods that inhibit and prevent the formation of inflammatory compounds. You have loads of delicious items from which to choose:

- ✔ **Fish:** Favour cold water oily fish, such as mackerel, herring, salmon, and fresh (not tinned) tuna.

- ✔ **Nuts and seeds:** Flaxseeds and walnuts are your best bets.

- ✔ **Seasonings:** Garlic, ginger, and turmeric contain anti-inflammatory compounds.

- ✔ **Vegetables:** Both onions and mushrooms damp down inflammation.

- ✔ **Fruit:** Find cooling compounds in berries, apples, mangoes, and apricots.

Cooking with the Best

You probably can't wait to start cooking with all these good-for-you ingredients now that you know how they care for your heart. Turn to the recipes in any part of this book and find plenty of ways to prepare these recommended foods. Start with fresh ingredients, and you end up with gorgeous flavour and dishes full of healthy fibre and plenty of antioxidants.

For maximum benefit, choose foods that aren't processed or refined. Such wholefoods contain a full complement of nutrients, in the right mix that nature intended. Antioxidants for instance work better together than alone.

For a gourmet touch, make an effort to use fresh herbs whenever possible, adding them to the recipes in the book to suit your taste. Use Figure 2-1 to help you spot the ones you're looking for at the supermarket. The common, less expensive herbs, such as coriander and basil, are sold in large bunches, while the dearer kinds come in little plastic boxes.

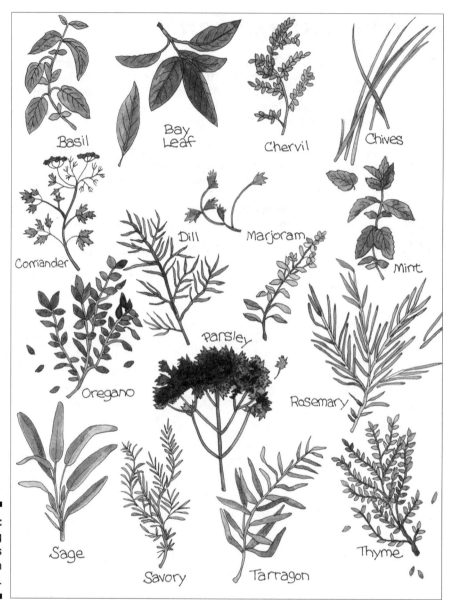

Figure 2-1:
Identifying
fresh herbs
to use in
recipes.

Chapter 3

Separating Fat from Fiction

· ·

In This Chapter

▶ Considering cholesterol-rich foods

▶ Looking at 'bad' foods

▶ Giving the thumbs up to nuts

▶ Putting heart-healthy foods on your shopping list

· ·

Cholesterol-friendly diets often focus on all the foods you shouldn't eat, rather than those you should. You can almost see the wagging finger when the subject of eggs or meat comes up and hear the 'tsk, tsk' over high-fat foods. But the truth isn't that simple. Different people inherit different genes and handle the nutrients in foods in different ways. For some people, certain 'forbidden' foods may even have redeeming virtues. For example, egg yolk contains lecithin, which lessens the effects of cholesterol, plus lutein and other beneficial heart-healthy nutrients.

This chapter shows you how to view cholesterol-containing foods realistically, so that you can include some of them in your meals. Fats are considered in terms of quality rather than just lumping them all together. Some are so good for you that they absolutely must feature on your menus to keep your heart healthy and your cholesterol balance in check. And if you have any worries about nuts and the fat they contain, we sort them out and put them into proper perspective.

Use the suggested 'good' foods in this chapter to write your own shopping list – a cholesterol-friendly diet is more versatile, and has more flexibility than most people expect!

Calming Down about High-Cholesterol Foods

So what about eggs and other animal sources of protein that contain ready-made cholesterol? Can you ever eat them again if you're watching your cholesterol balance? The answer, of course, is yes – if you do it the right way.

Normally, as you consume more cholesterol, your liver compensates and produces far less. But other factors, such as a high intake of fat, a lack of physical activity, and carrying excess weight – especially around the middle – can also lead to an elevated cholesterol level.

Looking at the bigger picture

Although remaining aware of the foods that contain pre-formed cholesterol and limiting their intake is a good idea, totally avoiding a food simply because it's high in cholesterol is the wrong way to go. Foods such as eggs and meat are very nutritious and supply important vitamins and minerals, so don't banish them altogether. Simply aim to eat them in reasonable quantities and make sure that you team them up with foods that contain little or no cholesterol.

Having an egg for breakfast two or three times a week is fine if the rest of the day you concentrate on eating fruits, vegetables, wholegrains, lean meats, poultry, and fish. Eating this way also gives you healthy oils and plentiful nutrients for reducing the risk of heart disease.

The Savoury Steak Salad with Tomato Dressing in Chapter 10 combines a small portion of meat with lots of vegetables – a mix of high- and no-cholesterol ingredients. And the single egg in the Creamy Apple Crumble in Chapter 21 owes no apology, because it earns its place by holding the crumble together.

Just because a dish contains no cholesterol doesn't give you permission to eat all you want. Meringues are made with only egg whites and no yolks, but that doesn't make them health foods. They're still high in sugar, although they make a better choice than a rich, cream-filled sponge cake. (For handy suggestions on healthy ways to include eggs at breakfast time, turn to Chapter 7.)

Taking stock of a risky combination: Cholesterol and saturated fat

Saturated fat intake is more predictive of heart disease than the amount of cholesterol you consume. Although dietary cholesterol can certainly increase levels of unhealthy LDL cholesterol (the type that deposits in arterial walls), for some people saturated fat has an even greater impact on blood cholesterol levels – especially if your intake of antioxidants is low. So a useful way to judge high-cholesterol foods is to see how much saturated fat they also contain.

Most dietary guidelines for heart health around the world, including those from the UK Department of Health, suggest keeping total fat intake to no more than around a third of daily calories, with no more than a third of these coming from saturated fat. These figures are difficult to use in practice unless you're a trained dietician, but food labels make it easier to find out how much saturated fat and cholesterol is present in a food product, although cholesterol isn't always labelled. The label also tells you how much saturated fat (and sometimes cholesterol) a typical single serving provides.

Some manufacturers also show Guideline Daily Amounts (GDAs), which express fat and saturated fat as a percentage of target maximum daily intakes. The GDAs for fat are 70 grams per day for women (of which no more than 20 grams is saturated fat) and 95 grams per day for men (with no more than 30 grams as saturated fat). In addition, limiting your intake of preformed dietary cholesterol to less than 300 milligrams per day is always a good idea. Cutting down on saturated fats naturally keeps dietary cholesterol intakes low. (Check out Chapter 1 for more about dietary cholesterol. Chapter 5 offers help on the intricacies of reading labels.)

For fresh foods that don't come with a label that details nutritional content, nutrition charts are available to give you the missing information. Table 3-1 gives you some telling figures for cholesterol and saturated fat content in an assortment of common foods that people usually associate with cholesterol worries, for better or worse. In terms of saturated fat, eggs and shellfish aren't so bad. A small study published in the *American Journal of Clinical Nutrition* in 1996 also shows that substituting prawns (a food high in cholesterol but low in fat) for beef or other high-fat foods in the diet does not adversely affect cholesterol levels.

Table 3-1   Cholesterol Content and Saturated Fat in Common Foods (per 100 grams or 100 millilitres)

Food Item	Cholesterol Content in Milligrams	Saturated Fat Content in Grams
Whole egg	391	3.2
Egg yolk	1120	8.7
Egg white	trace	0.0
Lean rump steak, grilled	76	2.5
Mince beef, extra lean, cooked	75	3.8
Streaky bacon, grilled	90	9.8
Back bacon, grilled	75	8.1
Chicken breast without skin	90	1.5
Cheddar cheese	97	21.7

(continued)

Table 3-1 *(continued)*

Food Item	Cholesterol Content in Milligrams	Saturated Fat Content in Grams
Cream cheese	95	29.7
Parmesan, grated	93	19.3
Feta cheese	70	13.7
Whole milk	14	2.5
Semi-skimmed milk	6	1.1
Skimmed milk	3	0.1
Single cream	55	12.2
Double cream	137	33.4
Crème fraîche	113	27.1
Whole milk yogurt	11	1.7
Low-fat yogurt	1	0.7
Coconut milk, canned	0.0	0.2
Butter	213	52.1
Olive oil	0.0	14.3
Prawns, boiled	280	0.2
Safflower oil	0.0	9.7
Brazil nuts	0.0	16.4
English walnuts	0.0	5.6

Derived from: McCance and Widdowson's The Composition of Foods, 6th Edition. Food Standards Agency, 2002.

Getting the Fat Story Straight

Although the quantity of fat you eat still counts, the kind of fat you eat is enormously important. This section introduces you to the various types of fat as well as a human-made version known as trans fatty acids.

Some fatty foods are actually an essential part of ways of eating that are associated with lower cholesterol. You're about to find out which fatty foods these are.

When low-carb diets raise cholesterol

Low-carb diets encourage people to replace starchy foods and sweets with protein foods. Low-carb diets such as the South Beach Diet recommend lean meats, fish, and low-fat dairy products, but some people embrace the advice about eating more protein and start loading up on red meat and cheese, which are high in cholesterol as well as saturated fat.

Certain individuals can manage such an increase in dietary cholesterol; their bodies produce less cholesterol in response, resulting in no change in their original cholesterol levels. But for individuals who are sensitive to dietary cholesterol, and have no need for additional saturated fat, dramatically increasing the intake of cholesterol and saturated fat can cause cholesterol to rise rapidly to dangerously high levels. The take-home message is, if you follow a low-carb way of eating, have your cholesterol levels monitored regularly to know if the foods in your low-carb diet are affecting your cholesterol balance.

Introducing the fatty cast of characters

All fats are not created equal. Most fats are a combination of the three basic types of fatty acid – saturated, polyunsaturated, and monounsaturated – but in different proportions. When in doubt about the makeup of an oil you have in your kitchen, take a look at Figure 3-1, which tells you at a glance the makeup of many of the most common cooking oils. Each oil has a different effect on cholesterol levels. Cook with those high in monounsaturated and polyunsaturated fatty acids to control cholesterol.

Every molecule of fat is composed of a glycerol backbone and three chains of fatty acids (carbon and hydrogen atoms linked together) that stick out from it to form a shape similar to a capital E. The difference between each type of fat is in the composition of these chains. Some have more hydrogen atoms than others. When a chain has all the hydrogen atoms it can hold, it's considered saturated. When one hydrogen atom is missing, the fat is monounsaturated, and when two or more hydrogen atoms are missing, the fat is – you guessed it – polyunsaturated. When a fatty acid chain contains fewer hydrogen atoms than it is able to hold, the fat becomes liquid at room temperature.

Saturated fats

Foods high in saturated fatty acids are generally solid at room temperature. Butter, for example, is mostly saturated fat, which is why it comes in blocks and not in a bottle! You find saturated fat in the following foods:

✔ Fatty meats, meat products (pasties, pies, sausages, burgers), and poultry skin.

✔ Full fat dairy foods such as cheese, milk, cream, and animal fats such as butter, lard, ghee, and suet.

✔ Cakes and biscuits made with hard animal fats.

✔ A few plant foods, notably coconut oil and palm oil.

Although coconut has received a bad name because of its saturated fat content, it mainly contains fatty acids such as caprylic and lauric acid that the liver uses as a fuel. Consuming small amounts of these doesn't have a major adverse effect on your blood cholesterol balance. When eating a diet containing a lot of coconut oil, any increase in LDL cholesterol is counter balanced by a higher level of HDL. If you use coconut oil for cooking, select virgin coconut oil, which isn't artificially solidified (a process known as *hydrogenation*). Processed forms of coconut oil are odourless and contain partially hydrogenated trans fats that do have a harmful effect on your cholesterol balance. (See the section 'A twist in the plot: Trans fatty acids' later in this chapter for more info.)

Eating excess saturated fats can raise levels of the unhealthy LDL cholesterol and total blood cholesterol levels, but you can help to offset this effect by eating plenty of antioxidant-rich fruit and vegetables.

Monounsaturated fats

Monounsaturated fat is the mainstay of the well-studied Mediterranean diet that experts associate with a lower risk of heart disease. Good sources of monounsaturated fatty acids include these foods:

✔ Olives and olive oil

✔ Rapeseed oil

✔ Nuts such as macadamias, cashews, walnuts, peanuts, and almonds

✔ Avocados

Monounsaturated fats lower your 'bad' LDL cholesterol levels, reduce the likelihood of LDL cholesterol oxidation (which makes it easier for plaque to accumulate in arteries), and stabilise or even raise your 'good' HDL cholesterol levels.

Macadamia nuts contain an exceptionally high proportion of monounsaturated fats. 81 per cent of their oil is monounsaturated, compared with 77 per cent for olive oil, 60 per cent for rapeseed oil, and 62 per cent for avocado oil.

Polyunsaturated fats

Foods high in polyunsaturated fatty acids are generally liquid at room temperature, and they come in two types: the omega-6s and the omega-3s. For heart health, a diet needs to provide the right proportion of each. (See the section, 'Embracing essential fatty acids' in this chapter.) Primary sources of polyunsaturated fats are the following:

- ✔ Vegetables oils such as sunflower, safflower, soya, sesame, and corn oils
- ✔ Oily fish
- ✔ Nuts and seeds

Consuming polyunsaturated oils reduces LDL cholesterol levels, and helps to lower total cholesterol levels.

Comparing different fats

These three basic forms of fat – saturated, polyunsaturated, and monounsaturated – all belong in your diet. The question is, in what proportion? Some guidelines, designed to lower LDL cholesterol, recommend reducing total fat to between 25 per cent and 35 per cent of total calories, with monounsaturated and polyunsaturated fats making up the majority of the calories. Keep saturated fat to less than 10 per cent of calories, and ideally to less than 7 per cent in order to reduce cholesterol – particularly LDL cholesterol.

Different fats and oils used in cooking contain about the same amount of calories. One tablespoon of butter provides 108 calories, and one tablespoon of olive oil contains 119 calories.

These proportions should cause no problems to you as a cook. Any recipe with 30 per cent calories from fat tastes rich and delicious. However, if you eat out a lot, you're likely to eat dishes with far higher fat content if you're not careful. Figure 3-1 compares the fat content of different fat sources.

Fat is the flavour carrier in food. If you attempt to follow a very fat-restricted diet, making food tasty is much more of a challenge. The lowest you can go and still keep foods such as soups and stews appealing is about 15 per cent calories from fat.

	Cholesterol mg/Tbsp ☐	Saturated Fat ■	Other Fats ☐	Monounsaturated Fat ☐	Polyunsaturated Fat ☐
Rapeseed oil	0	6%	31%	←1%	62%
Safflower oil	0	9%	78%	1%→	12%
Sunflower oil	0	11%	69%		20%
Corn oil	0	13%	62%		25%
Peanut oil	0	13%	33% 5%		49%
Olive oil	0	14%	9%		77%
Soybean oil	0	15%	61%		24%
Macadamia nut oil	0	16%	←3%		81%
Chicken fat	11	30%	22% 1%		47%
Lard	12	41%	12%		47%
Beef fat	14	51%	4% ←1%		44%
Palm oil	0	51%	10%		39%
Butter (fat)	33	54% 4%	12%		30%
Coconut oil	0	77%	2%→	15%	6%

Figure 3-1: Comparing the dietary fats.

A twist in the plot: Trans fatty acids

A century ago, food manufacturers came up with a process known as *hydrogenation* to make liquid vegetable oils turn solid at room temperature. For an idea of what hydrogenation involves, take a look at the fatty acid chains in Figure 3-2. Hydrogenating an unsaturated vegetable oil that's missing hydrogen atoms adds hydrogen atoms back in so that a more rigid structure forms.

Thanks to the advent of hydrogenation, new partially hydrogenated fat products came into the world, known as shortening, or margarine. By the 1930s, food manufacturers began to use the partially hydrogenated fats on a large scale. The advantages to both producer and customer were that a product such as margarine or shortening acts like butter but is less expensive. Hydrogenated fats also have a long shelf-life.

But partially hydrogenated fats have a problem. Hydrogenation causes an unnatural twist in the double bond in their centre. The name for these misshapen characters is trans fatty acids. The easy way to think of trans fatty acids is that they are TRANSformed.

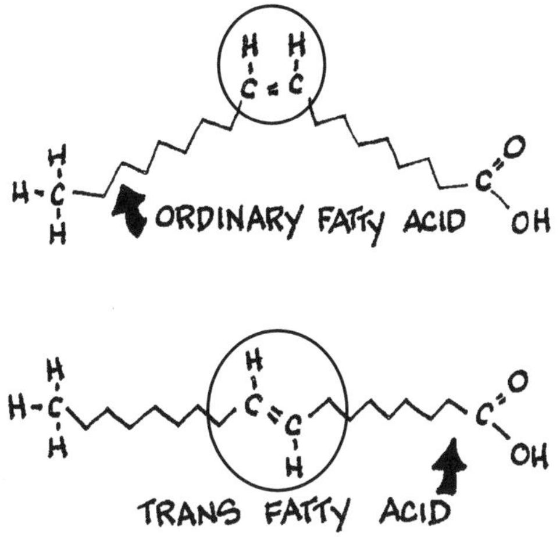

Figure 3-2:
Ordinary
and trans
fatty acid
chains.

Trans fats can still participate in the many important functions that fat normally performs throughout the body, but their behaviour is defective. They impair the functioning of cell membranes and the immune system and may have an impact on hormone synthesis. In terms of heart health, trans fats make platelets in the blood more sticky, increasing the likelihood of unwanted blood clotting, leading to heart attack or stroke. They also interfere with the body's ability to regulate blood pressure and the muscle tone in the walls of your arteries. These deformed molecules also raise total cholesterol, and they increase the unhealthy LDL cholesterol while lowering the good HDL cholesterol. This combined effect on the ratio of LDL to HDL cholesterol, an important indicator of the risk of heart disease, is double that of saturated fat.

According to a 2007 study on trans fatty acids and heart disease published in the journal *Circulation*, people with the highest red blood cell levels of trans fats are three times more likely to have a heart attack than those with the lowest levels – even after taking age, smoking, and other dietary and lifestyle cardiovascular risk factors into account. In the UK, the Scientific Advisory Committee on Nutrition recommends intake of trans fats that are equivalent to less than 5 grams per day. Recently, low-fat spreads have been reformulated, meaning that they now contain a lower level of trans fats, and thanks to manufacturers making voluntary reductions in their use of trans fats, average intakes in the UK are now down to less than 2.5 grams per day, although some people actually consume ten times this amount! In the Mediterranean diet, which experts associate with heart health, trans fats hardly feature at all, so there's still room for improvement!

To cut out trans fats from your diet, you have to cut down on eating the huge number of processed and packaged foods that contain hydrogenated fats, such as:

✔ Pastry, pies, and pasties

✔ Convenience foods such as ready meals

✔ Cake and cake mix

✔ Biscuits and crackers

✔ Chocolate bars

✔ Hard margarine and vegetable shortening

✔ Fast food such as burgers, chips, and milkshakes

✔ Takeaways such as fish and chips, Chinese, and Indian

✔ Other deep-fried foods including restaurant meals

✔ Pizza bases

✔ Crisps and other savoury snacks

Trans fats don't have to be included on food labels, but they can lurk in other ingredients that do have to appear, such as:

✔ Partially hydrogenated vegetable oil

✔ Hydrogenated vegetable oil

✔ Shortening

Trans fats can hide in other foods too, including the following:

✔ Crackers

✔ Fast foods fried in oil, such as doughnuts and French fries

✔ Butter-flavoured popcorn

Embracing essential fatty acids

Polyunsaturated fats are divided into two groups: the omega-6 fatty acids and the omega-3s. You mainly find omega-6s in vegetable oils, and omega-3s in oily fish, some nuts and seeds such as walnuts and linseeds, but also green leafy vegetables and rapeseed oil. Another name for these acids is *essential fatty acids* (EFAs). They are workhorses, doing all sorts of important jobs in the body. The EFAs provide the raw material for building cell walls and help convert food into energy. They also make up a major portion of your brain. And that's only the beginning of the long list of their many functions.

Essential fatty acids also play a vital role in preventing heart disease. The omega-6 fatty acids may even slow down the production of cholesterol. The omega-6s and the omega-3s work together, in opposing ways, to keep your circulatory system healthy.

Your body uses essential fatty acids to make hormone-like compounds, called *prostaglandins*. Some omega-6s produce a type called Series 2 prostaglandins, which make the blood stickier and promote inflammation. Balancing these effects, the omega-3s generate Series 3 prostaglandins that block the actions of the Series 2. The omega-6 fatty acids also promote high blood pressure, but the omega-3 fatty acids in fish oil counteract this effect by lowering an elevated blood pressure. Omega-3-rich fish oils also help to keep arteries more fully open and help prevent an irregular heartbeat.

When omega-3 fatty acids replace saturated fat in the diet, they lower blood levels of the very harmful small particles of LDL cholesterol by increasing their particle size, and also have beneficial effects on metabolism of HDL cholesterol.

Trouble in paradise: Overconsumption of omega-6 fatty acids

The balance of omega-6 fatty acids in your diet compared to omega-3s is very important for heart health. Since earliest times, humans evolved on a diet providing omega-6s and omega-3s in a ratio of about 1:1. Even 100 years ago, before the advent of processed oils, the ratio was only slightly higher at perhaps 2:1. However, these days, the modern Western diet consists of EFAs in a ratio of between 10:1 to as high as 20–25:1, in favour of the omega-6s. This ratio can encourage blood clots, inflammation, and abnormal cholesterol balance.

Increasing your intake of omega-3s

The great majority of people eating a diet full of refined and processed foods have relatively low intakes of omega-3. Another reason for the lack of omega-3s is the push towards eating low-fat and even non-fat foods. At one time, doctors even warned people off butter and recommended vegetable oils and spreads instead. Unfortunately, most commercial vegetable oils and spreads contain a predominance of omega-6 fatty acids. Few people also increased their intake of omega-3s from nuts and fish to maintain the proper EFA balance.

You're likely to need to eat more of the following EFA-rich foods:

- ✔ Oily, cold-water fish such as salmon, sardines, mackerel, trout, pilchards, fresh tuna, and herring
- ✔ Walnuts
- ✔ Flaxseed or linseed oil
- ✔ Wild game such as venison, pheasant, grouse, and wild duck

However recent evidence suggests that the type of fatty acids in vegetable sources may not have the same benefits as those in fish.

Not consuming enough omega-3 essential fatty acids can increase the risk of heart disease. Aim to eat 2 to 4 portions of oily fish a week, although women who may have a future pregnancy should stick to 2 portions to reduce their exposure to potential toxins.

Butter wannabes

Doctors often recommend margarine and vegetable oil spreads for lowering cholesterol because they're made with oils that are low in saturated fat. The various types differ in nutritional benefits, and if you take flavour into consideration, no single one is perfect.

Here are some points to keep in mind if you want to cook with these products:

- Avoid margarines made with hydrogenated fats.

- Vegetable oil spreads made with a mix of essential fatty acids are fine if you spread them on toast, but in a frying pan, some very low fat spreads may dissolve into a watery mess.

- Butter substitutes function well as an ingredient in homemade baked goods.

In Chapter 22, the Chewy Oatmeal and Raisin Bites give you a chance to bake with a vegetable oil spread.

Some vegetable oil spreads contain sterols and stanol esters, natural plant substances that closely resemble animal sterols such as cholesterol. These compounds are made from soya beans or pine tree pulp and help to lower cholesterol levels. They block the absorption of cholesterol in the digestive tract in a similar way to some drugs. Clinical trials have shown that for people with elevated cholesterol, consuming these products can reduce bad LDL cholesterol by 10–15 per cent, when they also follow a diet low in fat. These spreads, however, can be quite costly and you need to eat the recommended dose, which can be 2 to 3 servings a day (or 1 mini drink), for maximum effect.

Chewing the fat over healthy oils

So which fats are best for cooking and for health, when you consider flavour as well as nutritional composition? If you want to cut back on saturated fat and trans fats, the final list of acceptable oils (which do not include the poor-quality processed oils) is quite short. We recommend the following cooking oils for the recipes in this book:

- **Olive oil:** Use as a primary cooking fat and for salad dressings.

- **Rapeseed oil:** A good source of monounsaturated fats and omega-3 fatty acids, and low in saturated fat. Rapeseed oil is also good value for money, because it's cheaper than olive oil, and has a very mild flavour. This oil is often for sale as 'blended vegetable oil' or just 'vegetable oil', and so check the ingredients list to ensure that the product is rapeseed oil.

- **Safflower oil:** Use in cooking and baking, when you want a mild flavour.

- **Sesame oil and other gourmet nut oils such as almond and hazelnut:** These oils are good as flavour condiments.

Cooking with a smidgeon of butter for flavour is fine as long as you're not eating a lot of saturated fat in other foods.

Nibbling on Nuts – in Moderation

Here's some good news! You can eat nuts. In fact, having some nuts as a snack and using nuts in your cooking is actually good for your heart. Eating just 30 grams of plain (unsalted) nuts a day can lower total and LDL cholesterol. Clinical studies have shown that diets containing walnuts, almonds, or macadamia nuts decrease both total and LDL cholesterol, while also having a beneficial effect on good HDL cholesterol levels.

Thirty grams of nuts is usually about a handful – 14 walnuts, 18 medium cashews, and 22 almonds.

Welcoming little nutritional packages

The high level of monounsaturated fats and essential fatty acids in nuts is an important factor in their beneficial effects. Other reasons include the high amounts of protein, fibre, vitamin E, magnesium, and potassium they contain.

Nuts are also rich in the amino acid, arginine. The body uses arginine to produce nitric oxide, a relaxing compound that can dilate blood vessels.

Eating nuts rather than doughnuts

All sorts of new research is proving that eating nuts lowers the risk of heart disease. Research published in the *British Journal of Nutrition* in 2006 shows that the risk of coronary heart disease is 37 per cent lower for those who consume nuts more than four times per week compared to those who never or seldom consume nuts, with an average reduction of 8.3 per cent for each weekly serving of nuts. Studies also suggest that nut eaters tend to weigh less than those who rarely eat these delicious snacks, because their fibre and protein content suppresses appetite. So what are you waiting for?

Stock up on the following nuts and nibble away:

- ✔ Almonds
- ✔ Brazil nuts
- ✔ Cashews
- ✔ Chestnuts
- ✔ Hazelnuts
- ✔ Macadamias
- ✔ Pecans

✔ Pine nuts

✔ Pistachios

✔ Walnuts

Peanuts also have their benefits, but they don't go on the A list because they are often salted, covered in chocolate, or dipped in sugar. But plain roasted peanuts and peanut butter (look for healthy types) are just fine.

Bringing Cholesterol-Friendly Foods into Your Kitchen

The first step in filling your kitchen with heart-healthy foods is to take a hard look at the items you normally buy and do some editing. Hunt through your fridge and freezer and explore the dark recesses of your cabinets. Consider the foods you have on hand and go from there.

Taking stock of the foods you have to hand

Even if you're already on the right track when it comes to cooking with healthy foods, you can probably find room for improvement. Check the ingredients you have to hand and throw out old stand-bys that don't serve your health. Here are some questions to ask as you poke around your kitchen:

✔ Are the produce drawers in your refrigerator nearly empty?

✔ Do you see vegetables that are red, orange, purple, yellow, and green?

✔ Is there a colourful display of fruit on the kitchen counter?

✔ Are the breakfast cereals, breads, and crackers made with whole grains?

✔ Do you have a stockpile of biscuits, cakes, and sweets?

✔ What oils do you have for cooking?

✔ Where are the nuts?

You get the idea. Look for whole, minimally processed fresh foods. Stock up on the good sources of soluble fibre, nutrients, and healthy fats that we recommend in this chapter and in Chapter 2.

When you cut out foods that contain trans fats, hydrogenated oils, and loads of salt, you give yourself a bonus because these are typically present in processed and fast foods that are missing important nutrients.

Rewriting your standard shopping list

Why not add these healthy foods to your shopping list, and thank yourself for years to come:

- ✔ Peas, beans, and lentils of all sorts, including canned and dried types.

- ✔ Berries such as blackberries, strawberries, blueberries, and raspberries. Frozen berries are fine if the ones you want aren't in season.

- ✔ Olive or rapeseed oil.

- ✔ Flaxseed oil.

- ✔ Rolled oats.

- ✔ Green leafy veg such as spinach and broccoli. Try bags of salad if you're short on time.

- ✔ Lean mince or poultry such as chicken or turkey breast.

- ✔ Dried fruit, seeds, and unsalted nuts such as Brazils or walnuts.

- ✔ Wholegrain bread and oat-based breakfast cereals or barley.

- ✔ Canned fresh, frozen, smoked salmon, or other oily fish such as mackerel, herring, sardines, and pilchards.

- ✔ Low-fat dairy milk and yogurt, soya milk or yogurt, and tofu.

Of course, dozens of other foods benefit the heart (as you can see in the recipe chapters), but these food items are a good place to start.

Chapter 4

Controlling Cholesterol When Eating Out

. . . .

. . . .

Sometimes you don't feel like cooking, or you simply don't have time to fuss in the kitchen. Life is often this way for some people, it seems. According to research carried out by Halifax Financial Services in 2008, Brits spend a total of £86 a month, or £62,610 over a lifetime, dining in restaurants and ordering takeaway foods.

Even if you do eat out regularly, you can still watch your cholesterol. The number of healthy options on menus is on the rise, and by remembering the tips in this book you can spot the more nutritious foods on the menu and avoid the deep-fried chocolate bars. Eating out is arguably even good for your heart – it lets you relax and reduce your stress levels while someone else does the cooking and takes the strain!

This chapter walks you through ordering breakfast, lunch, and dinner in a variety of restaurants, and gives you several tips on how to keep yourself well nourished when travelling for business and on holiday. Even away from home you can continue to eat many of the foods that help you control your cholesterol balance.

You won't find much here about ordering in upmarket restaurants and five-star hotels, however, because the chefs in these kitchens turn out such a wide variety of foods that you can always find something healthy, or request personal options such as leaving out the mayonnaise or sauce. The real challenge is finding something good for your heart, body, and soul in your local eatery. Read on.

Avoiding Greasy Spoon Cafés at Breakfast Time

Coffee shops and fry-up cafés sell breakfasts made to order and served quickly, pouring your eye-opening coffee for you even before you sit down. If you have breakfast out once in a while, don't worry too much about what you eat. Enjoy the treat – go ahead and order the eggy bread, scrambled eggs, and bacon. But for the rest of the day, trim your fat intake and fill up on wholegrains, fruits, vegetables, legumes, fish, and lean meats. If you eat breakfast in restaurants all the time, however, take a long, hard look at what's on the breakfast menu to ensure that it's good for your health.

Look for simple, nourishing foods, such as muesli and fresh fruit, and wholegrain cereals such as porridge, oat bran cereal, and wholewheat cereals. Avoid less healthy options such as pancakes, waffles, Danish pastries, and doughnuts made with white flour and sugar – these foods lack fibre and nutrients important for heart health. Breakfast meats such as bacon and sausage are high in saturated fat and loaded with salt, and so have them only once in a while. Try a bowl of wholegrain cereal with semi-skimmed milk and a sliced banana, dried fruit, or berries, or yogurt and fresh fruit plus some crunchy rye toast. Granted, your breakfast may not seem as entertaining as those that some people around you are eating, but then, you're not at a party.

If you're tempted to order strips of sizzling streaky bacon opt instead for grilled lean back bacon, which is lower in fat than regular streaky; combine it with a wholewheat bread roll for the wholegrain; and half a grapefruit for antioxidants. Such a meal is satisfying and far better for your health.

Breaking your fast the healthy way

You can eat most standard breakfast foods as long as you choose the healthy versions. The following sections give you specifics about the most heart-friendly items in each category.

Cereals

Have a high fibre, preferably wholegrain cereal, such as unsweetened muesli, Shredded Wheat, Kashi, Weetabix, or oat bran flakes, rather than one loaded with sugar, which unfortunately is true of many breakfast cereals. Top the cereal with semi-skimmed or skimmed milk.

Beware of granolas, which may contain as much fat and as many calories as a dessert.

In the hot cereals category, oatmeal tops the list for its cholesterol-lowering soluble fibre, but keep these two points in mind:

  ✔ Choose the regular, old-fashioned kind that digests slowly and keeps blood sugar from rising rapidly. Choose in preference to instant oatmeal, in which the grain is chopped into little bits and has a very high glycaemic index. (Chapter 1 has more information about the glycaemic index.)

  ✔ Stay away from flavoured oatmeal products because they're sure to contain loads of added sugar.

Eggs

Poached and boiled eggs are both good for high-quality protein prepared without fat. When you poach an egg, the white of the egg protects the yolk, the only part of the egg that contains cholesterol, and keeps the cholesterol from oxidising. Oxidised cholesterol is the kind that is more likely to lead to an accumulation of plaque, narrowing the arteries and setting the stage for a heart attack or stroke.

Stay away from scrambled eggs because the yolk and cholesterol come in direct contact with a very hot cooking surface and easily oxidises. Frying eggs also exposes the yolk to direct heat. And needless to say, Eggs Benedict coated in buttery hollandaise sauce is definitely off limits!

And if you've made up your mind that you're never going to eat egg yolks again because you know they're high in cholesterol, you can always try asking the waiter to make you an egg white omelette. However, egg white omelettes need some jazzing up, because they taste bland and your omelette now doesn't have the satisfying fat that the yolk provides. Also order some lean back bacon or a bit of smoked fish, such as salmon, to put together a tasty breakfast that also supplies enough energy to last until lunch.

Rolls, muffins, and toast

Order rye toast for a grain that contains phytonutrients, a class of substances that have many health benefits including acting as antioxidants. To watch your fat intake, request that the toast is served dry, not slathered in spread, but with butter on the side that you can add if you want.

Think twice before you order a healthy-sounding bran muffin. Bran muffins are likely to have a high sugar and fat content, despite all that fibre. In fact, virtually all muffins normally served in restaurants are just cake in another form.

Potato cakes and hash browns

Spuds are a source of potassium, which helps lower blood pressure. But order them plain boiled rather than roast or chipped. Chipped potatoes are often frozen products that restaurants buy in bulk, and may contain partially hydrogenated oils, which increase blood levels of cholesterol.

Breakfast meats and fish

For the taste of pork, have lean back bacon that is lower in total fat and saturated fat than streaky bacon. If you want fish, try kippers, smoked salmon, or gravadlax (cold-cured salmon). Savour these on a slice of wholegrain toast trimmed with sliced, raw red onions that thin the blood and counteract inflammation, fresh sliced tomatoes for heart-protective lycopene, and olives with their healthy monounsaturated fats.

Fresh fruit

Instead of getting your fruit from juice, why not ask for one of the following:

✔ A grapefruit half (if taking medications, check the drug information sheet within the pack for potential interactions, especially if you're taking a statin drug to lower cholesterol levels).

✔ A slice of refreshing cantaloupe or honeydew melon.

✔ A bowl of soluble-fibre-rich canned prunes (gets the bowels moving!)

✔ A banana.

✔ A bowl of berries such as strawberries.

If the only fruit on the menu is tinned fruit, or you decide you want the canned prunes, ordering tinned fruit occasionally is fine. Eat the fruit and try to select versions tinned in juice rather than syrup.

Whole fruit provides fibre and more nutrients than fruit juice, is more filling, and less harmful to the teeth.

Hot drinks

If you need your morning caffeine, order black or green tea for the phytonutrients these drinks contain. (See Chapter 2 for more info about phytonutrients.) These beverages can also help wean you from the need to consume large amounts of coffee to get going. Black tea contains about a third less caffeine than coffee, and green tea contains only half the amount in black tea. Caffeine stresses the adrenal glands and the heart muscle as the chemistry it triggers sends your body into high gear. You can also try fruit or herb teas and soya milk.

Black and green teas contain phytonutrients that help keep blood vessels functioning normally, reduce chronic inflammation (which is now considered a risk factor for heart disease), and function as antioxidants, preventing the 'bad' LDL cholesterol from shifting to its dangerous oxidised form. (Chapter 24 gives you details on the health benefits of these teas.)

But if only a cup of java coffee will do, limit yourself to one or two cups in total for the day. As you find out in Chapter 24, research shows that drinking a lot of unfiltered coffee can raise cholesterol. Unfiltered coffee contains a substance called *cafesterol*, which is the strongest dietary cholesterol-raising agent known. Filtering removes cafesterol from brewed coffee, however. So, if you're one of the millions of people who line up in the morning at trendy coffee places for an order of gourmet coffee, take care over the brewing method and extra ingredients you choose. Have cappuccino made with skimmed milk to reduce saturated fat and skip those sweet concoctions, often laced with stuff such as caramel syrup, which these shops are always inventing. These beverages, although delicious, can add hundreds of calories to your daily intake before you've even had your first meal.

Instead of having a rich coffee drink, save the calories and fat for actual breakfast foods and have your coffee as plain as possible.

Eating on the hoof

You're on the road, spending the night in a hotel, and you wake up hungry. Making your way to the hotel lobby, you find the free breakfast buffet that comes with the price of the room. The table holds an array of sweet rolls, sugar-coated cereals, white toast, sweetened orange juice, together with jams, margarine, and non-dairy creamer for your coffee. Or perhaps you're faced with an array of fried black pudding, fried bread, greasy eggs, and fatty bacon? What a way to start the day!

A meal of these breakfast foods certainly gets your blood sugar up and running, but this menu is not one you need for heart health. When faced with a hotel buffet, concentrate on the healthier foods that sometimes show up:

- ✔ Have the brown or wholemeal toast, which is, in part, made with wholegrains. Smear it with a little honey if you want something sweet, but not the margarine if it contains trans fats.

- ✔ Grab the Shredded Wheat – which has no sugar and is a wholegrain – before someone else does.

- ✔ As well as a small glass of fruit juice, take a portion of the whole fruit, usually apples or bananas or fruit salad. These fruits give you fibre and cause your blood sugar to spike less. (Few hotel guests take these, so you don't have much competition here.)

- ✔ Have your morning caffeine in the form of tea, a source of antioxidants.

If you'd rather not rely on the hotel breakfast buffet to supply a healthy breakfast, here are some suggestions for taking your breakfast along with you when you travel:

✔ Oranges, grapes, apples, and bananas travel well, but peaches don't. Dried fruits, such as dates, apple rings, and halves of apricots, are also good choices.

✔ Pack some low-fat cream cheese to get you through your first morning meeting. Have this with crunchy, wholegrain crackers or rye crispbread.

✔ Bring along a small jar of nut butter (you can buy macadamia, almond, walnut, and Brazil nut butters in health food stores) and have this with wholegrain bread and baked goods, including those made with the recipes in Chapters 6 and 20. This mini-meal can supply you with enough fuel to last until lunch.

If the hotel breakfast buffet fails the healthy test and you forgot to pack any nutritious foods, slip around the corner to the local café and order some of the recommended breakfast foods listed in this section.

Seeking Out Nourishing Lunch Breaks

Of all the eating-out scenarios, the lunchtime workday meal presents the most challenges if you're watching your cholesterol balance. You have limited time to eat and have to rely on whatever restaurants are within walking or short driving distance of your workplace. Consequently, you're eating at the local coffee shop, a sandwich outlet, a deli, or a casual chain or franchise restaurant. You can find many heart-healthy foods on the menus of these eateries. Here are some suggestions:

Business lunches with guys don't have to include steak and chips

Somewhere between the martini lunch and when real men decided not to eat quiche, food for males became irrevocably associated with all that's meaty and fat. Business meetings are held in restaurant-bars that specialise in steaks and ribs. Serious man's food is the order of the day. It takes an independent male indeed to go against this trend. What do you do in such a situation?

Plan ahead and show your alpha-male leadership. Know in advance exactly what you're going to order so that you aren't tempted to go along with the gang. In a clear, loud voice, order the grilled fish. Have that salad, dressing on the side, so the others can see that you're a man with a plan. Men who eat healthy lunches and skip dessert also earn a fast pay-off compared with their companions who load up on heavy food: they find it easier to stay awake and clear-headed during the afternoon meetings, while their competition is dozing off.

✔ Make soup your first choice at lunch. Lunch outlets can't deep-fry it or add much sugar, so when you have soup for lunch, you're already way ahead of the game. The stock still contains all the vitamins and minerals of the various ingredients that have cooked in it in the process of making the soup. Many soups give you at least a serving of vegetables, a good step toward your daily quota. Served hot, soup is a satisfying mini-meal on chilly days. And many soups are bulky, filling you up but with fewer calories. Good choices are fish, bean, lentil, tomato, and mixed vegetable soups.

✔ Lunching on crispy salad is a fine choice. Salads are usually low in fat (not counting the dressing of course!), and the vegetables are raw and full of nutrients. Salads contain fibre foods that help steady blood sugar. Ingredients such as onions and garlic have a blood-thinning action. Colourful salads in particular give you a variety of heart-protective antioxidants.

✔ Grilled chicken atop a mixed greens salad makes a lean, complete meal.

Avoid salads that feature fatty meats, fried noodles, cheese, and lots of oily croutons, such as chef's salad, Chinese chicken salad, and Caesar salad.

✔ Choose the fruit salad with low-fat or regular fat cottage cheese.

✔ Request wholemeal bread instead of white. Eating two slices gives you two servings of wholegrains, a good way to lower your risk of heart disease. (Chapter 20 tells you all about the health benefits of wholegrains.) Or request rye bread or pumpernickel, also made with a good proportion of rye flour, to increase the variety of grains in your diet.

✔ Enjoy sandwiches spread with a little mustard rather than mayonnaise to cut fat and calories. You can also request your sandwich dry and order a small portion of low-fat salad dressing to spread on the bread.

✔ Having oily fish for lunch is a great idea. Fish is also a protein food that can provide you with energy for several hours, especially important if you have a busy afternoon ahead. Here's what to look for on menus in specific types of restaurants:

Putting the 'break' back into lunch break

The midday meal is called a lunch 'break' for a reason. It's also a time to rest and recharge your batteries. One way to give yourself respite is to lunch in a restaurant. Healthy items to order include a soup and salad, baked or grilled fish, chicken stir-fry, spaghetti marinara, and side orders of vegetables, or even sushi, vegetable noodles, or tomato-based pasta sauces. Have a cup of tea, sugar-free drink or smoothie, or – better still – drink water, and skip dessert (and wine). And remember, if you do order a typical dinner item at midday, ask for a small-sized portion so you don't load up on calories and need an afternoon nap.

Ordering for the shy and unassertive

When you're in a restaurant, requesting something special is perfectly acceptable, especially for reasons of health. You're the customer, and if your waiter ends up a bit disgruntled that's fine. Besides, many restaurants these days have a policy of accommodating health-conscious guests and some even display the fat and energy content of dishes if you ask for it. Even if you feel timid, press on and speak up! Here are some things you can request to eat more nutritious foods and cut calories:

- A substitution of one food for another, replacing potato salad with fresh fruit, or onion rings and chips with plain, cooked vegetables with no butter.

- Lunch or dinner composed of only healthy appetisers and vegetable side dishes.

- Several vegetable side dishes with your main course.

- An appetiser-size serving of a main course.

- Your meal cooked with a minimum amount of fat.

- A two-egg omelette made with one yolk.

- Salad dressing and gravy on the side, so that you can limit the amount you eat.

- A half-portion.

- A doggie bag, so you can eat part of your meal now and save the rest for another meal.

- No mayonnaise and no cheese.

- A glass of iced water or a cup of herbal tea.

- Information about the following: what kind of fat or oil the food you want to order is made with, whether the major ingredients are fresh or pre-packaged and frozen, and how the dish is prepared.

- **Coffee shops:** Tinned tuna and tinned salmon are the usual offerings. A tuna salad sandwich is a better choice than egg salad or roast beef to control cholesterol, but the best way to have your tinned tuna or salmon is unadorned as part of a green salad. Dress this with vinaigrette rather than mayonnaise. If such a salad is not on the menu, ask whether the cook can assemble one for you.

  Instead of eating fish with tartar sauce, which contains fatty mayonnaise, enjoy fish with a sprinkling of malt vinegar or a squeeze of lemon juice. These acidic condiments nicely complement the oiliness of fish.

- **Family restaurants:** Many of these establishments offer fish dishes prepared with health in mind. The menus may include items such as low-fat grilled white fish, for example sea bass, haddock, or cod, and salads topped with grilled or baked salmon.

- **Delis:** Smoked and marinated fish – salmon, trout, and herring – are standard items. Enjoy some on a piece of rye or a bagel, with some coleslaw on the side. You may also see cream cheese mixed with smoked salmon, which is delicious but high in saturated fat. Opt for low-fat versions. You can also find sandwiches filled with lean beef, chicken, pastrami, ham turkey, prawns, crayfish, smoked salmon, low-fat cream cheese, chargrilled vegetables, hummus, olives, gherkins, chilli, avocado, rocket, spinach, or peppers.

- **Fast food places:** Fish sandwiches in fast food restaurants sound like a healthy lunch to order, but typically the fish is deep-fried and covered in batter, not a heart-healthy choice at all. Perhaps try the beanburger with salad or other vegetarian options.

Doing Do-able Dinners

Finding healthy foods on dinner menus is usually fairly easy. From the soups and salads to the poultry and fish, you can assemble a delicious meal and still control cholesterol. Just don't order too much and then eat it all simply because you're paying for it.

If you know in advance that a restaurant's menu is a minefield of deep-fried foods, suggest another restaurant to your family or friends. You don't want to go to a place where everyone is chomping fried chicken and you're eating a green salad and baked filet of sole.

Eating traditional British food

Traditional British food tends to veer towards the unhealthy with lots of fat and pastry that plays havoc with your cholesterol balance. Fish and chips, Cornish pasties, steak and kidney pudding, pork pies, and Eccles cakes all make wonderful treats, but aren't good for you if they pass your lips every day. When you do succumb, select small portions and leave as much pastry on your plate as you can. Instead of apple pies, treacle tarts, and sponge puddings along the lines of spotted dick and jam roly-poly, opt for baked apples or fresh fruit instead. Look for some cholesterol-friendly options in Part VI of this book.

Fast food contains highly processed ingredients that are also low in nutrients. Even recent attempts by fast-food chains to introduce grilled chicken sandwiches and healthier salads don't compare with the healthier versions you can find in the average coffee shop or café, especially if you eat all the dressing or sauces provided with it. And if you want a reality check on the consequences of consuming burgers and chips, watch the award-winning film *Super Size Me*. A fit and healthy youngish man decides to eat fast food every meal for a month and also stops all exercise to find out how this lifestyle affects his health. He gains lots of weight, his cholesterol soars, and his system takes a full year to recover from the damaging effects of his experiment.

Exploring ethnic restaurants

Go for it! Step into that dimly-lit Indian restaurant. Sidle up to a sushi bar. Pop into that new Thai place around the corner. These restaurants offer traditional dishes; the time-tested, nourishing foods that have sustained peoples over the centuries. Typically, ethnic dishes include a wide variety of ingredients, including legumes, nuts, seeds, exotic vegetables and fruits, and unusual grains, spices, and herbs. Recipes for these dishes evolved as cooks found ways to prepare whatever foods were available locally, both wild and cultivated. Such dishes often contain good amounts of plant foods, which are high in fibre and phytonutrients, a trustworthy formula for creating heart-healthy meals. Just avoid dishes with rich, creamy, buttery, cheesy, or oily sauces, or ask for a little to be served on the side so you can choose how much you eat.

Chapter 5

Gearing Up for Healthy Cooking

. . . .

In This Chapter

▶ Finding healthy foods in supermarkets and health food shops

▶ Deciphering food labels

▶ Getting ready to cook

. . . .

A s you move towards a healthier way of eating to control cholesterol, changing how you shop for food and how you prepare it comes with the territory. This chapter guides you through the changes you need to make when shopping and cooking. Whether you're an expert or a timid beginner, you may still need to stock up and even tool up to start preparing more healthy meals.

The following sections give a guided tour of supermarkets and health food shops to show you where to buy cholesterol-friendly foods. We also give you some tips for sorting out what food labels are really telling you. This chapter also suggests some kitchen items that facilitate low-fat cooking and help save you time and labour. Of course, you can probably manage using your normal cooking routine, but making some changes helps to make preparing healthy meals much easier and increases the likelihood that you'll eat them.

Gathering Healthy Ingredients

Begin a new era of treating yourself well by having on hand only those foods that support heart health and cholesterol balance. Imagine a kitchen containing only fresh, quality ingredients so that whatever you choose to eat is good for you. By following the advice in this chapter, you can have such a kitchen.

You can find many of the recommended foods in your regular supermarket, but you may also need to visit health food shops and perhaps ethnic food shops or delicatessens for certain special items. You're about to discover a new way of shopping for food that is both satisfying and entertaining.

Rediscovering your supermarket

In this section we take you on a virtual tour of the place where you usually do your food shopping. Your current routine may take you to the deli section first to pick up luncheon meats and cheese, and then to the freezer section for handy, frozen vegetables and ice cream. But you can just as easily make your way to more nutritious foods. Here's how.

Shopping around the edges of the shop

While the aisles in grocery shops are filled with row upon row of boxed, bottled, and canned foods, which are mostly processed or refined products, the perimeter of supermarkets is where fresh and natural food is displayed. Make the edges of the markets your turf! Here's where you find the majority of foods with the most nutrients.

- Head for the produce section for fresh vegetables and seasonal fruits, making sure to buy a variety of produce and things you haven't eaten for a while. How about some berries, spinach, kale, asparagus, artichoke, avocado, mangoes, and sweet potatoes?

- While you're in the produce department, treat yourself to fresh herbs and other flavouring staples such as onions, fresh garlic, chillies, and root ginger.

- In the chilled section, look for milk and plain yogurt with a lower fat content, as well as low-fat and gourmet cheeses.

- In the dairy section, look for omega-3 enriched spreads containing olive or rapeseed oil to use on toast, or those that contain cholesterol-lowering sterols.

- Take home a carton of orange juice that contains some pulp for extra fibre.

- Check the meat section for turkey breast (a handy form of low-fat protein), pork tenderloin, and skinless chicken breasts. Also look for lean mince and other lean cuts of meat.

- Purchase fresh fish fillets and whole fish if you trust the quality. Otherwise, shop at a dedicated fishmonger. (Chapter 14 gives you guidelines on shopping for fish.)

- The deli section isn't off limits! Select reduced-fat turkey slices, lean back bacon, smoked salmon, marinated herring, and soya versions of breakfast meats such as vegetarian bacon and sausages.

- When you do buy eggs, favour brands that state on the label 'rich in omega-3', a type of fat that helps prevent the formation of clots and inflammation. (See Chapter 1 for an explanation of how inflammation plays a role in the development of heart disease. For more on omega-3s, check out Chapter 3.)

Touring the aisles

Supermarket aisles do harbour some healthy foods, such as wholegrain items and dried or canned beans. Make a point of strolling down the aisles to take a fresh look at what's available. You're sure to find many of the recommended items on the following list:

- ✔ In the cereal section, pick up some rolled oats.

  Stay away from all the instant hot cereals because they quickly raise blood sugar.

- ✔ Choose wholegrain brown rice, wild rice, bulgur wheat, barley, kidney beans, and lentils.

  Don't buy beans where you suspect turnover is slow. If overly dried out, they're past their prime and take forever to cook. Canned beans are an alternative but only if they aren't canned with sugar or salt.

- ✔ Bring home a bottle of olive oil – don't buy too large an amount because it can go off through the process of oxidation. Better to buy little and often.

- ✔ Look for all-fruit spreads that contain no added sugar.

- ✔ Poke around the baked goods section for wholegrain pittas, muffins, bagels, breads, and crackers. Corn tortillas are also a wholegrain product.

- ✔ Buy almonds, walnuts, macadamias, Brazil nuts, and nut butters (including peanut butter if you can find a brand that doesn't include hydrogenated oils).

Heading for the health food shop

If you haven't shopped for 'health foods' recently, you're in for a treat. The typically small and cluttered health food shop that used to smell faintly of medicinal herbs has evolved into a glamorous food emporium that offers a vast range of fresh produce, meats, and even fish, as well as a wealth of nutritious packaged and frozen items.

Health food shops carry an exotic and gourmet range of foods fit for a queen, but fortunately these stores also carry many tried and tested staples. You're sure to locate here many items that you probably can't find at the supermarket. But that's not to say that your usual supermarket doesn't sell some of them. Times are changing, and many superstores are beginning to offer healthy alternatives in response to customer demand. Here are some tips to help you with your shopping:

- ✔ Health food shops offer the full range of vegetable oils, from extra-virgin olive oil to rapeseed, safflower, and sesame seed oils. You can also find gourmet walnut, macadamia, and almond oils in health food shops.

Organic produce: Clean greens and more

Going organic means eating foods that are produced using organic farming practices and which have received minimal processing. These practices are proven and sustainable methods of producing food in harmony with nature, without the use of pesticides, antibiotics, hormones, artificial fertilisers, genetic manipulation, irradiation, or undue exposure to environmental pollution. Instead, farmers use traditional methods of pest control and crop rotation, grow green manure crops (such as clover), carefully time their sowing, and allow land to lie fallow. Organic farming is good for the planet, and also good for you. It results in products that are full of flavour, vitamins, and minerals, and which contain the lowest possible amounts of artificial chemicals.

The Soil Association (www.soil association.org) is the UK's leading environmental charity and international authority promoting sustainable, organic farming. The Association checks standards and certifies over 70 per cent of the organic foods sold in the UK to ensure that they are free of unwanted agricultural chemicals and genetic modification. Visit its consumer website, www.whyorganic.org, for an organic directory in which you can search for a variety of organic outlets, including box schemes that deliver fresh, organic fruit and vegetables to your door. The website's healthy eating section explains why organic is better for your health and includes seasonal recipes and nutritional advice. It even helps you search for places to enjoy an 'organic' holiday.

To limit your intake of pesticides:

✔ Eat a variety of fruit and vegetables.

✔ Wash all produce and peel them – remember government advice to peel and top carrots before eating.

✔ Buy organic produce whenever possible.

✔ Look for flaxseed oil found in the chilled section of the shop. (You need to store it in your fridge, too.) Shops sell flaxseed oil in opaque containers to protect its fragile fats from damage by light (the nature of flaxseed oil causes it to go rancid quickly). Purchase a small, 225 millilitre bottle so that you can use all the contents within a month.

✔ Look for frozen or dried soya mince (checking the salt content first), soya ice cream and soya milk, as well as vegetarian versions of common foods such as tinned soya chilli and quorn products.

✔ Spend a few minutes exploring any bulk bins that contain a variety of wholegrains, flour, legumes, nuts, seeds, oat bran, and dried fruits, such as dates, figs, prunes, apple rings, apricots, cherries, and cranberries. This is the thriftiest way to buy such ingredients, and you can scoop up just the amount you need. These staples are usually fresh because of their high turnover.

✔ Health food stores often offer wholegrain breads made with exotic low glycaemic index grains such as spelt, as well as wheat-free and gluten-free loaves. Also check out wholegrain pastas made with brown rice, spelt, quinoa, wholewheat, and buckwheat.

Buckwheat noodles, called soba noodles, are good with Chinese sesame sauce, which is made with sesame paste, soya sauce, rice wine vinegar, honey, sherry, fresh coriander, and chilli oil. This dish is good topped with toasted peanuts.

✔ All sorts of wholegrain breakfast cereals that don't contain trans fatty acids and added sweeteners are available in health food shops. Some are made with unusual grains such as spelt and quinoa. Try them all and never find breakfast boring again.

✔ Health food shops offer a full range of natural sweeteners, including date sugar, pure maple syrup, agave syrup (from the spiky, Mexican succulent used to make tequila), and raw honey, which are healthier than pure white sugar.

✔ Freezer sections contain such useful items as lower fat versions of frozen dinners, vegetables, sorbet, fish, and berries.

Figuring Out Food Labels

In the UK, manufacturers have adopted front of pack food labelling, which focuses on fat, saturates, sugars, and salt – all things that concern people who are trying to prevent heart disease. You may see traffic light coding, guideline daily amounts, or a combination of the two.

✔ **The traffic light system** shows you at a glance whether a food you're thinking of buying contains a high (red), medium (amber), or low (green) amount of fat, saturates, sugar, or salt. The label tells you how much of these substances is present in a given serving, stated in grams. If that part of the label is red, you know the food is high in something that you're trying to cut down on. The food is fine as an occasional treat, but keep an eye on how often you eat it and stick to smaller portions. If that part of the food label has an amber background, the food isn't high or low in these unhealthy substances and is mostly an okay option, but do try to go for 'green' when you can. Green means that the food is low in fat, saturated fat, sugars, and salt, and is the healthiest option.

The traffic light system isn't foolproof, however, because a food such as fresh salmon, which is high in healthy oils, has its fat content highlighted on a red background, and yet most people benefit from eating more oily fish! This system also doesn't show you how much of a substance is present as a percentage of the daily recommended amount.

✔ **Guideline daily amounts** show you how much of a substance a portion of the food provides as a percentage of an adult's guideline daily amount. These labels also provide information on calories, sugars, fat, saturates, and salt. So, if you're trying to cut back on salt or fat, select the product that provides the lowest percentage of your GDA. For more information on how to use GDAs, visit the www.whatsinsideguide.com website.

The drawback of this system is that it helps to be good with numbers – not everyone finds them as easy to use as the traffic light system.

Labels can mislead you, for example:

✔ A food low in fat may contain high amounts of sugar.

✔ Low-fat does not necessarily mean low-calorie.

✔ Simply because a food is low in fat doesn't mean it's necessarily good for you. Even small amounts of trans fats are harmful, and the pack doesn't always mention the level, so you need to look for partially hydrogenated fat on the label.

✔ In the UK, food labels don't have to provide information on the amount of cholesterol present in the food (though they do have to in some other countries, such as the US).

Labelling nutrition facts

Most labels show typical nutritional values in 100 grams of a food, and also how much is present in a typical serving. Figure 5-1 shows an example of a GDA-type food label for a pre-packed low-fat vegetable stew.

Vegetable Stew				
NUTRITION INFORMATION			GUIDELINE DAILY AMOUNTS	
Typical values	per 100g	per 300g serving	Woman	Men
Energy - kJ	240kJ	720kJ		
- kcal	85 kcal	255 kcal	2000	2500
Protein	5g	15g	45g	55g
Carbohydrate	4.4g	13.2g	230g	300g
of which sugars	1.1g	3.3g	90g	120g
Fat	2.2g	6.6g	70g	95g
of which saturates	1.0g	3.0g	20g	30g
Fibre	1.5g	4.5g	24g	24g
Sodium*	0.2g	0.6g	2.4g	2.4g
*Equivalent as salt	0.5g	1.5g		

Figure 5-1: A typical GDA-type food label showing details of nutritional content.

Figure 5-2 shows an example of a traffic light system food label. The label indicates that the food has low (green) amounts of fat and saturates, high (red) amounts of sugar, and medium (amber) amounts of salt: green indicates a healthy option, amber an okay option, and red a less healthy option.

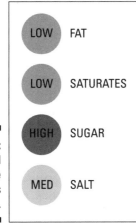

Figure 5-2:
A typical
multiple
traffic lights
food label.

Similarly to the nutrition labels, the nutritional information at the end of each recipe in this book gives you the actual amount of various nutrients per serving. It tells you the number of grams of fat, carbohydrate, and protein and also includes the specific amounts of cholesterol, sodium, and dietary fibre as well. When you decide on the number of grams of these various dietary components you want to aim for in your meals, you can use these recipe tabulations to help you add up your tally for the day.

Looking at what's a little and what's a lot

Get into the habit of checking labels. As well as helping you compare prices and pack weights, labels tell you the nutritional value of what you're buying with ingredients listed in descending order of weight.

When checking labels for *sugar* content, a good general rule is that per 100 grams of food (or per serving if a serving is less than 100 grams):

- ✔ **2 grams** of sugar or less is **a little** sugar.
- ✔ **10 grams** of sugar or more is **a lot** of sugar.

When checking for *fats*, remember that the type of fat is important. Some saturated fats can raise cholesterol levels, and so for a healthy heart cut back on products containing lots of saturated fats such as pies, pastries, butter, cheese, cakes, and biscuits. Monounsaturated fats (those found in olive oil and rapeseed oil, for example) don't increase the risk of heart disease, and moderate intakes of polyunsaturated fats may even lower the risk of a heart attack.

When checking labels for *total fat* content, a good rule is that per 100 grams of food (or per serving if a serving is less than 100 grams):

- ✓ **3 grams** of total fat or less is **a little** total fat.
- ✓ **20 grams** of total fat or more is **a lot** of total fat.

Whereas, for *saturated fats*:

- ✓ **1 gram** of saturated fat or less is **a little** saturated fat.
- ✓ **5 grams** of saturated fat or more is **a lot** of saturated fat.

The *salt* (sodium chloride) content of food is also important because over two-thirds of the sodium we eat comes from processed foods, including canned products, ready-prepared meals, biscuits, cakes, and breakfast cereals, where it enhances flavour, retains moisture, and helps products last longer on the shelf. Unfortunately most of us eat too much salt, and excess is linked with high blood pressure. Checking labels of products and avoiding those containing high amounts of salt is vital for keeping on top of your salt (sodium) intake. A good rule is that, per 100 grams of food, or per serving if a serving is less than 100 grams:

- ✓ **0.1 grams** of sodium or less is **a little** sodium.
- ✓ **0.5 grams** of sodium or more is **a lot** of sodium.

Salt is made up of sodium and chloride. When reading labels, multiply those giving salt content as 'sodium' by 2.5 to get the table salt content. For example, a serving of soup containing 0.4 grams of sodium contains 1 gram of salt (sodium chloride).

Adults should have no more than 6 grams of salt or about 2.5 grams of sodium a day. You can easily replace salt with herbs and spices because it doesn't take long to retrain your taste buds. Adding lime juice to food stimulates your tastes buds and decreases the amount of salt you need, too.

Aim to eat no more than 6 grams of salt per day – around one level teaspoon – and preferably much less.

Studying the label lingo

Labels geared to the health-conscious market are usually better at announcing what the food inside does *not* contain, but you need to read all the info on the labels, especially if you're watching your cholesterol. Although labels aren't allowed to mislead, some claims, such as 'lite' or 'reduced salt' have no legally agreed definitions, although new EU regulations are looking into this. In the meantime, double-checking with the actual nutrition information panel on packs is always a good move. For example, look for:

✔ Fat free (should contain less than 0.5 grams of fat per 100 grams/100 millilitres).

✔ Low fat (should contain less than 3 grams per 100 grams or 1.5 grams per 100 millilitres).

✔ Low sodium (should contain 40 milligrams or less per 100 grams/100 millilitres).

✔ High fibre (should contain 6 grams or more per 100 grams/100 millilitres).

✔ Sugar free (should contain less than 0.2 grams per 100 grams/100 millilitres).

✔ Low sugar (should contain less than 5 grams per 100 grams/100 millilitres).

✔ Low calorie (should contain 40 kilocalories or less per 100 grams/100 millilitres).

✔ Unsweetened (should have no added sugar).

✔ Reduced calorie products should contain at least 25 per cent fewer calories than the standard version.

Preparing to Cook

Even if you're someone who cooks with spontaneity and passion, bringing a semblance of order to the process can't hurt. Having all the ingredients and cooking tools ready to go in advance helps prevent a kitchen crisis and leaves you free to enjoy the pleasures of cooking. (In French cooking, the name for this divine state of preparedness is *mise en place.*) Why should TV chefs have all the fun, with their vast support staffs setting up everything in advance? Here's the drill:

✔ Put on your apron, roll up your sleeves, and check that clean dish towels and paper towels are within arm's reach.

✔ Warn everyone not to anger the cook and resolve to stay calm while cooking. A study in the *Journal of the American College of Cardiology* found that expressing anger accelerates the progression of atherosclerosis (hardening and furring up of the arteries).

✔ Clear your work surface of clutter and have a chopping board ready to use.

Keep items you use often close to where you usually use them. Store cookware you rarely use – perhaps that pasta machine – in the back of the cupboard or on a high shelf.

✔ Choose a recipe if you haven't already done so, and take a quiet moment to read thoughtfully through the entire instructions. You can avoid surprises and perhaps better organise your cooking procedure.

✔ Assemble all the ingredients that the recipe requires. For accuracy, give your full attention to measuring key ingredients, such as oil and spices.

✔ Wash and prepare produce and cut fruit and vegetables according to recipe instructions. Trim meats, and wash and prepare poultry. (Depending upon the recipe, sometimes preparing certain ingredients while others are cooking is a more efficient approach.)

✔ Keep a pan of hot, soapy dishwater nearby or fill the sink, where you can put dirty bowls, mixing spoons, and the like as you finish using them. In this way you have a jump-start on cleaning up the kitchen and your equipment ready to use again if you need it for another step in the recipe.

After you've finished cooking and the delicious results are yours to enjoy, sit down at a table to eat your meal slowly in order to fully appreciate this chance to nourish yourself, and think about how much better off your body and cholesterol levels are for the care you've put into choosing the most healthy ingredients.

Part II
Mastering the Beneficial Breakfast

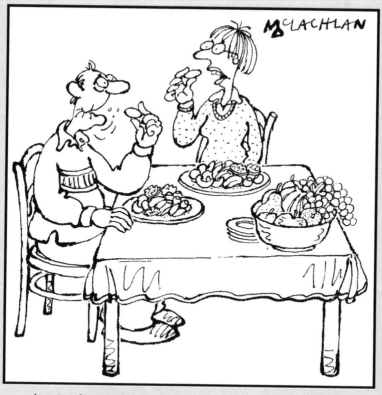

'I think you'd appreciate having nuts for breakfast in the mornings if you put your teeth in!'

In this part . . .

*T*he three chapters in this part focus on breakfast, a meal that's typically full of foods that raise cholesterol. But don't worry – you can discover lots of clever ways to start your day with heart-healthy dishes that are so tasty they're destined to become part of your morning routine.

This part explains why some carbohydrates are ideal for controlling cholesterol, and ensures that you have some protein while limiting your intake of saturated fat. And yes, it helps you unscramble all the advice out there about eating eggs. This part concludes with ideas for quick breakfast recipes to make sure that you can always obtain a meal to keep you going until lunch and that's also good for your cholesterol balance.

Chapter 6

Enjoying a Wholesome Breakfast with Wholefoods

Breakfast is the most challenging meal of the day when it comes to eating in a cholesterol-friendly way. So many standard breakfast items are missing nutrients that are good for your heart and contain loads of fat and sugar that contribute to obesity.

The recipes in this chapter enable you to take a fresh look at breakfast foods based on grains, identifying those items that are the most nutritious and providing healthy versions of French toast and pancakes. You can still enjoy these treats and take care of your arteries if you adjust the traditional recipes.

Sorting Out Starches and Sweets

When touring the aisles at your local supermarket, avoid the baked goods and cereals made with refined grains, sugars, and added fat. Hands off those Danish pastries, crêpes, toastable tarts, and cereals that can lead to high blood sugar, weight gain, and eventually heart problems when they form your usual breakfast. The good news, though, is that nutritious, wholegrain cereals, and baked goods are now showing up more often.

Adding wholefoods

Avoiding refined white flour and white sugar takes commitment, because white foods are so prevalent. You need to act like a sleuth and read those package labels closely. Planning what to eat for the day ahead also helps keep you away from these products. You stand to benefit if you replace just half the refined carbs you normally eat with unrefined wholegrain foods. Here are some actions to take:

✔ When you go shopping, search out wholewheat bagels, muffins, and wholegrain and multigrain breads. More and more manufacturers now provide these alternatives. Also, request wholewheat and wholegrain breads when you're eating breakfast out.

✔ Look for cereals made with wholegrains and those that contain no partially hydrogenated vegetable oils or added sugars. Unsweetened muesli is a winner.

✔ Have a big enough breakfast at home so that you're not tempted to eat from the snack trolley at work or stop for a fast food breakfast. Assemble what you plan to eat for breakfast the night before so that everything is ready to prepare quickly next morning.

✔ Carry nutritious snack foods with you when you're away from home. Then, when you feel hungry, you don't cave in and buy something starchy and sweet. Bring along almonds, macadamias, fresh cherries, grapes, crunchy vegetables and a natural yogurt dip, or salads with low-fat soft cheese and hummus.

Sowing your oats

Oats are one of the few grains that manufacturers leave unrefined with germ and bran intact. Several years ago, this homey breakfast staple suddenly became a must-have health food for its ability to lower cholesterol. Other foods, such as legumes, now share the spotlight, but a bowl of oatmeal still ranks as one of the healthiest choices you can make for breakfast. Bring on the porridge!

Oat bran contains soluble fibre, the kind that lowers cholesterol. Oats are also a good source of vitamin E, folate, iron, copper, and zinc, and they're very high in manganese and protein. According to one study, published in the *American Journal of Clinical Nutrition* in 2002, oats are far better than wheat for lowering cholesterol and for improving blood lipids and lipoprotein profiles. The researchers had 36 men, aged 50 to 75 years, consume two large servings of oat cereal or wheat cereal daily for 12 weeks. For those eating oats, levels of 'bad' LDL cholesterol declined without lowering 'good' HDL cholesterol or raising triglycerides. But for those consuming wheat cereal, LDL cholesterol, the ratio of LDL to HDL cholesterol, and triglycerides all increased (see Chapter 1).

Experts recommend that your intake of soluble fibre is between 5 and 10 grams a day. Please see below a list of foods where you can find it:

- ✔ Oat bran
- ✔ Dried split peas
- ✔ Strawberries
- ✔ Cooked rolled oats
- ✔ Apples
- ✔ Barley
- ✔ Beans
- ✔ Pears

Eat home-made porridge or muesli for breakfast, and sneak oatmeal, oat flour, and oat bran into your meals in other ways, too. For example, you can include them in recipes for muffins, pancakes (see the recipe for Pancakes with Pecan Nuts and Maple Syrup in this chapter), and meat loaf. Even oatmeal cookies count, too! (See the Chewy Oatmeal and Raisin Bites recipe in Chapter 22 for an especially nutritious version.)

Watching your sugar intake

Sugar supplies calories and contributes to excess weight which, in turn, increases your risk of coronary heart disease – especially if you have a raised cholesterol level.

If you're not careful, breakfast can include more sweet foods than any other meal of the day. Replacing some of that sugar with more wholesome sources of sweetness – and that doesn't mean artificial additives – is always a good idea, because these supply some nutrients such as vitamins and minerals, instead of the 'empty' calories of table sugar.

Try these natural sweeteners; each one has special benefits:

- ✔ **Maple syrup:** The natural sap of the maple tree, this syrup contains small amounts of calcium, potassium, magnesium, manganese, phosphorus, and iron, as well as trace amounts of B vitamins. Maple is also just the right flavour to complement many breakfast foods.

- ✔ **Honey:** You need less honey to sweeten a dish because honey is sweeter than table sugar. Hunt for local honey at farmers markets. Some honeys even have medicinal properties, such as Manuka honey, which is antibacterial.

✔ **Date sugar:** This form of sugar is dried, ground dates. Like dates, date sugar is loaded with nutrients such as niacin, potassium, and calcium. Buy this whole food sweetener in natural food stores and try it sprinkled on the Cranberry Fruit Pudding in this chapter. If you can't find date sugar, you can easily make it by drying dates and chopping them in a blender. You can also buy date sugar as a syrup.

✔ **Agave Syrup:** Made from the juice of the blue agave, this syrup is sweeter than honey, though less sticky. The sweetness comes mainly in the form of fructose (fruit sugar), which has less impact on blood sugar levels than glucose. As a result, the glycaemic index is lower than other natural sweeteners (see Chapter 1 for more on the glycaemic index). Another advantage is that, unlike honey, agave syrup dissolves readily in cold drinks such as iced tea.

All products containing sugar can contribute to tooth decay, and so go easy on intakes. Ideally, wean yourself off sugar so you don't look for added sweetness at all.

For information on the quantity of honey and maple sugar needed to replace white sugar, see Chapter 22, about baked desserts.

Going for Cholesterol-Friendly Breakfast Recipes

Sample these wholegrain recipes for a real treat. They taste more like gourmet specialties than sober health food. The fruit pudding is so yummy that it also works as a dessert, and the baked apples, cloaked in mango chutney, are just right for a change of pace.

Keeping artificial sweeteners out of the pantry

The recipes in this cookbook give you ways to prepare dishes made with natural, unrefined, and unprocessed foods. We avoid artificial substances whenever possible, and the recipes don't call for any human-made sweeteners or sugar substitutes.

People use chemical substances to replace real foods, such as maple syrup and honey, and they do cut calories. However, the way of eating that we present in this book, with the emphasis on plant foods and lean meats, already provides you with a way to do this. In addition, portion control (another good way to cut calories) is one of the cornerstones of this cholesterol-controlling diet (see Chapter 1).

☞ *Cherry-Studded Three-Grain Porridge*

Let this porridge inspire you to try other healthy versions, too. The toasted millet has a great, popcorn-like flavour, while the barley and oats provide plenty of soluble fibre. Dried cherries, which you can buy in health food shops and some supermarkets, contain powerful antioxidants – but you can replace them with cranberries if you prefer. Serve this mix of hot cereals for weekend breakfasts and enjoy leftovers on weekdays when you're short of time. To reheat the porridge, scoop some into a bowl, pour a little milk over the cereal to loosen it up, and zap the cereal in the microwave for 1 minute. Top with a little honey or maple syrup if you like.

Preparation time: *30 minutes*

Cooking time: *45 minutes*

Serves: *4*

50 grams millet	*30 grams dried cherries or cranberries*
50 grams pearl barley	*40 grams rolled oats*
840 millilitres water	*2 tablespoons oat bran*

1 Put the millet in a bowl of water and briefly swish it around to remove excess starch. Pour out the now cloudy water, repeat the rinsing, and pour out the water again. (Any remaining moisture on the grains evaporates in toasting.)

2 Distribute the millet in a saucepan on medium heat. Stir frequently with a wooden spoon until the grains dry and begin to give off a sweet, toasted scent, after about 2 minutes. Remove the saucepan from the heat and transfer the millet to a small bowl.

3 Put the barley in a bowl of water and briefly swish around to remove excess starch. Pour out the water, repeat the rinsing, and pour out the water again. (The barley does not require toasting.)

4 Put the water in the pan used to toast the millet and place over a medium high heat. Bring the water to the boil. Add the millet, barley, and dried cherries. Turn the heat to low and simmer the grain mixture, partially covered, for 15 minutes. Stir the grains once or twice during the process.

5 Add the oats and oat bran and continue to cook the grains on low for 30 minutes, stirring frequently, especially towards the end so it doesn't stick to the pan as it thickens. Add additional hot water when necessary for desired porridge consistency. Serve warm.

Go-With: *Serve with your choice of lean bacon, smoked salmon, or toasted nuts and flaxseed oil for added nutritional value.*

Per serving: *Calories 162; Fat 2g (Saturated 0g); Cholesterol 0mg; Sodium 3mg; Carbohydrate 34g; Dietary Fibre 5g; Protein 5g.*

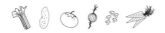

✎ *Pancakes with Pecan Nuts and Maple Syrup*

These elegant pancakes supply soluble fibre in the oat flour and bran and provide you with a small serving of nuts. The recipe also calls for wheatgerm, a highly nutritious part of wheat, which is normally removed when the grain is refined. This replenishes what was taken away from the plain wheat flour, which is refined. In this way, you have the lightness and delicate flavour of the refined flour plus the nutrients.

Preparation time: *20 minutes*

Cooking time: *15 minutes*

Serves: *4*

55 grams chopped pecan nuts

2½ millilitres unrefined safflower oil

180 millilitres maple syrup

60 millilitres orange juice

125 grams unbleached, plain flour

60 grams oat flour

1½ teaspoons baking powder

¼ teaspoon salt

2 tablespoons oat bran

1 tablespoon wheat germ

1 egg

420 millilitres buttermilk (see the tip at the end of the recipe)

2 tablespoons unrefined safflower oil, plus extra for greasing the griddle

1 Make the syrup: Heat the pecans and 2½ millilitres safflower oil in a small pan over medium-high heat, stirring frequently, until you can smell the pecan's fragrance (after around 2 minutes). Add the maple syrup and orange juice and stir to combine. Set aside.

2 To make the batter, sift together twice the plain flour, oat flour, baking powder, and salt. Add the oat bran and wheat germ to the flour mixture and mix with a fork. In a smaller bowl, whisk the egg. Add the buttermilk and safflower oil to the egg and whisk to combine. Gradually whisk the egg mixture into the dry ingredients, just until no lumps remain.

3 Heat a nonstick frying pan or griddle over medium heat. Dip a folded paper towel in the safflower oil and lightly coat the cooking surface. Spoon about 60 millilitres of the batter into the frying pan for each pancake. Cook for 1 to 1½ minutes, or until a few bubbles form on the top of the pancake and the underside is golden brown. Using a spatula, flip the pancakes over and cook for an additional 30 seconds, until they're just cooked through.

4 To make another batch, first lightly re-oil the cooking surface if necessary. Keep the pancakes and ovenproof serving plates warm in a low oven (120 degrees). Serve with the warm pecan, orange, and maple syrup mixture.

Tip: *For thicker pancakes, reduce the buttermilk to 300 millilitres.*

Per serving: *Calories 577; Fat 22g (Saturated 3g); Cholesterol 58mg; Sodium 424mg; Carbohydrate 87g; Dietary Fibre 5g; Protein 13g.*

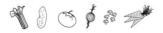

☺ Cranberry Fruit Pudding

This breakfast pudding is packed with fruit that's good for your heart, and makes a nice change from porridge. Raisins, cranberries, apples, and prunes are all rich sources of antioxidants and soluble fibre, which both help to lower LDL cholesterol levels. Traditional English puddings are usually made with cream and lots of sugar but this recipe is far lighter and topped with date sugar, which is simply dried, ground-up dates. You can enjoy this warm or cold the next day, with milk or yogurt.

Preparation time: *20 minutes*

Cooking time: *45 minutes*

Serves: *8*

8 chopped pitted prunes

60 grams dried cranberries

75 grams seedless, dark raisins

240 millilitres water

2 cored and chopped medium-size apples, such as Granny Smith (peeled, if you want)

1 sliced banana

25 grams sliced raw almonds

4 slices multigrain bread (bread that contains oats preferred) cut into 2-centimetre cubes

240 millilitres semi-skimmed milk

½ teaspoon vanilla essence

1 teaspoon allspice

2 tablespoons date sugar (see the tip at the end of the recipe)

1 Preheat the oven to 200 degrees. Put the prunes, cranberries, and raisins, along with the water, in a medium-size pan. Bring to the boil and then remove from the heat.

2 Stir in the apples, banana, almonds, and bread. Transfer the bread mixture to a greased 20-centimetre square baking dish.

3 In a small bowl, combine the milk, vanilla, and allspice. Pour the milk mixture over the fruit and bread. Sprinkle the top of the pudding with the date sugar.

4 Bake for 40 minutes, or until the apples have softened and the pudding is firm and golden brown. Enjoy it warm immediately or serve it cold the next day, with milk or yogurt.

Tip: *You can find date sugar in health food shops or make your own by processing dried dates in a blender. Muscovado or Jaggery are suitable alternatives.*

Tip: *Drizzle some of the syrup from the preceding 'Pancakes with Pecan Nuts and Maple Syrup' recipe over this pudding for a special treat.*

Per serving: *Calories 172; Fat 3g (Saturated 0g); Cholesterol 2mg; Sodium 79mg; Carbohydrate 38g; Dietary Fibre 4g; Protein 3g.*

Baked Apples with Turkey Sausage and Mango Chutney

This unusual European breakfast provides a mini-meal of carbohydrate, fat, and protein. Look for low-fat turkey sausage meat or use turkey mince, which is becoming more widely available. To decorate the apples before baking, cut away narrow strips of the apple skin using a citrus zester or apple peeler.

Special tools required: *Citrus zester or an apple peeler*

Preparation time: *15 minutes*

Cooking time: *45 minutes*

Serves: *4*

100 grams mango chutney	*4 tart apples such as Granny Smith*
1 tablespoon maple syrup	*100 grams low-fat turkey sausage meat*
360 millilitres water	

1 Preheat the oven to 180 degrees. Put the mango chutney, maple syrup, and water in a shallow 20-centimetre square baking dish just large enough to hold the apples. Stir the glaze with a fork to combine. Set aside.

2 Core each apple through to the bottom, and then replug the end with a bit cut off the core. Enlarge the cavity until it is about 2 centimetres across. Using a citrus striper, cut lines through the apple skin at intervals, starting at the stem end and running from top to bottom. The apples end up with 5 or 6 stripes.

3 Stuff each core opening with a quarter of the sausage meat, mounding it on the apple tops. Drizzle a teaspoon of glaze over the exposed sausage.

4 Put the baking dish in the oven. Baste the apples after 10 minutes and several times during baking. Bake until the apples are tender and the glaze has thickened, about 45 minutes.

5 Remove the apples from the oven and allow them to sit for 5 minutes. Spoon any remaining glaze in the dish over the apples. Serve warm.

Tip: *A loaf pan is handy for baking small to medium-size apples, the narrow width helping to hold the apples upright and in place.*

Go-With: *Serve the apples with sautéed polenta. You can purchase polenta ready-made, and then all you need to do is slice and sauté. (See Chapter 8 for more about ready-made polenta.)*

Per serving: *Calories 161; Fat 2g (Saturated 0g); Cholesterol 8mg; Sodium 172mg; Carbohydrate 36g; Dietary Fibre 4g; Protein 5g.*

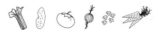

French Toast with Blueberry Sauce

This French toast – which some people know fondly as 'eggy bread' – contains fewer yolks and less fat than the usual French toast, but still tastes like you're having breakfast in Paris.

Preparation time: *15 minutes*

Cooking time: *20 minutes*

Serves: *4*

2 eggs

2 egg whites

240 millilitres skimmed milk

½ teaspoon vanilla essence

Zest of one lemon

8 slices day-old bread, cut in half on the diagonal (wholegrain or multigrain preferred)

Unrefined safflower oil for coating the frying pan

180 millilitres plus 1 tablespoon blueberry or apple juice (unsweetened)

1 tablespoon cornflour

350 grams fresh or frozen blueberries, thawed

2 tablespoons maple syrup

1 In a large shallow dish with sides, whisk the eggs and egg whites. Add the milk, vanilla, and lemon zest, and whisk to combine.

2 Working in batches, submerge some of the bread triangles in the egg mixture for several seconds until soaked. Turn the slices over and let them sit until the bread is saturated. Cook this batch, as follows, and then repeat with all the bread slices until all the bread is soaked then cooked.

3 Lightly oil a nonstick frying pan or griddle with the safflower oil. In batches, cook the bread triangles in a single layer over medium heat. Cook for 3 to 5 minutes until brown, turn the slices over, and cook for an additional 2 to 5 minutes, or until the French toast begins to brown and the centres are cooked through. Transfer the cooked French toast to a platter and cover loosely with aluminium foil to keep warm while you continue to cook the remaining soaked bread.

4 Meanwhile, using a fork, combine 1 tablespoon of the fruit juice and the cornflour in a small bowl. Set aside.

5 In a small pan, warm the blueberries, fruit juice, and maple syrup until the liquid simmers. Add the cornflour mixture and continue to simmer the sauce, stirring frequently, until it thickens after about 3 minutes.

6 Serve the French toast immediately, topped with the blueberry syrup.

Per serving: Calories 316; Fat 6g (Saturated 1g); Cholesterol 108mg; Sodium 352mg; Carbohydrate 55g; Dietary Fibre 6g; Protein 13g.

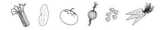

Chapter 7

Making a Healthy Cooked Breakfast

Most traditional cooked breakfasts are undeniably tasty, but come with lots of protein inside. Protein turns breakfast into a complete and satisfying meal, but can also bring saturated fat and cholesterol to your table as unwanted guests. The trick is to factor the meat and eggs you have for breakfast into your plans for lunch and dinner. That way, you can still have a good breakfast and feel well fed without compromising your cholesterol intake for the rest of the day.

This chapter discusses many protein options, including eggs. We also give you several tempting breakfast recipes that make use of savoury breakfast fish and meats. Enjoy!

Making a Point of Eating Protein

If you start the day with just a piece of dry toast and a cup of black coffee, you may crave a Danish pastry by 10 a.m. That's because your body converts the carbohydrates in the toast to energy in about an hour and a half – and then runs out of fuel. But protein takes longer to metabolise, at least two hours, and so it takes over when the toast energy conks out, giving you more lasting energy. A small amount of fat is good, too, because it burns even more slowly to provide your next energy boost, after about three hours. There, you've made it to lunch!

You may think that you don't need a serious breakfast, but you have good health reasons not to eat a skimpy, high-carb breakfast consisting of sweetened cereal or white toast and sugar-laden jam. A habit like that can increase the risk of heart disease, in several ways:

- ✓ Having a breakfast that's full of sugar and starch may lead to weight gain when a morning snack becomes a necessity.

- ✓ Feeling hungry can fill your morning with stress; as your brain tunes out, fatigue takes over, and consequently, things start to go wrong. Stress is a known factor for heart disease.

- ✓ Eating high-carb breakfasts can, over time, lead to a cluster of problems, including insulin resistance, elevated triglycerides, and in some individuals a raised cholesterol level.

Cracking Up on Eggs

Eggs are a part of many traditional cooked breakfasts, but they contain a significant amount of pre-formed cholesterol, which increases with the size of the egg. Small hens' eggs contain about 157 milligrams (although this size is rarely on sale in supermarkets, you may find them in farmer's markets), medium eggs 187 milligrams, large eggs 213 milligrams, and extra-large eggs up to 290 milligrams. Because most guidelines recommend that healthy people with normal cholesterol consume no more than 300 milligrams of cholesterol per day, eating one egg, whatever the size, takes a large bite out of this daily quota. If you already have a high LDL cholesterol and/or cardiovascular disease, limiting your intake of preformed cholesterol to no more than 200 milligrams per day is a wise idea. This means that you can work only one medium egg into your diet per day, assuming that you also avoid virtually all other sources of cholesterol for the rest of the day.

When eggs appear in most recipes, including those in this book, this usually means large eggs. To reduce the cholesterol content, simply substitute a smaller egg, such as in the Coddled Eggs with Sautéed Mushrooms recipe later in this chapter; and then add more mushrooms. However, use some caution when baking, because reducing the egg content can ruin the recipe.

The relationship between egg consumption and heart disease isn't as simple as the tidy rules in this chapter suggest, however. No study has ever shown that healthy people who eat more eggs have more heart attacks than those who eat fewer eggs. For instance, a study published in 1999 in the *Journal of the American Medical Association*, involving almost 120,000 healthy men and women over many years, found that people eating up to one egg a day have no higher risk of heart disease or stroke than those eating less than one egg a week. More recent studies, such as one involving over 21,000 male physicians published in 2008, confirm that eating one egg a day doesn't increase the risk of heart disease.

Eggs also contain nutrients such as folate, vitamin B6, and vitamin B12 that lower the risk of heart disease. These are known to lower elevated blood levels of homocysteine, a risk factor for heart disease (as described in Chapter 1). And although egg yolk contains cholesterol, it also contains vitamin E, which protects the cholesterol from oxidation. Vitamin E also helps to make cholesterol less 'sticky' and less likely to accumulate as plaque in artery walls. In addition, eggs contain a particular fat, called *sphingomyelin*, which appears to lower the absorption of cholesterol from your intestines.

Still, if your cholesterol is elevated, are eggs good for you? The answer is yes – if you limit cholesterol from other sources, and don't combine them with lots of butter, bacon, and cheese. And of course, you can eat the egg white, which contains no cholesterol, anytime.

The cholesterol in egg yolk becomes oxidised during the cooking process to a greater or lesser extent, depending on how you cook it. You want to keep this oxidation to a minimum, because oxidised cholesterol can lead to narrowed arteries. Exposure to oxygen, light, and heat oxidises the cholesterol, and this is exactly what happens when you scramble eggs. You break the yolk and maximise its exposure to the air, light, and the hot cooking surface. Frying an egg is only slightly better because the yolk is still exposed to high heat.

To minimise the oxidation that occurs as an egg cooks, use a cooking method that doesn't require high heat and keeps the yolk encased in white. Here are three classic ways of preparing eggs that protect the yolk:

- ✔ **Soft-boiling** an egg in its shell by placing it in cold water in a small saucepan, bringing to the boil, and letting it simmer gently for 4 minutes.

- ✔ **Poaching** an egg by breaking it into liquid and cooking it gently just below the boiling point for three minutes. The temperature is just right when the surface of the poaching liquid shows slight movement.

- ✔ **Coddling** an egg by placing it in an individual container that you cover and set in a larger pan of simmering water, which you then place on the stovetop or in the oven at very low heat. The warmth of the water bath slowly cooks the egg.

Instead of cooking an omelette with some filling, have poached eggs instead, garnished with the filling. (See the recipe for Poached Eggs and Bacon in Tomato Sauce later in this chapter.)

Eating egg whites is no yolk

Eating only the egg whites enables you to avoid the cholesterol, which is all in the yolks, but deprives you of most of the protein, vitamins, and minerals. However, if you have good reason to avoid the cholesterol in eggs, you can easily separate the whites from the yolks yourself if you follow this illustration. Then sample the Scrambled Egg Whites with Tomato and Feta recipe later in this chapter.

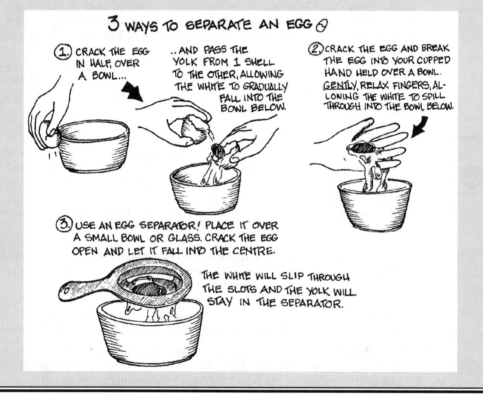

Expanding Your Breakfast Protein Options

Don't think that toast, cereal, and eggs are the only foods you can eat for breakfast. Instead, take a tip from the Japanese and Scandinavians who start the day with fish. Or try out some vegetarian products – those breakfast soya or quorn-based 'meats' that look and taste almost like the real thing – with your toast or cereal, or soya milk and yogurt. And don't forget nuts, so good on top of yogurt or sprinkled over pancakes along with the syrup (Chapter 8 tells you more about nuts).

Adding some fish

Anytime is a good time to eat fish, even as you have your first cup of coffee. The oils in fish are good for the heart in so many ways – from reducing triglycerides and normalising cholesterol levels to preventing blood clots. However, if all these reasons aren't enough to convince you to bite down on a herring or kipper early in the morning, and you need more convincing, why not sample the following fish dishes. This list starts with mild fish and builds up to the stronger stuff.

- ✔ Smoked trout, available packaged in the deli section of most supermarkets.
- ✔ Smoked salmon, the top choice for flavour and omega-3 content.
- ✔ Kippered herring, a hearty favourite of the Scots that you may want to try after getting your feet wet with other fish (avoid kippers and other smoked fish with added colourings, though).
- ✔ Marinated herring in wine with raw onions – popular in Scandinavia and widely available in supermarkets. Delicious – and wine and onions provide heart health benefits, too!
- ✔ Sardines – they're great on toast, for which you can find a recipe later in this chapter.

Dark, dense rye breads and pumpernickel go well as a neutral background for the richness of the fish. But watch your portion sizes. One slice of bread is enough!

Enjoying low-fat breakfast meats

Sometimes nothing but a piece of crisp bacon or sausage does as an accompaniment to eggs, and yet such meats are often high in saturated fat. To solve this dilemma, look for brands of sausage that contain reduced fat, especially turkey sausage. Choose back bacon, which is leaner than streaky bacon and, of course, have only modest portions of these tasty treats.

Vegetarian soya and quorn-based lookalikes are another option. Try a few different brands because some are only marginally better than eating cardboard, whereas others are quite delicious and easy to imagine coming straight from the farm. These products are low in fat and contain no cholesterol, but remember – soya masquerading as meat is still a highly processed food and not as nutritious as the original soya bean.

Surprising Yourself with Hearty Breakfast Recipes

The following recipes give you the chance to sample tasty scrambled eggs made with only egg whites, and to try your hand at poaching eggs. You can also sample some fish for breakfast when you use the recipe for sardines. And finally, treat yourself to potato cakes with some soya protein masquerading as bacon – a meal in itself, and a great way to start the day.

Scrambled Egg Whites with Tomato and Feta Cheese

Use this quick and easy recipe as a template for making egg-white scrambled eggs. The key is to include ingredients that have exceptional flavour and to include a little fat. Egg whites, which are lean and bland, need some help. In this recipe, the feta cheese, which is so salty and pungent you need only a small amount, balances the acidity of the tomato. Other combinations, such as asparagus and cheddar cheese, work just as well.

Preparation time: *5 minutes*

Cooking time: *3 minutes*

Serves: *1*

1 teaspoon olive oil	*Whites of 2 eggs*
1 spring onion, cut crosswise into small slices	*Freshly ground black pepper*
1 medium, fresh tomato, diced and de-seeded	*10 grams feta cheese*

1 In a small nonstick pan, heat the oil over medium heat. Add the spring onions and tomato to the oil long enough to coat them, and then add the egg whites. Cook for about 2 minutes, stirring regularly, until the whites start to become firm. Season to taste with pepper.

2 With the heat off, crumble the feta cheese on top of the scrambled egg mixture and cover to melt the cheese a little. Serve immediately.

Per serving: *Calories 134; Fat 7g (Saturated 2g); Cholesterol 9mg; Sodium 236mg; Carbohydrate 9g; Dietary Fibre 2g; Protein 10 g.*

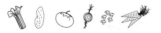

Poached Eggs and Bacon in Tomato Sauce

Try this breakfast dish, in which the poached eggs nestle in a heart-healthy tomato sauce. For this recipe, you can even poach the eggs the night before to save you time in the morning. Lean back bacon is added to boost the protein content of the dish.

Preparation time: *15 minutes*

Cooking time: *15 minutes*

Serves *4*

10 millilitres white vinegar

½ teaspoon salt

4 eggs

8 slices lean back bacon (smoked or unsmoked)

250 grams fresh tomato-based pasta sauce/ salsa, (available in deli sections of supermarkets), or a good brand of commercial tomato passatta

4 thin slices wholemeal bread

1 Pour water to a depth of 2½ centimetres into a deep, small saucepan, add the vinegar and salt, and bring to the boil. Lower the heat so that the water barely bubbles. One at a time, break the eggs into a small bowl and slip into the water. Cover the pan, or start to spoon the water over the eggs. Cook for 3 to 5 minutes until the white has just set and the yolk has filmed over.

2 Remove each egg with a slotted spoon and drain on a paper-towel-covered plate. Keep the eggs warm by covering the plate loosely with aluminium foil.

3 In a nonstick frying pan, dry-fry the back bacon until brown, cooking for 2½ minutes on each side. Meanwhile warm the sauce/salsa in a small pan and toast the slices of bread.

4 Assemble each serving by placing 1 slice of toast on a warmed plate. On top of this, place 2 slices of the bacon, slightly overlapping. With a slotted spoon, remove 1 egg from the pot and place on top of the bacon. Pour a quarter of the tomato sauce over and around the toast, drizzling a little over the egg. Serve immediately.

Tip: *You can poach the eggs the night before and store, covered, in the refrigerator. To warm the poached eggs, bring water to a gentle simmer in a medium-size pot. Trim any ragged edges from the eggs and, using a slotted spoon, gently lower each into the water. Reheat for 1 minute.*

Go-With: *This dish tastes even better accompanied by a fresh salsa.*

Per serving: *Calories 271; Fat 11g (Saturated 3g); Cholesterol 240mg; Sodium 1,458mg; Carbohydrate 22g; Dietary Fibre 3g; Protein 21g.*

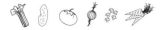

⏱ Coddled Eggs with Sautéed Mushrooms

Coddling gently cooks eggs at a moderate temperature and enables you to time the cooking of the yolk carefully, keeping it slightly runny and less oxidised. The mushroom-parsley base provides a simple mix of just a few flavours to appeal to a delicate morning appetite, and mushrooms are also good sources of chromium, a mineral that helps your body process glucose properly. Cook the eggs in 7½-centimetre ovenproof ramekins or use egg coddlers, special containers with tight-fitting lids.

Special tools required: *4 ovenproof ramekins (7½ centimetres wide) or egg coddlers*

Preparation time: *10 minutes*

Cooking time: *30 minutes*

Serves: *4*

1 teaspoon olive oil for coating the ramekins

1 teaspoon butter

100 grams button mushrooms, trimmed and diced

1 tablespoon finely chopped fresh parsley

Freshly ground black pepper

4 large eggs

60 millilitres (4 tablespoons) semi-skimmed milk

1 Preheat the oven to 180 degrees. Using the corner of a paper towel dipped in oil, wipe the inside of each ramekin to coat the bottom and sides with oil to help prevent the cooked eggs from sticking.

2 Melt the butter in a small frying pan set over medium heat and add the mushrooms and parsley. Sauté, stirring occasionally, for 7 minutes until the mushrooms soften. Season to taste with the freshly ground black pepper. Divide the mushroom mixture among the 4 ramekins.

3 Crack the eggs, one at a time, into a small bowl before carefully slipping each egg into a ramekin. (Cracking the eggs into a bowl first is helpful in case any egg yolks break.) Add 1 tablespoon of the milk to each ramekin. Season with pepper to taste.

4 Cover each filled ramekin with a square of aluminium foil so it fits loosely and not too tight. Set the ramekins in a shallow baking dish and add hot tap water to the dish so that it comes halfway up the sides of the ramekins. Bake for 20 minutes for softly set eggs or 5 minutes longer if you prefer firmer eggs. (After you remove the eggs from the oven, they continue to cook for a minute or two.)

5 Remove the ramekins from the hot-water bath and pat dry. Remove the foil and serve immediately.

Per serving: *Calories 107; Fat 7g (Saturated 2g); Cholesterol 216mg; Sodium 73mg; Carbohydrate 3g; Dietary Fibre 1g; Protein 8g.*

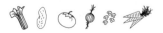

Savoury Fish and Egg White Scramble

Experts associate eating 2 to 3 servings of oily fish a day with a 50 per cent lower risk of fatal coronary heart disease, compared with those who don't eat fish. This egg recipe provides a tasty way to get this benefit in your breakfast. Whole egg omelettes aren't a good idea on a cholesterol-controlling diet, because the high heat oxidises the cholesterol in the egg yolk, making it sticky and more likely to promote the formation of plaque on artery walls. By cooking up an egg-white type of omelette you can avoid this problem, and mixing them with fish adds a richness that the missing yolk had provided.

Preparation time: *2 minutes*

Cooking time: *5 minutes*

Serves: *1*

30 grams white fish, smoked trout, or fish such as halibut leftovers

1 teaspoon olive oil

Pepper

1 tablespoon parsley, chopped

Whites of 2 large eggs

1 Crumble the fish into small bits. Heat the olive oil in a nonstick omelette pan and add the fish. Heat the fish on a medium heat for 2 minutes, stirring occasionally. Season with black pepper to taste.

2 Add the parsley and pour the egg white over the fish. Gather the whites around the fish as they begin to set. Meanwhile, pre-heat the grill. After 2 to 3 minutes, place the pan containing the omelette under the grill to finish cooking the top for another minute. The egg is cooked when it becomes opaque but still has the tenderness of custard. Serve immediately.

Vary It! *For an elegant touch, as the omelette is cooking, toast thin rye bread cut from a square loaf. Then cut the toast into 4 equal triangles to create toast points as a garnish for the dish.*

Per serving: *Calories 126; Fat 7g (Saturated 1g); Cholesterol 23mg; Sodium 130mg; Carbohydrate 1g; Dietary Fibre 0g; Protein 14g. Analysis doesn't include toast.*

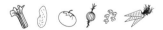

Sardines on Toast

Sardines and anchovies are both full of heart-friendly omega-3 oils. This recipe uses both types of fish for a stunning breakfast that's ideal for a lazy Sunday morning brunch. If you can't find fresh sardines, use a tin of sardines instead.

Preparation time: *5 minutes*

Cooking time: *15 minutes*

Serves: *4*

100 grams anchovy fillets in olive oil

Zest and juice of one lemon

8 fresh sardines, preferably with the back bone removed (ask the fishmonger to do this for you)

4 thin slices wholemeal bread

Rocket or parsley leaves to garnish

1 To make the anchovy sauce, mash the anchovy fillets in their oil and place in a small saucepan with the lemon juice and zest. Cook for 15 minutes until the anchovies dissolve into a paste. Pass through a fine sieve to remove the bones and zest.

2 Meanwhile, grill the sardines under a high heat for 3 to 4 minutes. Remove the backbone if still in place.

3 Toast the bread.

4 To assemble, place a slice of toast on a plate and drizzle with a little of the anchovy sauce. Place two sardines on top and drizzle over more sauce. Garnish with the rocket or parsley and serve immediately.

Vary It! *Instead of anchovy sauce, accompany the sardines with a simple tomato sauce made by sautéing some chopped tomatoes in a little olive oil.*

Per serving: *Calories 207; Fat 9g (Saturated 2g); Cholesterol 56mg; Sodium 1,159mg; Carbohydrate 12g; Dietary Fibre 1g; Protein 21g.*

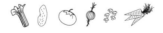

⌒ *Vegetarian Potato and Bacon Wedges*

These savoury, low-fat potato cakes usually gain plenty of enthusiastic praise from people who would never knowingly agree to eat bacon made from soya!

Special tools required: *Food processor (optional)*

Preparation time: *15 minutes*

Cooking time: *30 minutes*

Serves: *4*

2 large floury potatoes, peeled

½ medium onion

2 spring onions

1 red bell pepper

5 slices soya bacon

¼ teaspoon mixed, dried herbs

Freshly ground black pepper

2 tablespoons extra-virgin olive oil

1 Shred the potatoes by hand, using a metal grater, or use a food processor fitted with a grating disk.

2 Trim the onion and cut into thin slices. Trim and chop the spring onions. Trim the red bell pepper, remove the seeds, and slice into thin strips. Chop the soya bacon. Put all these ingredients and the mixed herbs in a large bowl and mix well.

3 Put the vegetable mixture in a medium-size pan and sauté the mixture in 1 tablespoon of the olive oil for 7 minutes, or until softened. Season with black pepper to taste. Set the vegetable mixture aside in a large bowl.

4 Transfer the potatoes to the bowl containing the vegetable mixture. Toss all ingredients to combine.

5 Put the other tablespoon of oil in a nonstick frying pan. Add one-half of the potato mixture to the pan. Using a spatula, press down on the vegetables to pack the ingredients. Cook on a medium heat for 10 minutes, or until the potatoes begin to turn brown on the bottom.

6 Using a spatula, cut a pie-shaped wedge in the potato mixture and turn over to brown the other side. Proceed to cut additional wedges until all the mixture has been turned over. If needed, add more oil during this process. Continue to cook until the vegetables are cooked and the potatoes are brown on the bottom. Season with pepper to taste. Keep wedges warm while cooking the remainder.

7 Repeat Steps 5 and 6 with the second half of mixture. Enjoy.

Per serving: Calories 204; Fat 7g (Saturated 1g); Cholesterol 0mg; Sodium 211mg; Carbohydrate 27g; Dietary Fibre 4g; Protein 9g.

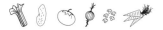

Chapter 8

Having Breakfast in a Jiffy

Toast and coffee is a quick breakfast, but it doesn't offer many nutritional benefits. To start your day with a healthy meal that sees you through until lunch, you need more than that. This chapter gives you some ideas on quick and easy breakfasts involving healthy fruit and nuts and even morsels such as last night's dessert or a jar of marinated herrings, which can form the basis of a healthy breakfast. Begin to think outside the box – the cereal box that is – to expand your breakfast food options beyond the usual suspects.

Eating even a small amount of nutritious food at home is far better for your heart than grabbing a fast-food, high-calorie, high-salt, refined-food meal on your way to work. Having a nourishing breakfast at home also helps reduce the allure of a mid-morning pastry snack. You may be surprised at how little time it takes to prepare a good breakfast, if you plan ahead.

Grabbing a Piece of Fruit

Research shows that making the effort to eat more fruit and veg can lower your risk of both heart attack and stroke. The UK Food Standards Agency recommends a minimum intake of 5 daily servings of fruit and vegetables as a general guideline. In fact, consuming as little as 3 or more portions of fruits and veg a day reduces the risk of fatal heart attack or stroke compared with individuals who eat less than 1 serving of fruit or vegetables a day. And for once, more is even better.

Make fruit at breakfast a habit, because it is an easy way to increase your fruit intake.

Thank heavens for the banana, the eat-on-the run breakfast food that comes in its own natural package. But don't stop there when looking for breakfast fruits. Stock up on all the delectable, sweet fruits that are an essential part of a healthy diet. Make a habit of eating fruit that supplies you with soluble fibre, the kind that lowers cholesterol, starting with apples and pears. Peaches, plums, and bananas are also a good source. Try to select the most colourful fruit because the pigments also function as nutrients (see Chapter 2). For instance, golden-reddish-orangey fruit, such as cantaloupe melons, papayas, and apricots, are a great source of betacarotene, an antioxidant that protects cholesterol and arteries. And when you have several options while shopping, buy pink grapefruit, blood oranges, and dark purple grapes rather than the less richly coloured versions.

If taken a statin drug, check with the drug information sheet before eating grapefruit.

Dried, frozen, and canned fruit all count too and can often be excellent breakfast foods – canned prunes or grapefruit, dried fruit compote, and thawed frozen berries, for example. Check out the recipe for Strawberry and Blackberry Sundae later in this chapter.

Squeezing a little fresh lemon or lime juice, fresh ginger, or ginger powder over melon helps to spark the flavour.

Another great fruit is kiwi, which is just the right amount for a breakfast portion. Kiwi is full of vitamin C, which your body must have in order to convert cholesterol into the bile acids that it then eliminates from your system. Other great sources of vitamin C, besides citrus, are berries, melons, and tropical fruit such as guava, papayas, and mangoes. (Figure 8-1 shows how to avoid the mango's single, enormous seed while you cut off all the bits you want to eat. Wait until you see a slice of diced mango with the skin turned inside out. Very fancy!)

Go for a variety of fruit to ensure that you benefit from a range of nutrients. If you haven't had, for instance, fresh pineapple in a while, now's the time to tuck in!

Raw fruit is much better than cooked. Excessive heat significantly damages the antioxidant capacity of fruit.

TWO WAYS TO CUT A MANGO...

1. SLICE THE MANGO IN HALF CUTTING AROUND ITS LARGE OVAL SHAPED PIT.

2. USE A PARING KNIFE TO SCORE THE FLESH OF EACH HALF WITHOUT CUTTING THROUGH SKIN!

3. TURN THE SKIN INSIDE OUT SO THE DICED PIECES STAND OUT!

CUT THE PIECES FROM THE SKIN.

.OR.

1. USE A VEGETABLE PEELER OR PARING KNIFE TO PEEL THE SKIN OF THE MANGO.

2. USE A CHEF'S KNIFE TO CUT THE MANGO IN HALF SLICING AROUND THE PIT.

3. CHOP OR SLICE THE FRUIT ON A CUTTING BOARD!

Figure 8-1:
Two different ways to cut a mango.

Being berry, berry good

Berries are great for breakfast, handy to eat by the spoonful, on their own, or on top of cereal. But these fruits also have a lot more going for them. The pigments themselves are powerful antioxidants. When you consume colourful berries, these nutrients go to work, protecting your 'bad' LDL cholesterol from oxidation so that plaque is less likely to accumulate in arteries. (Chapter 2 tells you more about these heart-healthy colours.) Berries also contain phytonutrients that dampen the chronic inflammation that contributes towards coronary artery disease.

Fresh berries are often expensive, especially when you buy them as speciality items out of season. However, when you consider the nutrients they provide, fresh berries are a bargain. Many supermarkets also sell frozen berries, often less expensive, and still full of nutrients because the berries are frozen soon after harvesting. But skip the frozen or canned berries that come in heavy, sugary syrup, to avoid excess empty calories.

Whenever possible, buy organic berries, fresh or frozen. Berries are high on the list of produce that is a source of pesticides in the diet. As a minimum, always gently but thoroughly wash berries just before eating. Washing berries and then storing them causes them to become waterlogged.

Here are some berries to put on your breakfast menu:

✔ **Blackberries** have almost as much antioxidant activity as blueberries (below). They're also a fairly good source of vitamin C, folate, vitamin E, potassium, and magnesium and an excellent source of manganese and fibre.

✔ **Blueberries** have more antioxidant power than just about any other fruit or vegetable, containing over two dozen phytonutrient pigments that join forces to quench free radicals (see Chapter 2 for more on these tiny molecules). Blueberries also provide modest amounts of vitamin C, folate, potassium, and vitamin A.

✔ **Raspberries** are also a good source of antioxidant power, especially black raspberries if you can find them. Like other berries, raspberries are also a good source of vitamin C and folate, and provide more fibre than most other fruits, thanks to all those tiny seeds.

✔ **Strawberries** contain about a third fewer antioxidant pigments than berries that are bluer, but still have more than many other kinds of fruit. They also provide vitamin C and some folate and potassium.

To store delicate berries, such as raspberries, place unwashed berries in a single layer in a shallow pan lined with paper towels, and store them in the refrigerator.

Eating whole fruit versus juice

Don't rely on fruit juice as your prime source of this major food category. Whole fruit is the only source that gives you all the fibre and nutrients you need, in the right combination. In comparison, juice is processed fruit, that's missing fibre and some nutrients. (Turn to Chapter 2 for details about specific fruits and what they provide.) One serving of fruit and vegetable juice is 150 millilitres, but can only count as one of your five-a-day fruit and vegetable requirement, however much of them you drink. If making a home-made smoothie from whole fruit, however, you can count the individual portions of fruit going into it.

Sliced oranges are more nutritious than orange juice. Both are a good source of vitamin C, but orange slices also give you valuable fibre and bioflavonoids, vitamins found in the pith and membranes of the orange. Bioflavonoids are especially concentrated in the white, soft stem that runs through the core. They strengthen the walls of your capillaries, which are the tiny blood vessels delivering oxygen to your tissues.

When you want orange juice, squeeze your own to ensure that it includes some pulp along with pith and membranes; or buy the home-style 'juicy bits' kind that contains a mixture of pulp and pith. Orange juice is a great choice when you want fruit juice because it's a good source of potassium and B vitamins.

Instant fruit combos

For something a little different to start your day, cut up a couple of different kinds of fruit, add some nuts or a herb, such as mint, and toss them together. Choose contrasting flavours, textures, and colours. Or combine a fruit with a small piece of cheese. Here are some ideas to get you started:

- Strawberries and bananas
- Blueberries and pears
- Yellow apple, red grapes, and almonds
- Peaches and mint
- Chopped apple and a wedge of low-fat cheddar cheese

Grape juice – especially red grape juice – is also a terrific source of antioxidants (see Chapter 2) and flavonoids, the nutrients given credit for the heart-healthy effects of red wine. Research now shows that consuming the non-alcoholic version of grape juice is also a good idea. Consuming a serving of fruit juice per day is beneficial, and can significantly reduce the susceptibility of LDL cholesterol to oxidisation, as well as improving the elasticity of arteries. Atherosclerosis, also known as hardening and furring up of the arteries, is less likely to develop in such an environment. In addition, grape juice slows the activity of blood platelets, reducing blood stickiness and the risk of an abnormal blood clot.

Read the labels of commercial fruit juices carefully before you take them home. Here's a checklist of what to look for and avoid:

- Select products that are made of 100 per cent juice.
- Avoid juice containing added sugar, which provides calories but fewer nutrients.
- Stay away from bottled juices that are labelled 'fruit drink'. They look like the real thing (in which the pigments are also antioxidants), but the juice drinks contain artificial colours and added sugar that do not function as nutrients.

If you come across luxury 100 per cent cherry juice or 100 per cent pomegranate juice, give them a try. Drinking them is a lot easier than dealing with the cherry and pomegranate seeds in these fruits, and both richly coloured juices help prevent heart disease. The antioxidant activity of pomegranate juice blocks the development of atherosclerosis, and the reddish-blue pigments in cherries have an anti-inflammatory effect. Chronic inflammation of the arteries (see Chapter 1) can contribute to the build-up of plaque.

The body absorbs fruit juice readily, causing a rapid rise in blood sugar. A spike in blood sugar can lead to an increase in risk factors for heart disease. (See Chapter 1 for more information.) To counteract this, have only small amounts of fruit juice at a time, about 150 millilitres, or one portion, especially if you're not having them together with solid food at the meal table. If you want more liquid, dilute the juice with water or soda water. Also, drink fruit juice slowly, so that it takes the same amount of time to consume as if you were slowly eating the actual piece of fruit.

One serving of juice is 150 millilitres, and can only count as one of your 5-a-day portions however much more you drink.

Starting Your Day the Nutty Way

For a long time, health messages have recommended staying away from fat, and so many people have cut back on the amount of nuts they eat and feel guilty when they do have a handful of almonds or peanuts. Although fat contributes 73 to 90 per cent of the calories in nuts, these fats are the healthy kinds that have beneficial effects on cholesterol balance. Nuts therefore deserve a place as staples in your kitchen because they supply protein, healthy fats, and many nutrients including selenium, magnesium, copper, folate, potassium, and vitamin E.

By the way, seeds such as sunflower, pumpkin, and sesame are also loaded with nutrients. They contain all the major building blocks (proteins, unsaturated fats, and a wide range of vitamins and minerals) of the plant they have the potential to sprout. Edible seeds provide B complex vitamins; vitamins A, D, and E; calcium; iron; potassium; magnesium; and zinc. In particular, sunflower seeds contain up to 50 per cent protein, and sesame seeds are high in calcium. Enjoy them raw, dried, roasted, or cooked and eaten as snacks, or tossed into salads, soups, and baked goods.

Seeds with the husks on have a long shelf life, kept in a cool, dry place in a tightly covered container, but store seeds without husks in a refrigerator, in a tightly covered container, and use within a couple of weeks.

Exploring the benefits of going nutty

Peanuts, almonds, and walnuts are the most frequently consumed nuts, with hazelnuts, cashews, pistachios, and macadamias next in popularity.

Nuts are just what the heart needs, for the following reasons:

- ✔ The commonly favoured nuts – peanuts, almonds, and walnuts – are high in polyunsaturated fat and low in saturated fat. Walnuts are a premier source of omega-3 fatty acids, another good thing.

- ✔ Many nuts are very high in monounsaturated fats, the cornerstone of the Mediterranean diet, which is associated with a lower risk of heart disease: peanuts contain 49 per cent; almonds 65 per cent; walnuts 23 per cent; and hazelnuts 78 per cent. Macadamia nut oil contains 81 per cent monounsaturated fat – the highest amount found in any food.

- ✔ In a small study published in the journal *Circulation* in 2002, snacking on almonds had positive results for healthy individuals with elevated cholesterol: participants consuming just 30 grams of almonds per day experienced significant reductions in the unhealthy LDL cholesterol and an improvement in the LDL:HDL ratio. Cholesterol levels improved even more in those consuming 75 grams of almonds a day, and these individuals also had a reduction in oxidised cholesterol.

- ✔ A study published in 2004 showed that eating just 20 grams of macadamia nuts per day significantly reduces both total and 'bad' LDL cholesterol levels. In fact, a review of all the evidence, carried out in 2005, found that eating 50 to 100 grams of nuts at least 5 times per week can significantly decrease total cholesterol and LDL cholesterol.

- ✔ Most nuts contain a good amount of *arginine*, an amino acid that the body uses as a building block to manufacture nitric oxide. Nitric oxide is a potent compound that dilates blood vessels, helping to prevent a blockage in arteries that may trigger a heart attack.

Adding an ounce of prevention to your breakfast

You benefit from eating even a small amount of nuts. The famous Nurses' Health Study, begun in 1976, considered 28 grams (1 ounce) of nuts to be a serving, not much if you really start nibbling. Yet the results showed that women who eat more than 5 servings a week have a significantly lower risk of coronary heart disease than women who rarely eat any nuts at all (see Chapter 3). So, make this amount part of your daily breakfast regime. Nuts taste great on all sorts of breakfast foods, from hot and cold cereal to yogurt sundaes. (See the Strawberry and Blueberry Sundae recipe later in this chapter.) Of course, the benefits don't increase indefinitely as you eat more nuts. They still provide lots of calories, and so enjoy them in moderation.

A small handful of nuts equals about 28 grams, which is about 6 walnut halves, 14 almonds, or enough peanut butter to smear on a piece of toast (about 2 tablespoons).

You can do worse than a peanut butter sandwich using wholegrain bread for breakfast. Peanuts, as well as other nuts, are a concentrated food source of protein, healthy fats, and many nutrients. Nuts are also a rich source of the B-complex vitamins, vitamin E, calcium, iron, potassium, magnesium, phosphorus, and copper. For starters, consider the following possible ways of adding nuts to your diet:

- ✓ Hunt for fresh ground peanut butter, which you can find at health food stores.

- ✓ Buy only brands of peanut butter that don't contain partially hydrogenated oil, a source of trans fatty acids, which you should avoid.

- ✓ Sprinkle some nuts in pancake and waffle batter before you start the cooking.

- ✓ Scatter nuts on hot cereal, cold cereal, and breakfast fruit-and-yogurt sundaes.

Perhaps you prefer to get your quota of daily nuts from nut butter. If so, browse through the nut section of a natural foods store, and you can find a luxurious assortment of nut butters, including delectable roasted almond and cashew. Or stay with classic peanut butter, but always read labels. Don't buy a peanut butter if the ingredient list includes added sugars or partially hydrogenated oils.

If the oil separates and is sitting on the top of the nut butter, don't pour it off. This oil is a good source of polyunsaturated and monounsaturated fatty acids (see Chapter 3). After you stir the oil into your nut butter, store the jar in the refrigerator, and the oil won't separate out again.

Preparing Breakfast in Your Sleep (Well, Almost)

Even if you wake up feeling groggy, some breakfasts are so quick and easy to put together that you can still give yourself something decent to eat. Here are some suggestions:

- ✓ Try tinned kidney beans rather than baked beans on rye toast. Warm the beans in a small pan set over a medium heat, stirring occasionally, and spoon the heated beans over the toast. Beans on toast is a time-honoured breakfast favourite and is jolly good for you. Beans can raise your HDL level and lower your LDL level, because they are a low glycae-mic index carbohydrate and contain fibre, particularly soluble pectin (see Chapter 2 for more on pectin).

✔ Start the day with whole rolled oat porridge that you cooked the night before. The oats taste fine the next morning if you heat them in the microwave. If you're committed to eating rolled oats for their soluble fibre every day, this strategy lets you bring them to the table in record time, day after day.

Choose whole rolled oat porridge in preference to flavoured instant hot breakfast cereals, which more rapidly raise blood sugar levels.

✔ Whip up a shake in a blender. Start with 2 large serving spoons of low-fat yogurt and add a cup of fruit, a couple of tablespoons of soya protein powder, and 60 millilitres of fruit juice.

✔ If you don't want bread, spread nut butter on slices of apple and pear, rye crispbreads, or rice cakes.

Grabbing Quick-and-Easy Breakfast Recipes

In addition to the recipes presented here, other recipes in this cookbook are quite acceptable for breakfast. After exploring the delicious recipes here, take a look at all the dessert recipes in Chapters 21 and 22. Instead of helping yourself to a Danish pastry, have a slice of nutritious Banana and Date Tea Loaf (see Chapter 22). Even the Chewy Oatmeal and Raisin Bites (also in Chapter 22) make a tasty breakfast along with your morning cuppa. If a serving is fine for dessert after supper, it can also fit into a cholesterol-controlling diet 12 hours later!

Herrings with Home-Made Dill Sauce

This is the way Norwegians, Swedes, and Danes start the day – with a helping of marinated herring – an excellent source of omega-3 fatty acids and monounsaturated fats. Herrings also contain a generous amount of vitamin D, necessary for the absorption of calcium; vitamin B12, which helps keep homocysteine levels in check (see Chapter 1 for more about homocysteine); and selenium, the trace mineral that works together with the important antioxidant, vitamin E. To make this dish, begin with a jar of pickled herring, normally served as an hors d'oeuvre with drinks. Select the version that also contains sliced onions, which make an appetizing addition to the mixture. Onions have an anti-inflammatory effect that protects the heart.

Preparation time: *15 minutes*

Serves: *4*

1 jar (350 grams) marinated herring with onions

1 tablespoon chopped fresh dill

1 tablespoon coarse-grained mustard

3 tablespoons low-fat sour cream

2 tablespoons reduced-fat mayonnaise

1 teaspoon lemon juice

Freshly ground black pepper

1 Empty the jar of marinated herring into a sieve and drain. Hold the sieve under the tap and gently rinse the fish with running water to remove the sharp flavour of the marinade.

2 Transfer the herring to a cutting board and cut the fish into narrow strips. Pat dry with paper towels.

3 Put the dill, mustard, sour cream, mayonnaise, and lemon juice in a medium-sized bowl and mix thoroughly to combine. Stir in the herring. Season with pepper to taste.

4 Serve with slices of dense rye bread or toast.

Per serving: *Calories 216; Fat 15g (Saturated 3g); Cholesterol 14mg; Sodium 484mg; Carbohydrate 9g; Dietary Fibre 0g; Protein 10g. (Analysis does not include bread.)*

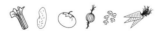

☉ Polenta with Basil and Tomato Sauce

The classic way of preparing polenta is to add it to a pan of boiling water and stir the mixture continuously for up to an hour, adding more hot water if necessary, until the grain absorbs the liquid and is thoroughly cooked. Polenta has superior flavour, which is great for breakfast if you prepare the polenta the night before. Follow the instructions on the pack and pour the cooked, thick polenta into a loaf tin; and when you're ready for breakfast, just cut off a slice. Alternatively, look for handy packs of polenta, packaged in see-through wrapping, in the grain section of specialty shops. Cut off slices of the ready-made polenta to make this recipe.

Preparation time: *5 minutes*

Cooking time: *10 minutes*

Serves *4*

20 millilitres extra-virgin olive oil

1 pack (600 to 700 grams) ready-made polenta, cut into 8 to 10 slices

1 tin (425 grams) chopped tomatoes

Handful fresh basil leaves, cut into strips

Freshly ground black pepper

1 Add a little olive oil to 2 large nonstick frying pans set over medium-high heat. Arrange half the polenta slices in each pan and cook until the under-surface begins to brown, after about 7 minutes. Lower the heat slightly if the oil begins to spatter.

2 Meanwhile, put the chopped tomatoes and basil in a small saucepan. Cook, covered, over a medium heat to desired consistency – around 10 minutes is ideal to lose that 'tinned' taste. Season with pepper.

3 Using a spatula, turn over the polenta slices and cook for an additional 5 minutes.

4 To serve, distribute polenta slices on serving plates and spoon the heated tomato sauce over each serving.

Tip: *Use plain ready-made polenta rather than the sun-dried tomato version, which can have an overly pungent, artificial taste.*

Tip: *If you like your polenta crispier, you can cook it for as long as 12 to 14 minutes per side, depending on the heat distribution in the pan.*

Per serving: *Calories 167; Fat 5g (Saturated 1g); Cholesterol 0mg; Sodium 600mg; Carbohydrate 28g; Dietary Fibre 4g; Protein 4g.*

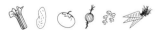

◯ Strawberry and Blackberry Sundae

What a fun way to eat foods that are good for you – layered in a sundae. Try this recipe to taste how berries, yogurt, cereal, and sliced almonds all come together. The Grape-Nuts contain crunchy wholewheat, a nutritious wholegrain, and malted barley – a source of soluble fibre and natural sweetness. Then go on to invent your own breakfast dessert.

Preparation time: *5 minutes*

Serves: *1*

4 strawberries, de-husked and cut in half

6 tablespoons plain low-fat bio yogurt

30 grams Grape-Nuts cereal

35 grams fresh or frozen blackberries

1 tablespoon sliced almonds, preferably toasted

1 Place 2 halved strawberries in the bottom of a parfait glass or a stemmed water glass that flares at the top.

2 Add half the yogurt and top with the cereal.

3 Add the blackberries and the remaining yogurt.

4 Top with the remaining 2 halved strawberries and sprinkle with the almonds.

Tip: *Try a little drizzle of honey if you find the plain yogurt a little too tangy.*

Vary It! *If you prefer, blueberries work just as well as blackberries in this recipe.*

Per serving: Calories 234; Fat 5g (Saturated 1g); Cholesterol 6mg; Sodium 250mg; Carbohydrate 40g; Dietary Fibre 5g; Protein 10g.

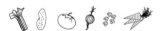

☞ *Walnut and Blueberry Yogurt Muffins*

This recipe includes as many healthy ingredients as possible. The soya flour and egg whites provide protein, oat flour and bran supply soluble fibre, the walnuts and safflower oil give you essential fatty acids while the blueberries add antioxidants. For a nutritious breakfast on the run, grab one of these muffins as you head for the door.

Preparation time: *20 minutes*

Baking time: *35 minutes*

Yield: *12 muffins*

140 grams wholewheat flour	*3 tablespoons oat bran*
60 grams oat flour	*60 grams walnuts, chopped*
40 grams soya flour	*375 grams low-fat plain yogurt*
2 teaspoons baking powder	*White of 1 large egg*
½ teaspoon baking soda	*3 tablespoons unrefined safflower oil*
½ teaspoon allspice	*2 tablespoons honey*
¼ teaspoon salt	*60 grams fresh blueberries*

1 Preheat the oven to 190 degrees.

2 Sift together in a large bowl the wheat flour, oat flour, soya flour, baking powder, baking soda, allspice, and salt. Add the oat bran and walnuts and stir to incorporate.

3 Put the yogurt, egg white, safflower oil, honey, and blueberries in a bowl and stir to combine.

4 Make a well in the centre of the flour mixture and pour in the yogurt mixture. Stir to moisten the flour and thoroughly mix.

5 Place paper muffin cup liners in a muffin baking tin. Spoon some of the batter, which is stiff, into each muffin cup, filling it three-quarters full.

6 Bake the muffins for about 35 minutes until the tops are golden brown.

Tip: *If you prefer a sweeter, richer-tasting muffin, substitute molasses or maple syrup for the honey and replace the blueberries with raisins or chopped dates.*

Vary It! *If you don't eat wheat, make these muffins with flour made from spelt, an ancient form of wheat that for many people is less allergenic. It behaves the same as modern wheat in baking.*

Per serving: *Calories 176; Fat 9g (Saturated 1g); Cholesterol 2mg; Sodium 297mg; Carbohydrate 21g; Dietary Fibre 3g; Protein 7g.*

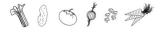

Part III
Making Your Day with Heart-Healthy Snacks and Starters

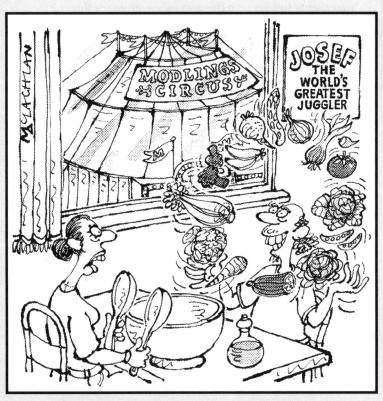

'OK-you've tossed the salad enough, Joseph.'

In this part . . .

This part gives you guidelines for making delicious stocks and suggests special cholesterol-lowering ingredients to toss into the pan as you prepare the various soups. Here, we help you to assemble salads and explain why favouring the most colourful ingredients is good (they're full of phytonutrients). The final two chapters in this part give you recipes designed for entertaining. (Yes, you can control your cholesterol and have good party nibbles and starters at the same time!) These delicious morsels are good for both your heart – and your guests.

Chapter 9

Preparing Simple and Hearty Soups

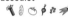
*1*f you think of soup as just water with a few added ingredients, anyone who can boil water can make a good soup. Making soup is simple because you don't need precise measurements, and it doesn't take too much time and effort because you don't have to watch the pot!

This chapter includes everything from simple first-course soup offerings to soups that are meals in themselves. These soups are short on fat and long on flavour and leave plenty of room for invention. Do some experimenting. You really can't go wrong with soup!

At a pinch, tinned soup is fine. For a quick lunch, a bowl of tinned lentil soup is far better for your heart than a pasty or sausage roll. But choose lower salt or sodium brands of soups (check the labels) to avoid increasing your blood pressure. Also favour low-fat and fat-free items to reduce calories and always avoid soup products made with hydrogenated oils that can contain trans fats (see Chapter 3 for more on these human-made fats), which have an adverse effect on cholesterol balance. Check the ingredient list on labels for contents.

If a label you're reading doesn't show the salt content, you can multiply the 'sodium' content by 2.5 to get the table salt content. For example, by multiplying the 1 gram of sodium in a serving of soup by 2.5, you find that it contains 2.5 grams of salt (sodium chloride). Try to limit your salt intake to no more than 6 grams per day.

Developing a Tasty Stock

A *stock* is the liquid remaining after certain ingredients are cooked in water and then strained out, and is valuable when cooking for low cholesterol. The goal is to make sure that the flavour of the added ingredients transfers to the stock. But that's not all that ends up in the liquid. Vitamins and minerals also migrate from the ingredients to make a healthy, nutritious brew. Bones contribute some calcium, needed to maintain healthy bones and a normal heartbeat, and a little protein; carrots contribute betacarotene, an antioxidant; and onions provide the phytonutrient quercetin, which helps to damp down inflammation (see Chapter 1). Well-skimmed stock is an excellent substitute for fat in certain dishes, providing concentrated flavour without the fat or calories. For instance, instead of sautéing vegetables, such as sliced courgette or runner beans, in oil, try cooking them in a small amount of savoury stock, instead.

Beef stock, too, is very handy when you want the robust flavour of meat in a soup or casserole dish, but without the saturated fat. In making beef stock, start with beef shank or chuck and marrow bones, and brown them first, in the oven or stock pan, to develop additional, rich flavours.

Add a teaspoon of cider vinegar or another type of vinegar to stock ingredients to extract more minerals from bones during cooking.

Fish stock has more limited uses, destined only for fish dishes, but in these, a full-flavoured stock can guarantee that the fish you're cooking turns out to be as satisfying as one covered in cream sauce. To make fish stock, start with fish trimmings (heads, tails, fins, bones) and add some vegetables, such as onion, carrot, and celery, and seasonings such as parsley, bay leaves, and peppercorns, plus white wine and a squeeze of lemon juice. Simmer for one hour.

Supermarkets sell tinned chicken and beef *broth*. A broth is made by cooking the meaty parts of chicken or beef in water, whereas a stock is made with the bones plus other ingredients, such as vegetables. Tinned broth can successfully replace home-made stock in recipes, especially when you add some flavourful vegetables and herbs.

Read on to find out how to make various stocks that are very tasty and relatively low in fat. Use these in the cholesterol-friendly soup recipes in this chapter or serve stock as a light and appetising starter to a meal.

Boiling up vegetable stock

This light, fresh-tasting vegetable stock adds complexity to the flavour of bean and vegetable soups and is essential when preparing vegetarian recipes. To make vegetable stock, start with finely chopped vegetables, which cook quickly. Put them in a pan of water, bring to the boil and simmer, covered, for ½ hour or more, until the vegetables are very tender. Use vegetable stock in dishes with short cooking times to keep the flavour of stock from deteriorating. For instance, vegetable stock is a good choice for the cooking liquid when preparing rice or risotto.

Onions, carrots, and celery are a must for making vegetable stock and are standards in chicken and beef stock as well. You can also add other vegetables, but do so with care. Although celery has little taste itself, scientists recently discovered that it contains chemicals that stimulate the newly discovered 'savoury' taste buds that detect a taste sensation known from the Japanese as 'umami'.

Think twice before adding veg that tends to dominate flavour or colour the stock, such as cabbage, broccoli, cauliflower, spinach, parsnips, turnips, asparagus, beetroot, and garlic (unless you're warding off vampires). The taste of red cabbage is just what you want in borscht, where it complements the beetroot, but is probably unwelcome in pea soup.

A good vegetable stock also calls for sprigs of fresh herbs such as parsley, thyme, a small bay leaf, and a single clove. Other options include marjoram, chervil, or a slice of fresh ginger. The French romantically call this little bunch of herbs a *bouquet garni*.

Virtually any stock, including vegetable, benefits from adding the rich flavour of mushrooms. Use whole mushrooms or just the trimmed stems from mushrooms you've prepared for another dish. Better yet, use dried ones, such as porcini, which are easy to keep on hand because they store for months. Look for bargain black mushrooms in Chinese markets. These mushrooms are dried shiitakes, shown in studies to lower cholesterol because they contain a specific amino acid that helps speed up cholesterol processing in the liver.

Fresh-made vegetable stock provides a savoury and robust setting especially suited for grains, beans, and a recipe's featured vegetables. The following procedures are all designed to ensure that you cook with the tastiest vegetables, and that you develop and extract the maximum flavour from them:

- ✔ **Use vegetables that are mature but not old and, ideally, in season.** Check Chapter 15 for information about what to look for when you shop for fresh produce.

- ✔ **Sauté or roast vegetables before adding them to the stock pot.** Lightly sauté the vegetables in olive oil until they begin to brown to ensure rich flavour and deepen the colour of the stock. Roasting really brings out the flavour and sweetness of Mediterranean vegetables such as tomatoes and peppers.

- ✔ **Purée vegetables before adding to the water.** When you *purée* vegetables, you finely mash them to a smooth, thick consistency. Press well-cooked vegetables through a sieve or purée them using a blender or a food processor fitted with a metal blade.

- ✔ **Begin cooking vegetables and meats in cold water.** This method draws juices from these foods and extracts the most flavour.

- ✔ **When straining out vegetables from a finished stock, press them against the sieve with the back of a spoon.** By pressing the vegetables, you can release more of the juices. The final broth is less clear but more flavourful.

☺ *Roast Vegetable Stock*

Roasting vegetables for a stock adds another prep step that requires little effort. But the flavour pay-off is big, reducing the need for salt and fat in the final dish.

Preparation time: *15 minutes*

Cooking time: *1½ hours*

Serves: *12 (3 litres in total; 250 millilitres each serving)*

2 large onions, quartered but not peeled	*5 sprigs parsley*
4 carrots, peeled and roughly cut	*2 sprigs fresh thyme*
2 celery stalks, roughly cut	*10 peppercorns*
2 parsnips, peeled and roughly cut	*120 millilitres white wine (optional)*
6 cloves garlic, peeled (optional)	*3 litres water*
2 tablespoons extra-virgin olive oil	

1 Preheat the oven to 200 degrees. Place the onions, carrots, celery, parsnips, and garlic (if desired) in a 23-x-30-centimetre roasting pan. Drizzle with olive oil and put the pan in the oven.

2 Roast, shaking the pan occasionally and turning the ingredients once or twice for about 45 minutes, or until the vegetables are nicely browned.

3 Using a slotted spoon, transfer all the ingredients to a stockpot. Add the parsley, thyme, peppercorns, white wine, if desired, and all but a couple of ladlefuls of the water.

4 Add the remaining ladlefuls of water to the roasting pan and, using a large spoon, mix it around, loosening the bits of vegetables that have stuck to the bottom. Pour this mixture into the stockpot along with the remaining water.

5 Bring the contents of the stockpot to the boil, partially cover, and reduce the heat so the mixture simmers gently, just sending up a few bubbles at a time. Cook for 30 to 45 minutes or until the vegetables are soft.

6 Strain, pressing the vegetables to extract as much juice as possible. The stock is now ready to use in other recipes, such as the liquid for cooking grains or as the base for a soup or risotto.

Tip: *Stock keeps fresh for 1 to 2 days, but you can extend its refrigerator life if you boil it after 2 days to destroy any bacterial growth. If there is a layer of fat on top of the stock, don't skim it until you're ready to use the broth. The fat helps protect the stock. You can also freeze stock, which keeps for 4 to 6 months at 0 degrees. Pack it in recipe-size quantities, using small containers so you can fill them nearly to the top. In this case, remove the fat before storing, because it tends to turn rancid even at very low temperatures.*

Tip: *You may need to inspect the 'juices' at the bottom of the roasting pan. If they are 'burned on', you don't want to add it into the broth.*

Per serving: *Calories 22; Fat 2g (Saturated 0g); Cholesterol 0mg; Sodium 8mg; Carbohydrates 1g; Dietary Fibre 0g; Protein 0g.*

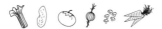

Creating chicken stock

You can derive a certain amount of satisfaction from having a good, homemade chicken stock at hand, an essential in any well-stocked kitchen (groan). When you're in the mood for soup, you already have a basic ingredient that you can trust for quality and content. Although chicken soup has a reputation as being fiddly to make, it really isn't a big deal. You can make stock just in the process of cooking chicken, which many people do at least once a week.

Making chicken broth from scratch

Gourmet cooks prepare a chicken broth, using a whole chicken, along with vegetables and herbs, cooking the ingredients for three hours or more and then discarding them, now robbed of their flavour and nutrients. An extra-rich chicken broth is the result. But if you can't bear to throw out what looks like food and you need a chicken stock in quicker time, here's an alternative.

Basic Chicken Stock

This recipe makes use of the classic ingredients for chicken stock, but at a push, only the onion and bay leaf are essential for a savoury chicken broth. This recipe also leaves you with the chicken pieces to use in another dish.

Preparation time: *15 minutes*

Cooking time: *1½ hours*

Serves: *12 (3 litres in total; 250 millilitres each serving)*

1 whole 1.3 to 1.8-kilogram chicken

1 onion, roughly cut, not peeled

1 carrot, roughly cut

1 small stalk celery, roughly cut

1 teaspoon cider vinegar

1 sprig fresh thyme or a pinch of dried thyme

1 small bay leaf

Several sprigs fresh parsley

3½ litres water

1 To shorten the cooking time, cut the chicken into parts.

2 Place the chicken, onion, carrot, celery, vinegar, thyme, bay leaf, and parsley in a large stock pot. Add the water.

3 Bring almost to the boil, partially cover the pot, and adjust the heat so that the mixture simmers gently, sending up a few bubbles at a time. Cook for 1½ hours, until the stock is richly flavoured.

4 Using tongs, remove the chicken from the pot and set aside to eat separately. Strain the stock, pressing on the vegetables to extract as much juice as possible.

5 Refrigerate the stock overnight so that the broth congeals and the fat rises to the top. Before using the stock, use a spoon to skim the chicken fat from the surface and discard.

Vary It! *To make beef stock, substitute meaty beef bones, such as shank, shin, or ribs. Add a couple of parsnips, a few sprigs more parsley, a couple cloves, 10 peppercorns, and more water if necessary. Cook for at least 3 hours.*

Tip: *Skinning the chicken prior to adding it to stock cuts down on the fat you need to skim later.*

Per serving: *Calories 12; Fat 1g (Saturated 0g); Cholesterol 5mg; Sodium 6mg; Carbohydrates 0g; Dietary Fibre 0g; Protein 1g.*

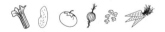

Minimising the saturated fat to lower cholesterol

Poultry and meats contain saturated fat, but you can prevent most of it from ending up in your stock. Follow these three easy tips to cut the fat and your cholesterol:

✔ Start with less fat in the first place, buying lean cuts, and trimming away any visible fat.

✔ When cooking stock, take care that the liquid doesn't reach a full boil. All that bubbling makes it easier for the molecules of fat to mix with the molecules of water. Fat that is dispersed like that is difficult to remove.

✔ When the stock finishes cooking, you can follow the process in Figure 9-1 to remove any excess fat.

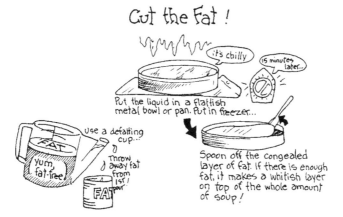

Figure 9-1: Cutting fat from your soup stock.

You can also keep some frozen homemade stock at hand and use it to replace salt or butter for a more heart-healthy recipe. Simply follow these easy steps:

1. **Reduce the stock until it's highly concentrated.**

2. **Freeze it in an ice cube tray.**

3. **Transfer the stock cubes to a freezer bag.**

4. **To enhance the flavour, pop a couple of cubes into the dish you're preparing – use each cube to replace ½ teaspoon of salt.**

Basing Soups on Hearty Ingredients

Select one of the cholesterol-controlling foods from Chapter 2 and build a soup around it. Add stock, flavourings, and a little garnish. This process is how we came up with the recipe for carrot soup in this section. Or, you can concoct a standard soup favourite, such as onion soup or lentil soup, which features some of the recommended vegetables and legumes. This chapter also includes yummy recipes for each of these soups.

You can also add heart-healthy foods that aren't part of the original ingredients without ruining the flavour. Vegetable soup welcomes lentils and beans, for example, and root vegetables, barley, and rice enhance turkey soup. These add-ons and others can make a good-for-you soup even healthier for your heart and add an interesting twist to an old recipe.

Featuring soluble fibre

All manner of legumes – beans, lentils, and peas – contain soluble fibre, as do certain grains and vegetables. Check the list of soluble fibre foods in Chapter 2 and consider these intriguing options you may otherwise overlook as ingredients for your soups:

- Apples
- Barley
- Brown rice, red rice, and even wild rice
- Butter beans
- Cannellini beans
- Lentils, red, yellow, brown, or green
- Okra
- Pears
- Soya beans
- Sweet potatoes

Crying over onion soup

Would you ever imagine that savoury, soul-satisfying onion soup is health food? Well it is, thanks to the anti-inflammatory action of compounds found in onions. That's good news, because inflammation is now known to play a role in the development of heart disease. For details about how this works, see Chapter 1.

Although classic French onion soup relies on butter and a generous topping of cheese, the version in this chapter relies on olive oil, red wine (which provides antioxidants), garlic (which also damps down inflammation), and less of the cheese typically called for, mellow Gruyère.

To avoid crying when chopping onions, use an onion chopper that encloses the onion as you activate the integral chopping blade. Alternatively, wear wrap-round sunglasses or swimming goggles!

Adding vitamins and minerals

Folic acid, vitamin B6, and vitamin B12 keep homocysteine in check, which is another factor in heart disease now coming to the fore. Wholegrains supply B6 and folate and also add texture. Next time you're cooking soup, toss in a small handful of one of these ingredients:

- ✔ Barley
- ✔ Brown rice
- ✔ Buckwheat
- ✔ Millet
- ✔ Quinoa

Poultry and meats are good sources and include vitamin B12, too!

Antioxidants are known to help prevent the accumulation of plaque in arteries. One of them, betacarotene, is also an orange-yellow pigment present in carrots and other orange-coloured foods. Boost the health potential of your soups with the following ingredients:

- ✔ Apricots (goes well with lamb)
- ✔ Carrots
- ✔ Dark leafy greens such as spinach and kale – the green in the chlorophyll covers over the orange betacarotene, but it's there
- ✔ Orange sweet potatoes
- ✔ Orange pumpkin and squash
- ✔ Sweet red pepper

Try the recipe for Curried Carrot Soup with Fresh Ginger later in this chapter and soak up the betacarotene in this golden-orange potage. The soup is garnished with fresh ginger root. To help you tackle the root, see the step-by-step guide in Figure 9-2. To store leftover ginger root, put it in a sealed plastic bag and keep it in your freezer until you need it again.

MINCING PEELED GINGER

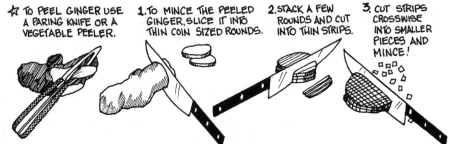

☆ TO PEEL GINGER USE A PARING KNIFE OR A VEGETABLE PEELER.

1. TO MINCE THE PEELED GINGER, SLICE IT INTO THIN COIN SIZED ROUNDS.

2. STACK A FEW ROUNDS AND CUT INTO THIN STRIPS.

3. CUT STRIPS CROSSWISE INTO SMALLER PIECES AND MINCE!

Figure 9-2: The proper steps for mincing ginger root.

Blending cream-less cream soup

The ingredients you leave out are also important in making a soup that fits into a cholesterol-friendly diet. Ingredients such as cream, for example, which is very high in saturated fat and calories, need replacing.

This section tells you how to prepare a creamy vegetable soup that doesn't contain any cream. The secret is to blend the vegetables until they're nearly smooth but still a little chunky and then add some mashed potato. In this section's recipe for Curried Carrot Soup with Fresh Ginger, the potato starch thickens the mixture, and because of the potato's off-white colour, the soup even looks a little creamy!

A few kitchen experiments with broccoli produced a ratio of vegetable, potatoes, and stock that gives the right texture for a satisfying cream-less cream soup: 4 measures vegetables to ½ measure mashed potatoes, plus 2 measures of stock. Try using a chicken stock made from leftover bones and dinner trimmings, or from the recipe given earlier in this chapter. Store fresh stock in the refrigerator overnight and scrape the congealed fat off the top before adding the stock to the pot.

Bad news/good news about low-fat sour cream

When producing low-fat sour cream, manufacturers add guar gum and other substances to replicate the mouth feel of full fat. Unfortunately, the resulting sour cream can feel more like gelatine than butter (you could try reduced-fat crème fraîche instead). However, the *guar gum*, a thickener made from legumes, is also a great source of soluble fibre known to lower cholesterol.

Here is the procedure to follow:

1. **Start with 4 measures of cooked vegetables, such as steamed broccoli, and blend them in a food processor fitted with a metal blade until nearly smooth.**

   Don't over-process the vegetable, or it becomes frothy, and the final soup feels like a broccoli milkshake in your mouth.

2. **Put 2 measures of chicken stock in a large soup pot, add the blended vegetables and ½ measure mashed potatoes, and whisk to combine.**

3. **Warm over medium heat for 15 minutes.**

4. **Season with freshly ground black pepper and serve.**

You can add other seasonings and ingredients, but this is the basic recipe. Try serving the cream-less cream of broccoli soup with a drizzle of hot sesame oil as a garnish. Divine – no one ever misses the cream.

Of course, the soup is still healthy with the sesame oil. All soups, including cream-less cream soups, need some fat. Without any fat, the broccoli mixture is nothing but a vegetable purée. To its credit, fat is a flavour carrier and provides some needed calories. Without a little fat, a vegetable soup is bland, and after you've eaten it, you're soon hungry again.

Going for guilt-free gourmet recipes

The following soups are proof that a healthy soup can still provide a real culinary treat. They're easy to make, and they're deliciously artistic in addition to having health benefits. They have enough substance to entrance your guests as well.

Curried Carrot Soup with Fresh Ginger

This satisfying soup is full of heart-healthy ingredients, including carrots, which provide soluble fibre to control cholesterol, and root ginger, which helps to damp down inflammation as well as helping to make blood less sticky. The recipe calls for Madras curry powder, which is relatively hot. Select a milder blend such as Korma if you prefer.

Special tools required: *Food blender*

Preparation time: *30 minutes*

Cooking time: *1 hour and 15 minutes*

Serves: *4*

1 large Spanish onion, coarsely chopped

2 tablespoons extra-virgin olive oil

Thumb-sized piece of ginger root, peeled and finely grated (see Figure 9-2)

1 tablespoon Madras curry powder

900 grams medium carrots (8 to 10), peeled and sliced horizontally into 1-centimetre pieces

1 large potato, peeled and diced

1 litre chicken stock (see the Basic Chicken Stock earlier in this chapter or use low-sodium, fat-free tinned chicken broth)

¼ teaspoon black pepper

60 millilitres low-fat soured cream

1 In a large saucepan, over a high heat, sauté the onion in the oil for 5 minutes, stirring occasionally. When the onion begins to give up its moisture and reduce in volume, lower the heat to medium.

2 Add to the onion all but 1 tablespoon of the ginger and the curry powder. Continue cooking the mixture for around 5 to 7 minutes until the onion is tender and translucent.

3 Add the carrots and potato to the onion mixture and cook for 15 minutes, stirring occasionally.

4 Add the chicken stock to the vegetables and bring to the boil over a high heat. Lower the heat and simmer, uncovered, for 30 to 40 minutes.

5 Remove the pan from the heat, allowing the soup to cool a few minutes before proceeding.

6 With a ladle, scoop some soup into a blender. Mix in batches, taking care when handling the hot liquid. Pour the puréed soup into a bowl.

7 Return the puréed soup to the pot. Season with black pepper. Warm the soup over a medium heat.

8 While the soup is reheating, combine the soured cream with the reserved ginger. Serve the soup immediately, with a dollop of ginger soured cream as a garnish.

Per serving: Calories 286; Fat 11g (Saturated 3g); Cholesterol 9mg; Sodium 254mg; Carbohydrates 41g; Dietary Fibre 8g; Protein 9g.

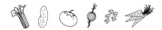

☺ Lentil Soup

In a heart-healthy diet, lentil soup is one of the staples. Lentils are a low-fat source of protein and contain soluble fibre that helps to lower cholesterol. Here's a Middle Eastern version, made with coriander, lemon, and spinach – the deep green of the leaves breaking up the beige-brown of the lentils. Along with the soup, serve a plate of slices of feta cheese and black and green marinated olives as accompaniments. Also provide wedges of lemon, called for in the recipe, so diners have the option of adding a squirt of lemon juice to the soup to accentuate the flavours even more.

Preparation time: *15 minutes*

Cooking time: *1 hour and 10 minutes*

Serves: *6 (generous servings)*

300 grams brown lentils	*15 grams fresh parsley, chopped*
2 litres water	*¼ teaspoon black pepper*
1 medium-size onion, diced	*⅛ teaspoon hot red pepper flakes or to taste*
5 cloves garlic, peeled and minced	*1 lemon, cut into wedges*
1 tin (175 grams) tomato paste	*Feta cheese (optional)*
1 teaspoon ground coriander	*Olives (optional)*
350 grams spinach, stems removed and coarsely chopped	

1 Place the lentils and water in a large saucepan and bring to the boil, covered. Reduce the heat to medium-low and cook the lentils for 30 minutes.

2 Add the onion, garlic, tomato paste, and coriander to the lentils. Cook the lentil mixture on medium-low for an additional 30 minutes. The lentils begin to dissolve and the soup becomes thick.

3 Add the spinach, parsley, black pepper, and pepper flakes. Continue to cook the soup for another 10 minutes on medium-low, to wilt the spinach and combine the flavours.

4 Serve with side servings of lemon wedges, feta cheese, and olives. Because this soup thickens on standing, add a little water to reheat the soup.

Per serving: *Calories 221; Fat 1g (Saturated 0g); Cholesterol 0mg; Sodium 70mg; Carbohydrates 40g; Dietary Fibre 15g; Protein 17g. (Olive and feta not included in analysis.)*

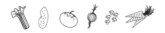

French Onion Soup

The classic recipe for French onion soup requires at least an hour to sauté the onions until they turn a rich brown, and then you melt cheese over the top of the soup under a hot grill. In this speedier version, you first bake the onions, which shortens the sautéing time, and you place a more modest garnish of cheese in the bottom of the soup bowl. You then pour the hot soup in over the cheese, which melts deliciously. *Voilà!* You're finished cooking and ready to enjoy all the same flavours as the classic version, but with less fat.

Preparation time: *15 minutes*

Cooking time: *1 hour and 50 minutes*

Serves: *6*

6 large Spanish onions (about 1½ kilograms)

4 tablespoons extra-virgin olive oil

6 garlic cloves, sliced

60 millilitres red wine

1 litre beef broth (if tinned, use the low-sodium and fat-free variety) (see the tip at the end of the recipe)

500 millilitres chicken broth (see the Basic Chicken Stock recipe earlier in this chapter or use tinned, low-sodium fat-free chicken broth)

Black pepper

6 medium slices wholegrain bread

75 grams grated Gruyère cheese

1 Heat the oven to 190 degrees. Peel the onions, cut them in half vertically, and cut each half horizontally into thin slices. Place the whole onions, with the skins on, in a roasting pan for an hour, until they begin to soften.

2 Remove onions from the oven and allow to cool for 5 minutes.

3 Heat the olive oil in a large saucepan over medium heat. Add the sliced onions and garlic. Sauté on medium heat until brown, but not burned, stirring occasionally, for about 20 minutes.

4 Add the wine and simmer until the wine is reduced to a glaze, about 3 minutes.

5 Gradually mix in the beef broth and chicken broth, scraping up browned bits from the bottom of the pan.

6 Turn the heat to medium-high and bring just to the boil; lower the heat to a simmer, so that the soup sends up a few bubbles at a time. Season to taste with black pepper. Simmer the soup until the flavours blend, about 15 minutes. At this point, you can cover and refrigerate the soup, if you want, to serve the next day. Reheat the soup before continuing.

7 Meanwhile, toast the bread and place 1 slice in each of 6 soup bowls. Top with 2 table-spoons of the cheese. Or use a grill and sprinkle the cheese on the bread and let the cheese melt as the bread toasts. Ladle the soup over the toast and serve immediately.

Tip: If using tinned beef broth and/or canned chicken broth, omit the salt seasoning.

Per serving: *Calories 283; Fat 16g (Saturated 4g); Cholesterol 15mg; Sodium 261mg; Carbohydrates 24g; Dietary Fibre 4g; Protein 12g.*

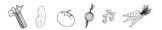

Leek and Mixed Vegetable Soup

Eating a minimum of 5 servings a day of fruit and vegetables is recommended for general good health. Lunching on vegetable soup is an easy way to start. This forgiving mixture of vegetables accepts all sorts of heart-healthy additions – leftover vegetables from last night's dinner, a handful of cooked beans, or some cooked brown rice or barley. Or enjoy it as is, a range of colourful vegetables and nutrients, tied together with the delicate flavour of leek – a soothing rainy-day dish with a hint of spring.

Preparation time: *10 minutes*

Cooking time: *25 minutes*

Serves: *4*

1.4 litres chicken stock (see the Basic Chicken Stock recipe earlier in this chapter or use tinned, low-sodium low-fat chicken broth)

1 leek, top trimmed, cut horizontally into 1-centimetre pieces and washed thoroughly to remove sand

1 carrot, cut horizontally into 1-centimetre pieces

1 celery stalk, cut horizontally into 1-centimetre pieces

1 courgette, quartered lengthwise and quarters cut horizontally into 1-centimetre lengths

1 butternut squash, quartered lengthwise and quarters cut horizontally into 1-centimetre lengths

1 small potato, peeled and diced

3 sprigs parsley, stems removed

1 tablespoon extra-virgin olive oil

¼ teaspoon black pepper

Pinch of red pepper flakes

1 Place all ingredients in a large saucepan and bring to the boil.

2 Lower the heat to medium and cook for 20 to 30 minutes, or until the vegetables are soft.

3 Serve the soup immediately, with a slice of wholegrain bread and a small wedge of quality cheese on the side.

Vary It! *For a soup with fuller flavour, at the beginning of the cooking process, add ½ teaspoon dried herbs, such as thyme, oregano, or basil, or a combination of these.*

Tip: *To give the vegetables in your soup some dignity, give each type a uniform cut rather than serving a hodgepodge of produce.*

Per serving: *Calories 177; Fat 6g (Saturated 2g); Cholesterol 6mg; Sodium 194mg; Carbohydrates 27g; Dietary Fibre 6g; Protein 7g.*

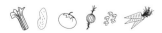

Bumping up Soup into a Meal

Turn to soup when you need a time-saving, complete meal in one. You can give yourself some protein, some carbohydrate, and some healthy fat just as if you sat down to a three-course meal. Because it's bulky, soup also lets you fill up sooner, on fewer calories. Try the following lunch suggestions for hearty soups that you can call dinner.

Inventing soup-and-sandwich combinations

A cup of soup and half a sandwich are just enough to satisfy your hunger and make a great lunch – the soup is warming, and the half sandwich filling. Here are some suggested combinations whose ingredients are good for your heart (you can find instructions for all the soup recipes in this chapter):

- Cream of Pumpkin Soup with sliced turkey breast with cranberry relish on wholemeal bread.
- Onion Soup with egg salad on French bread.
- Beetroot Soup with lean sliced beef with horseradish on rye bread.
- Corn and Sweet Red Pepper Chowder with salmon salad on pumpernickel.
- Cream-less cream of broccoli soup with sliced chicken breast on wholemeal bread.
- Lentil Soup with wholemeal pitta filled with Greek salad made from tomato, cucumber, and lettuce and garnished with feta cheese and olives.

Supping on substantial soup recipes

For some people, a simple little broth just won't do it. When children are hungry or you have a burly bloke to feed, your bowl of soup better look like a real meal. The two recipes in this section, Beef and Barley Soup and Chicken and Okra Cassoulet, fit the bill. And they both help you to control cholesterol and take good care of your heart, providing soluble fibre and a variety of nutritious vegetables.

Beef and Barley Soup

A winning combination: barley is a great grain for controlling cholesterol because it supplies soluble fibre, the mushrooms are also a good source of chromium that helps your body metabolise carbs, and this soup freezes well.

Preparation time: *15 minutes*

Cooking time: *2 hours and 30 minutes*

Serves: *6*

550 grams beef shin on the bone, trimmed of excess fat	*175 grams button mushrooms, trimmed, and quartered*
Black pepper	*1½ litres water*
3 tablespoons extra-virgin olive oil	*1 teaspoon dried thyme*
1 carrot, diced	*100 grams pearl barley, rinsed*
1 medium onion, diced	*1 tin (400 grams) chopped tomato*
1 stick celery, diced	*1 teaspoon unsalted butter or substitute*
	3 tablespoons chopped flat-leaf parsley

1 Season the meat to taste with black pepper. Heat 2 tablespoons of oil in a large saucepan and place the meat in the pan. Over a medium-high heat, cook the meat on all sides for about 15 minutes until seared and well browned. Remove the meat and set aside.

2 Add the remaining 1 tablespoon of oil to the pan and lower the heat to medium. Add the carrot, onion, celery and mushrooms, and cook for about 10 minutes until tender. To the vegetable mixture, add the reserved meat and the water.

3 Bring to the boil and adjust the heat to maintain a gentle simmer. Cover the pan and cook the soup for 1½ hours, until the meat is tender.

4 Add the thyme, barley, and tomato. Simmer the soup for an additional 30 minutes, until the barley is tender.

5 Remove the meat and shred into small chunks.

6 Skim any obvious fat from the surface of the soup. Return the meat to the soup. Add the parsley. Season to taste with black pepper.

Per serving: Calories 250; Fat 13g (Saturated 3g); Cholesterol 30mg; Sodium 117mg; Carbohydrates 20g; Dietary Fibre 5g; Protein 14g.

Chicken and Okra Cassoulet

Can you remember when you last ate some okra? Okra is an essential ingredient in this dish and gives you a serving of soluble fibre. Sausage is another essential ingredient, for the flavour. Use the real thing for sensational taste: smoked hard-cooked pork sausage such as chorizo. Before serving, skim the visible fat from the soup and enjoy a few slices of sausage. After all, this meal is your dinner. Or if you must go very lean, hunt around for a tasty brand of low-fat chicken or turkey sausage and use this instead. But the smoked pork sausage wins on flavour and satisfaction, hands down.

Special tools required: *Food processor*

Preparation time: *30 minutes*

Cooking time: *1½ hours*

Serves: *8*

1.1 kilograms chicken breast, skin removed

3 litres chicken stock (see the Basic Chicken Stock earlier in this chapter or use low-sodium, fat-free tinned chicken broth)

2 medium onions, peeled

2 green bell peppers, cored and seeds removed

3 sticks celery

60 millilitres olive oil

6 cloves garlic, minced

175 grams smoked pork sausage, thinly sliced (reduced-fat versions are available)

1 tin (400 grams) tomatoes, chopped

2 tablespoons tomato paste

450 grams fresh or frozen okra, cut into 1-centimetre pieces

1 tablespoon ground coriander seed

Hot pepper sauce

Cayenne pepper

Black pepper

Steamed rice

1 In a large saucepan, poach the chicken breast in the stock over a medium heat, uncovered, for 20 minutes, until cooked through. Remove the chicken and set aside the meat and the stock.

2 Meanwhile, roughly chop the onions, peppers, and celery. In a food processor fitted with a metal blade, finely chop the vegetables.

3 Heat the oil in a large, heavy-bottomed saucepan and add the garlic and the finely chopped vegetable mixture. Cook the vegetables on a medium heat for 10 minutes, stirring occasionally, until the onion is soft and translucent.

4 Add the sausage, tomatoes, tomato paste, and the reserved stock to the vegetables.

5 Bring the vegetable and sausage mixture to the boil and then reduce to a simmer.

6 Shred the chicken and add this to the pan, along with the okra and ground coriander seed. Season the soup to taste with the hot pepper, cayenne, and black pepper.

7 Simmer the cassoulet for 1 hour to combine the flavours. Ladle over steamed rice and serve. This soup tastes even better the next day.

Per serving: *Calories 340; Fat 18g (Saturated 5g); Cholesterol 76mg; Sodium 542mg; Carbohydrates 16g; Dietary Fibre 4g; Protein 30g.*

Inventing Soups with Tinned and Bottled Ingredients

Tinned soup, such as Cream of Tomato, Chicken and Leek, or mixed Vegetable, is handy to have around for emergencies. If high blood pressure is a concern, check labels and look for low-salt or low-sodium versions to avoid the copious amounts of sodium normally present in tinned soup

Doctoring tinned chicken broth

If you do resort to tinned chicken stock in some of the preceding recipes, choose a product that's virtually fat free and low in sodium. You can then work with it a bit, adding a healthy fat such as extra-virgin olive oil and not adding additional salt. Include some of the vegetables and herbs featured in the two stock recipes and season with freshly ground pepper to make the broth more interesting.

If using tinned chicken stock for Chinese cooking, add a few slices of fresh ginger, a couple of cloves of garlic, 1 spring onion, and a tablespoon or two of dry sherry.

Opening a tin of this and a bottle of that

Okay, so you don't have time to cook one of the recipes in this chapter from start to finish. You can still enjoy some homemade soup! Combining ready-made ingredients can lead to some surprising results. Try some of the following soups, which you can throw together in no time and with very little effort.

Try these heart-healthy selections, which include quantities to give you an idea of the ratio of ingredients. Feel free to adjust the amounts to suit your own taste, however, as you have fun experimenting with these soups.

✔ **Cream of Pumpkin Soup:** Using a food processor fitted with a metal blade, purée in batches the following ingredients: 400 grams of pumpkin soup (1 tin), 700 millilitres homemade chicken broth, 1 pear (peel, stem, and core removed), 120 millilitres whole milk, ½ tablespoon Madras curry powder (or if you prefer, ½ teaspoon cinnamon and ⅛ teaspoon nutmeg). Cook over a medium heat for 30 minutes, stirring occasionally, and serve. The pumpkin is a great source of antioxidant vitamin A, and the pear provides soluble fibre.

✔ **Sweetcorn and Red Pepper Chowder:** In a food processor fitted with a metal blade, process 225 grams of roasted sweet red peppers (1 jar) and 450 grams of frozen sweetcorn (1 bag) until the mixture has the consistency of apple sauce. Add enough home-made vegetable or chicken stock to obtain this consistency. Cook over a medium heat, and in 15 minutes you have a thick-textured, delicious lunch chowder, and the peppers provide you with antioxidants.

✔ **Salmon Potage:** Purée in a food processor fitted with a metal blade 400 grams (1 tin) of salmon (skin and bones removed), 480 millilitres semi-skimmed milk, and 1 teaspoon dried dill. Warm on a medium heat, stirring occasionally. Add pepper to taste. The salmon contains omega-3 fatty acids that lower cholesterol.

✔ **Beetroot Soup:** Combine over a medium heat the following ingredients: 900 grams of borscht (1 bottle) (or made up from 300 grams of Red Borscht Concentrate), 480 millilitres chopped fresh cabbage, 1 apple (diced), 1 potato (diced), and 1 tablespoon fresh dill. Cook for 30 minutes. Serve in individual soup bowls, each garnished with a tablespoon of reduced-fat soured cream.

Chapter 10

Savouring Super Salads for Everyday Meals

In This Chapter

▶ Looking for the freshest salad ingredients

▶ Fixing fantastic salads and dressings

▶ Converting a salad into a meal

Salads are a great way to get all sorts of ingredients that keep your heart healthy and lower cholesterol. Vegetables, fruits, and beans in salads provide special vitamins and minerals, as well as soluble fibre, while salad oils help balance the 'good' HDL and the 'bad' LDL cholesterol. (Check out Chapter 1 for more info on HDL and LDL cholesterol.) These dishes are also your chance to include some raw foods in your diet. In this form, they retain all their original nutrients and take longer to digest, so they tend not to raise blood sugar rapidly and help keep cholesterol at lower levels.

Browse through this chapter to find information on buying and storing produce and the basics on making salad. Experiment with the recipes for side salads, main course salads, and salad dressings. Treat yourself to the best ingredients you can find, particularly because you're eating them raw. Make your salads irresistible, and you're likely to eat more of these cholesterol-controlling foods.

Making Salads with the Best and the Brightest

Fresh salad produce contains the most nutrients, which begin to ebb the longer the fruit and veg sit around in your kitchen. Produce harvested when fully ripe is also the healthiest. When fruits and vegetables are picked before they're fully ripe, they don't have a chance to acquire the last uptake of nutrients, particularly minerals.

For really fresh produce, try growing your own in pots or in a border. For starters, buy potted chives and thyme to pinch off and add to salads. If you want to discover more, take a look at _Growing Your Own Fruit & Veg For Dummies_ (Wiley) by Geoff Stebbings.

Shopping for the freshest produce

Search out farmers' markets, street markets, and local greengrocers in your area for local produce, and have a chat with the person managing the fruit and veg section in the supermarket where you shop. Ask which items are local and which come from abroad. Of course, during winter months the supply of local produce is limited in northern climates, making buying fruits and vegetables from other regions a necessity. Supplement your supply with frozen fruits and vegetables, which are processed soon after harvesting and retain a good proportion of their original nutrients.

Handling fruits and veg with care

Although many fruits and vegetables do just fine in the vegetables compartment of refrigerators, some foods require special care. Here's a quick review of the needs of certain items:

- ✔ Tomatoes don't ripen properly in the fridge, and so they don't get juicy and sweet. They require temperatures above 10 degrees Celsius. To ripen tomatoes, leave them sitting on the kitchen counter, not in the sun, and when ripe, eat them within a day or two. Refrigerating tomatoes, even ripe ones, causes them to lose flavour and become mushy.

- ✔ Use asparagus as soon as possible after you buy it and store it in the refrigerator. Stand stalks upright in a tall container filled with $2^1/_2$ centimetres of water. Cover the asparagus tops loosely with a plastic bag.

- ✔ Ripen avocados at room temperature. After they're ripe, you can transfer them to the vegetable drawer of your refrigerator.

✔ To keep a bunch of herbs fresh, trim the ends off the stems and place in a tall glass of cold water to which you add a pinch of sugar. Store this in the refrigerator. Trim the ends and change the water as necessary. You can also revive wilted sprigs by moistening the herb with a fine mist of water and chilling the herb briefly.

Looking at the colour of your produce

Plenty of research shows that colourful fruits and vegetables are full of phytonutrients (which in many cases are also the pigments themselves) plus nutrients that are good for you just like vitamins and minerals. But what's also clear is that combining a variety of phytonutrients in one meal multiplies their beneficial effects. A mix of foods in different colours contains much more antioxidant power, enhances blood vessel protection, and proves more effective at lowering cholesterol. You can read more about the specific phytonutrients in Chapter 2.

The recipe for Colourful Coleslaw that appears later in this chapter is a great way to sample one of these nutrient cocktails. Here are some other ways to add colourful fruits and veg to your salads:

✔ Sweet peppers come in five colours – green, red, orange, yellow, and purple. Buy one of each. Core and slice these, and cook in olive oil flavoured with sliced clove garlic. Serve as part of an antipasto.

✔ If you need some citrus in your salad, add pink grapefruit or blood oranges, which have flesh that is red, purple, or burgundy. They are less acidic than regular oranges and have a subtle taste of raspberry.

✔ If you're making coleslaw, add some purplish-red cabbage along with the green, but remember that raw red cabbage has a peppery taste.

✔ Shred orange carrots and slice red radishes into your standard lettuce salad. Make the salad with red leaf lettuce.

✔ When you want raw onions in a salad, add red onions rather than yellow onions for a touch of colour and milder flavour. Red onions are at their best raw; when cooked, they become watery and lose their colour.

Tossing Together Your Basic Salad

Making a salad is simple. In fact, two of the following recipes – the Beetroot, Pear, and Chicory Salad and the Fennel, Orange, and Avocado Salad – feature just three main ingredients. Some fine-tasting oil and vinegar add the finishing touch. The individual flavours of each ingredient are there to savour separately and also to complement each other.

Leading with lettuce

When creating a salad, start out with an interesting lettuce. The familiar iceberg has its uses when you want crunch and something juicy – it's 96 per cent water – but experiment with other, more interesting leaves to spruce up your next salad. Try the following:

- **Rocket:** With its pungent, spicy flavour, this lettuce bites back. Rocket is excellent combined with sweet or bitter leaves as the first course for an Italian meal. For a treat, top rocket with a few toasted walnuts and a well-trimmed slice of Prosciutto or some shaved Parmesan cheese.

- **Curly endive:** This lettuce is good with a full-bodied dressing, especially a sweet one, which balances the green's slightly bitter taste.

- **Radicchio:** Serve this rather bitter-tasting lettuce raw, braised, grilled, or wilted, perhaps with a splash of vinegar and oil.

- **Red leaf lettuce:** This lettuce has frilly-edged leaves that are delicate in texture and flavour. Enjoy this lettuce mixed with other greens and with a mild dressing.

For really crisp lettuce, wash it under cool running water, shake off the excess moisture, blot with paper towels, and refrigerate for about an hour before you use it to make a salad.

Vitamin K, present in leafy greens and other vegetables, helps the blood to clot. It acts as an antidote to the drug, warfarin, which is often prescribed for heart patients as a blood thinner. If you're one of these patients, you need to combine the two items safely, by ensuring that your intake of foods rich in vitamin K remains steady and you have your clotting times checked regularly. This way, the opposing actions of these two substances stay in balance.

Making the best-dressed list

Salad dressings are an opportunity to eat cholesterol-friendly vegetable oils. Polyunsaturated and monounsaturated oils lower LDL, and monounsaturates raise HDL as well. (For more on LDL and HDL, see Chapter 1.) For optimal health, go one better and use unrefined versions of these oils, to avoid trans fatty acids and to retain nutrients stripped off during the refining process.

The way to differentiate between refined and unrefined oils when you go shopping is that the refined oils are basically all the same pale yellow colour. They're also flavourless. In contrast, unrefined oil has the colour and flavour of the food it was made from, such as the green oil made from olives. Always look for high-quality oils that say 'unrefined' on the label.

Stocking up on quality oils

You don't need a wide variety of oils for making salad dressing, but you do need the best. Many vegetable oils have distinctive flavours, and so sample different brands to find the ones you really like. Here are the different kinds of oils to consider:

- **Extra-virgin olive oil:** Your best option, for flavour, texture, and health, olive oil contains monounsaturated fats, which lower LDL and raise HDL, just what you want.

  Like tea, olive oil contains polyphenols, antioxidants that protect LDL from oxidation, meaning that it's less likely to contribute to the formation of arterial plaque. Monounsaturates in olive oil also lower high blood pressure.

- **Safflower oil:** You can use this oil in salad dressings although it has a heavier, oilier feel in the mouth than olive oil.

- **Toasted sesame oil:** Imparts an Asian flavour to a salad.

- **Avocado oil**: Rich in monounsaturated fatty acids, this oil has a lovely green colour and makes a great tasting salad dressing.

Treating yourself to specialty nut oils

Gourmet nut oils add a delectable flavour that is so distinctive, you need only add a couple of teaspoons. Try the following:

- **Walnut oil:** Brings a depth and richness of flavour even to simple greens. It also contains omega-3 fatty acids, which lower cholesterol.

- **Macadamia nut oil:** If you add this to any dressing that you're preparing, you boost your intake of monounsaturated fatty acids, which are abundant in this oil.

- **Almond oil:** Delicious as a dipping oil for bread, as well as in salad dressings and baked goods.

- **Hazelnut oil:** Adds a depth of flavour to salad dressing and, like olive oil, is high in monounsaturated fat (75 per cent of total fat in the nut).

Flavouring your dressing

To build a dressing, start with the oil and add other tasty ingredients. Garlic is a good place to start. Research shows that regularly consuming garlic helps to raise the healthy HDL cholesterol and lower the harmful LDL cholesterol. Include garlic, raw or cooked, in your meals and aim for 1 to 3 cloves a day. Raw onions can also raise HDL cholesterol.

The flavour of garlic mashed through a garlic press is ten times stronger than garlic that's minced only with a knife. Mashed garlic is also more therapeutic. Crushing releases more *allicin*, a phytonutrient that lowers cholesterol, thins the blood, and widens blood vessels. After you mash the garlic, set it aside for 10 to 15 minutes to allow its medicinal properties to develop.

The first step in making an oil and vinegar dressing is to decide how acidic you like it. (Some people use equal amounts of oil and vinegar and find the bite of the dressing just right. Others prefer a 3 to 1 ratio of oil and vinegar, as you find in the recipes in this chapter – feel free to adjust these amounts if you like.) Next, add a small amount of flavourings, such as a little mustard and a pinch of herbs, until you come up with a dressing that hits the spot.

When you use one of the less acidic vinegars, such as balsamic or rice wine vinegar, you need less oil to balance the tartness and thereby save calories. To judge the acidity and flavour of a dressing accurately, dip the edge of a lettuce leaf in the dressing and sample this – don't taste with a teaspoon.

Consider adding these ingredients to your dressing for flavour:

- Dijon or wholegrain mustard
- Minced shallots for a mild onion flavour
- Fresh herbs, such as mint, oregano, basil, or dill
- Vinegars flavoured with tarragon, sherry, or chilli peppers

Dried herbs have a more intense flavour than fresh herbs. When a recipe calls for 1 teaspoon of dried, and you prefer fresh, add 3 teaspoons of fresh herbs.

Going beyond the regular green salad recipes

Salads are good on their own and are also useful to serve with dinner. The following examples are good ones to have in your repertoire. The coleslaw in particular goes well with all types of meat and fish.

⌒ Colourful Coleslaw

You can tell this salad is full of antioxidants because it's also full of colour, most notably the orange in the carrots and the red in the tomatoes. The cabbage, with its reddish-purple hue, contains *anthocyanins* (powerful phytonutrient antioxidants) and almost twice the vitamin C found in green cabbage. Eating such foods plays an important role in controlling cholesterol. In a small study conducted at Western General Hospital in Edinburgh, consuming 200 grams of raw carrot every day for 3 weeks resulted in a significant and lasting reduction in total cholesterol.

To prepare this coleslaw, either use a food processor to shred the cabbage and carrots or do it the old-fashioned way and burn some calories as you shred the vegetables by hand using a grater.

Special tools required: *Food processor (optional)*

Preparation time: *15 minutes*

Serves: *8*

½ cucumber, peeled

½ small head of red cabbage, shredded

2 carrots, peeled and shredded

2 medium tomatoes

3 tablespoons safflower oil

3 tablespoons flavoured rice wine vinegar

Black pepper

1 Cut the cucumber once lengthwise and cut each piece in half again lengthwise. Dice each cucumber spear into small cubes. Put in a large bowl and add the shredded cabbage and carrots.

2 Cut the tomatoes into small 1-centimetre pieces and add to the other vegetables.

3 In a small bowl, mix together the safflower oil and wine vinegar. Pour the dressing over the cabbage mixture.

4 Toss to combine and season to taste with black pepper. Serve for lunch with a sandwich or with fish for dinner.

Per serving: *Calories 71; Fat 6g (Saturated 0g); Cholesterol 0mg; Sodium 17mg; Carbohydrate 6g; Dietary Fibre 2g; Protein 1g.*

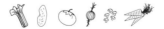

○ *Sliced Tomatoes with Avocado Dressing*

This recipe provides the full range of healthy oils, including monounsaturates and polyunsaturates as well as omega-3 fatty acids in the flaxseed oil. It also specifies vine-ripened tomatoes because they contain more nutrients and are more flavourful.

Special tools required: *Food processor*

Preparation time: *10 minutes*

Serves: *4*

1 medium avocado	*1 tablespoon sherry vinegar*
1 shallot, minced (1 tablespoon)	*Black pepper*
60 millilitres olive oil	*450 grams vine-ripened tomatoes, sliced*
1 tablespoon fresh flaxseed oil (see the tip at the end of the recipe)	

1 Cut the avocado in half lengthwise. Rotate one half and remove. Use a large spoon or the tip of a knife to remove the seed from the other half. Cut each avocado in half lengthwise and peel the skin. Put the avocado in a food processor fitted with a metal blade.

2 Add the shallot, olive oil, flaxseed oil, and sherry vinegar. Process until smooth. This recipe makes about 180 millilitres dressing, enough for 450 grams of tomatoes, plus 60 millilitres of dressing left over.

3 Season the dressing to taste with black pepper.

4 Arrange the tomatoes on individual salad plates. Garnish each with 2 tablespoons of avocado dressing.

Tip: *Check that the flaxseed oil is still fresh by sampling a bit. It should have a flavour faintly reminiscent of butter.*

Per serving: *Calories 246; Fat 24g (Saturated 4g); Cholesterol 0mg; Sodium 11mg; Carbohydrate 10g; Dietary Fibre 5g; Protein 2g.*

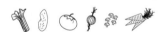

☺ *Beetroot, Pear, and Chicory Salad*

This recipe shows that using the perfect combination of ingredients makes it easy to prepare an elegant dish. This salad gives you juiciness, crunch, sweetness, and the heartiness of a root vegetable, and it comes out a festive magenta colour.

Preparation time: *15 minutes*

Cooking time: *1 hour*

Serves: *6 as a side salad with dinner, or 2 for a lunch main course*

3 raw beetroot	*3 tablespoons unrefined safflower oil*
1 firm dessert pear (such as William or Bosc)	*1½ tablespoons balsamic vinegar*
1 head chicory, plus optional 6 additional chicory leaves as garnish	*Black pepper*

1 Preheat the oven to 200 degrees. Wash the beetroot, wrap them in aluminium foil, and put them on a baking sheet. Cook for about 1 hour, until you can easily pierce the beetroot with a thin-bladed knife. Remove from the oven and cool for about 20 minutes. Peel the beets, dice them, and place them in a large bowl.

2 Dice the pear and add to the beetroot. Cut the chicory crosswise into thin slices and add to the bowl.

3 Whisk together the oil and vinegar in a small bowl and pour over the salad.

4 Toss all the ingredients together. Season to taste with black pepper.

5 Distribute the salad among individual salad plates or transfer the salad to a serving bowl. Garnish with optional chicory leaves, the wider end tucked under the edge of the salad.

Vary It! *Combine equal parts of diced beetroot and diced apples and toss with a low-fat mayonnaise dressing seasoned with mustard and fresh dill.*

Tip: *This dish is one to eat soon after making it, rather than letting it sit overnight.*

Per serving: *Calories 89; Fat 7g (Saturated 1g); Cholesterol 0mg; Sodium 20mg; Carbohydrate 7g; Dietary Fibre 1g; Protein 1g.*

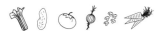

↻ Rocket Salad with Barley and Chickpeas

This salad, which has an Italian accent thanks to the rocket and marinated artichoke hearts, makes a great buffet offering or a tasty dish that goes well with lasagne. It also gives you another way to include barley – a good source of soluble fibre – in your meals. Cook the pearl barley from scratch or prepare it the night before for dinner and make extra to have this salad the next day for lunch.

Preparation time: *10 minutes*

Serves: *6*

300 grams cooked pearl barley (see the tip at the end of the recipe)

1 jar (350 grams) marinated artichoke hearts, drained

1 tin (425 grams) chickpeas, rinsed

1 bag (200 grams) washed salad greens that include rocket, or a mix of rocket and red leaved lettuce

2 tablespoons balsamic vinegar

6 tablespoons extra-virgin olive oil

2 tablespoons lemon juice

Black pepper

1 In a large bowl, mix together the pearl barley, artichoke hearts, and chickpeas. Add the salad greens and toss with the barley mixture.

2 Whisk together the vinegar, oil, and lemon juice. Drizzle over the salad and toss.

3 Season to taste with black pepper and serve immediately.

Tip: *To prepare barley from scratch, begin with 200 grams of grain and cook according to package instructions. The cooking process takes about 45 minutes and yields around 300 grams of grain.*

Tip: *This dish tastes best if you chill the artichoke hearts and chick peas. If you don't want to serve it right away, throw together and chill the barley, artichokes, chickpeas, and dressing, and then just add the salad greens and toss to coat right before serving. Then, the salad is cool, crisp, and full of flavour.*

Per serving: *Calories 267; Fat 17g (Saturated 2g); Cholesterol 0mg; Sodium 246mg; Carbohydrate 27g; Dietary Fibre 6g; Protein 5g.*

☺ Fennel, Orange, and Avocado Salad

The oranges in this salad are roughly cut, with the membranes left intact. That way, you get the full benefit of the bioflavonoids – antioxidants that strengthen capillary walls – contained in the membranes. The oranges also provide tartness that balances the creamy avocado. And the fennel offers crispness and a refreshing, liquorice-like flavour.

Preparation time: *10 minutes*

Serves: *4 as a side salad, or 2 for a light lunch*

1 small bulb Florence fennel, trimmed	*3 tablespoons extra-virgin olive oil*
1 navel orange, peeled	*1 tablespoon balsamic vinegar*
1 avocado, peeled and stoned	*Black pepper*

1 Cut the fennel bulb in half lengthwise and then crosswise in thin slices.

2 Separate the orange into segments and slice these into 1-centimetre chunks, including the membranes and the soft white part that runs through the middle of the orange.

3 Cut the avocado into 1-centimetre chunks. Gently combine the avocado, orange, and fennel together in a large bowl.

4 Mix together the olive oil and the balsamic vinegar in a small bowl and drizzle over the salad. Toss together gently with a wooden spoon to avoid cutting into the soft avocado. Season to taste with black pepper and serve.

Tip: To cut the avocado into chunks, first cut the avocado in half lengthwise. Rotate one half and remove from seed. Use a large spoon or the tip of a knife to lift out the seed from the other half. Cut each avocado in half lengthwise and peel the skin. Cut the avocado flesh into chunks.

Per serving: Calories 195; Fat 17g (Saturated 3g); Cholesterol 0mg; Sodium 32mg; Carbohydrate 13g; Dietary Fibre 6g; Protein 2g.

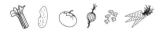

☙ Spinach and Walnut Salad with Ruby Grapefruit

Spinach is a world-class vegetable in terms of nutrition. It's loaded with vitamins and minerals that are good for your heart, including the antioxidants betacarotene, vitamin C, and alpha-lipoic acid; folic acid, which helps lower homocysteine levels; and potassium, which is associated with lower blood pressure. In addition, researchers focusing on fruit and vegetable intake in over 75,000 women taking part in the American Nurses' Health Study found that consuming more green leafy vegetables and citrus fruit lowers the risk of experiencing a stroke. This salad contains both. These benefits aside, wait until you experience the mix of textures and flavours in this salad – the richness of toasted walnuts balances the juiciness of tart grapefruit. Most people definitely want seconds!

Preparation time: *20 minutes*

Cooking time: *3 minutes*

Serves: *6 as a side salad for dinner, or 2 for lunch*

50 grams walnut halves	*3 tablespoons extra-virgin olive oil*
1 head chicory, trimmed and washed	*1 tablespoon red wine vinegar*
1 ruby grapefruit, peeled	*1 small shallot, minced*
700 grams baby spinach, washed and stems removed	*½ teaspoon Dijon mustard*
	Black pepper

1 In a small nonstick frying pan, toast the walnuts over a medium heat until they begin to brown and become fragrant (between 3 and 7 minutes – keep an eye on them and stir a few times). Transfer to a bowl and set aside.

2 Slice the chicory crosswise in thin slices and put it into a large bowl.

3 Separate the segments of grapefruit and cut into bite-size chunks. Add the grapefruit, spinach, and walnuts to the bowl with the chicory.

4 In a small bowl, whisk together the olive oil, vinegar, shallot, and mustard. Pour over the salad.

5 Gently toss all the ingredients together. Season to taste with black pepper.

Tip: *This recipe nicely complements the Beetroot, Pear, and Chicory Salad in this chapter. Serve both on a buffet.*

Per serving: *Calories 157; Fat 12g (Saturated 1g); Cholesterol 0mg; Sodium 101mg; Carbohydrate 9g; Dietary Fibre 4g; Protein 4g.*

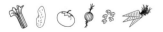

Salads That Start with Protein

Salads, like soups, are forgiving dishes that let you add all manner of extra ingredients. Take advantage of this and include more vegetables, fruits, and nuts in your salads. You can also turn a simple salad into a complete meal just by topping it with lean protein.

Making nutritious salads isn't hard. Simply add healthy titbits that you probably already have in your kitchen cupboards or refrigerator. Here are some possibilities:

- Open a tin of beans, such as kidney, butter beans, chickpeas, or cannellini. Drain the beans in a sieve, rinse them with water, and sprinkle them in a salad.

- Toss in some nuts, such as pecans, walnuts, macadamias, or sliced almonds, and add some seeds such as sesame and sunflower. You can even add trail mix – a combination of dried fruits and nuts – which is available from health food shops.

- To increase soluble fibre, include apples, carrots, green beans, lentils, Brazil nuts, or barley.

- Add slivers of chicken breast from last night's dinner.

- Enlist recently leftover cooked vegetables to join the salad.

- Garnish your salad with a small cluster of purple grapes.

- Use the tins or jars of artichokes, olives, and marinated sweet red peppers that you were saving for guests.

Avocados earn an A

Avocados make a great addition to salads. Yes, they're high in fat, but it's the healthy, mono-unsaturated kind. Like the oil in olives, the fat in avocados protects your arteries. In an Australian study of middle-aged women, eating avocados daily for three weeks improved the ratio of 'good' HDL cholesterol to 'bad' LDL cholesterol more effectively than following a low-fat diet.

Avocados contain a greater proportion of soluble fibre than most fruit and vegetables, and they're especially rich in a powerful antioxidant,

glutathione. They also contain another helpful compound, betasitosterol, a plant-based substance that reduces the amount of unhealthy LDL cholesterol absorbed from food and lowers triglyceride levels as well.

You may need to let avocados ripen after you bring them home from the shop. To do this, put the avocados in a paper bag with an apple, set this on your kitchen sideboard, and keep them there for 2 to 3 days.

Hot salads for cool nights

Salads aren't only for eating in the heat of the day. A salad can make a great main course, especially when topped with chicken, fish, or some sort of meat right out of the pan or fresh off the grill. The sizzle in such foods is just what a quiet leaf of lettuce needs.

Try mixing greens salad with seafood such as large grilled scallops, smoked salmon, or prawns. Tart it up with exotic fruits such as mango slices and add nuts such as toasted sliced almonds. This is a great way to include shellfish in a cholesterol-controlling diet. By including them in a salad, you don't need a large serving of these cholesterol-containing foods to feel like you've had a satisfying dinner.

The advantage of using a salad as the base for animal protein is that a small 100–120-gram serving of beef, chicken, or shellfish can fill you up.

Recipes for main-course salads

The three recipes that follow are meals in themselves, providing servings of protein, plus vegetables and trimmings. Add some wholegrain bread toasted with olive oil and herbs, and finish with one of the fruit desserts in Chapter 21 for gourmet eating at home.

Wholesome Chicken Salad

This festive salad is a great meal to make for family and friends on a weekend afternoon, and a good reason to start up the barbecue grill. If you prefer to keep this dish vegetarian, skip the chicken and add more sweetcorn and beans. These two foods contain complementary amino acids, the building blocks of protein, which when combined provide high-quality protein.

Special tools required: *Blender*

Preparation time: *25 minutes, plus at least 3 hours for marinating the chicken*

Cooking time: *40 minutes*

Serves: *6*

Marinade:

2 fresh, red chilli peppers, deseeded

6 large cloves garlic

2 teaspoons ground cumin

Juice of one lemon

240 millilitres water or vegetable stock

Salad:

6 skinless, boneless chicken breasts

3 ears of corn on the cob, husks removed (or a large tin of cooked sweetcorn)

1 tin (425 grams) black beans, no added salt, drained

1 small head of iceberg lettuce, shredded

Dressing:

120 millilitres extra-virgin olive oil

3 tablespoons red wine vinegar

2 tablespoons balsamic vinegar

1 tablespoon fresh coriander, chopped

Juice of ½ lime

Black pepper

1 In a blender, purée the chilli with the garlic, cumin, lemon juice, and water or vegetable stock.

2 Arrange the chicken breasts in a shallow dish and spread both sides with the chilli marinade. Refrigerate, covered, for a minimum of 3 hours.

3 Meanwhile, if using fresh corn on the cob, bring a large pot of water to the boil and add the cobs of corn. Cook on a high heat for about 12 minutes until tender, and allow to cool. Working on a cutting board, slice off the corn with a knife. Collect the corn in a bowl and manually break up any strips into individual kernels. Add the black beans to the cooked fresh (or tinned) corn and mix.

4 In a small bowl, whisk together the olive oil, red wine vinegar, balsamic vinegar, coriander, and lime juice. Season the dressing to taste with black pepper. Pour over the corn and bean mixture and toss to combine.

5 Heat a grill or grill pan and cook the chicken breasts for about 10 minutes per side (depending on the thickness of the chicken), until no pink meat remains. Cut the chicken across the grain into slices. Season to taste with black pepper.

6 To compose the salad on individual plates, first arrange a handful of lettuce. Top with a sixth of the corn and bean mixture. On top of this, arrange a sliced chicken breast, and serve.

Per serving: *Calories 429; Fat 22g (Saturated 4g); Cholesterol 73mg; Sodium 80mg; Carbohydrate 25g; Dietary Fibre 7g; Protein 33g.*

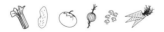

Savoury Steak Salad with Tomato Dressing

You can have steak for dinner on occasions, even though it's a red meat and contains higher amounts of saturated fat. Just limit the amount of saturated fat you have in other meals that day and limit the portion, which is easy to do when you combine steak with lots of vegetables in a salad such as this one. The dressing for this salad is based on a purée of grilled tomatoes, making it leaner than most oil dressings. Grilling the tomatoes is essential to produce this rustic, full-flavoured dressing, a tomato-red sauce flecked with bits of slightly charred and smoky tomato skin. This dressing is also good served warm over grilled chicken and fish.

Special tools required: *Collapsible metal steamer, food processor*

Preparation time: *60 minutes, plus 2 hours or more for marinating the steak*

Cooking time: *55 minutes*

Serves: *4 (dinner-size salads)*

3 tablespoons red wine	*120 millilitres extra-virgin olive oil*
3 cloves garlic, peeled and chopped	*8 button mushrooms, cleaned and sliced*
2 sprigs parsley or other herb, stems removed and chopped	*2 sweet red bell peppers, cored, seeded, and sliced*
450 grams lean steak	*225 grams green beans, trimmed*
Black pepper	*2 teaspoons red wine vinegar*
450 grams tomatoes, trimmed and cut in half horizontally	*12 leaves red leaf lettuce, washed and torn into pieces*
4 large shallots, trimmed and chopped	

1 In a shallow baking dish, combine the red wine, 1 clove of garlic, and the parsley. Stir to combine. Place the steak in the marinade and turn over to coat both sides. Season with pepper. Refrigerate, covered, for 2 hours. Remove the steak 20 minutes before cooking to bring to room temperature.

2 Turn on the grill. Arrange the tomato halves, cut side up, on a grill tray and grill 10 centimetres from the heat for 15 minutes. Turn the tomatoes over about half way through cooking and allow the skin to blister and slightly char.

3 In a frying pan, cook the shallots in 1 tablespoon of the olive oil on a medium heat for about 5 minutes until they just begin to go translucent. Add the mushrooms and continue to cook for an additional 3 minutes. Transfer to a bowl, cover to keep warm, and set aside.

4 Add the red peppers to the same pan along with 1 tablespoon of olive oil. Cook on a medium heat, stirring occasionally, for about 10 minutes, until they begin to soften and brown.

5 Meanwhile, place a collapsible metal steamer inside a medium-size pot with a tight-fitting lid. Add just enough water so that it comes to slightly below the bottom of the steamer. Place the green beans in the steamer and cover the pot. Cook on a medium heat for about 4 minutes, until the green beans turn bright green and are still a little crunchy. Turn off the heat and remove the lid.

6 In a food processor fitted with a metal blade, add the grilled tomatoes, red wine vinegar, and the remaining 2 cloves of chopped garlic. Begin puréeing, slowly adding the remaining olive oil by drizzling it through the processor tube. Season this salad dressing to taste with black pepper.

7 Barbecue or grill the steak for 4 minutes per side for medium rare. Transfer the steak to a plate, cover loosely with aluminium foil, and let it rest for 5 minutes for residual cooking and to distribute the juices evenly. Place the steak on a cutting board and slice across the grain.

8 Put the lettuce in a large bowl and drizzle with three quarters of the dressing, setting the remaining dressing aside. Toss the salad. To compose the salad, divide the dressed lettuce among 4 dinner plates. Spoon the shallot-mushroom mixture over each. Arrange the green beans on this and then the sweet peppers. Top with slices of steak. Drizzle a stripe of the remaining tomato dressing across each salad.

Per serving: Calories 474; Fat 33g (Saturated 6g); Cholesterol 63mg; Sodium 66mg; Carbohydrate 19g; Dietary Fibre 5g; Protein 26g.

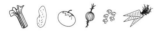

Salad companions

Salad needn't stand alone. If you enjoy your salad with a slice of baguette and butter, try spreading bread, preferably wholemeal, with mashed avocado instead. That way, you avoid the saturated fat in butter. And because having red wine is good for the heart, why not also enjoy a glass along with your salad?

Tuna Salad Niçoise

Salad Niçoise is one of the great classic salads, inspired by the produce of summer in Provence, France, and the fish that swim in the Mediterranean Sea. It embodies many of the ingredients that make the Mediterranean style of eating so good for the heart. Classic Salad Niçoise involves the preparation of many ingredients, including hard-boiled eggs, which we leave out here. This recipe is a shortened version of this dish, but is still a satisfying mix of flavours, and takes less time to prepare. Enjoy this mini-meal for lunch.

Special tools required: *Collapsible metal steamer*

Preparation time: *10 minutes*

Cooking time: *5 minutes*

Serves: *1 (generous lunch salad)*

120 grams French green beans, cut into 2-centimetre lengths

1 tin (175 grams) light tuna chunks, packed in water

1 tablespoon capers

2 tablespoons extra-virgin olive oil

2 teaspoons balsamic vinegar

2 teaspoons Dijon mustard

Black pepper

1 Using a medium-size saucepan with a tightly fitting lid, insert a collapsible metal steamer and enough water to partially fill the area beneath the steamer platform. Add the green beans, cover the pot, and steam for about 3 minutes, until the beans are slightly tender and bright green. Transfer the green beans to a sieve and rinse under cold water to stop the cooking and retain the colour.

2 Put the beans in a large bowl. Add the tuna and break into small chunks. Add the capers and combine all ingredients.

3 In a small bowl, whisk together the olive oil, vinegar, and mustard. Drizzle over the tuna mixture. Toss lightly with a wooden spoon. Season to taste with salt and pepper.

Vary It! *If you want to make enough of this salad to serve 4 people, here's what to do. Use 3 tins of tuna and simply double the amounts of all the other ingredients. Add some sliced steamed red-skin potatoes, 1 red bell pepper (trimmed, seeds removed, and sliced), and a handful of cherry tomatoes. Also beef up the dressing with a handful of basil leaves, chopped, and, if you're not watching your sodium, 6 minced anchovies. Garnish the salad with marinated olives, available in gourmet markets.*

Per serving: Calories 518; Fat 29g (Saturated 4g); Cholesterol 108mg; Sodium 1224mg; Carbohydrate 13g; Dietary Fibre 4g; Protein 50g.

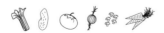

Chapter 11

Creating Mouth-Watering Starters for Special Occasions

*P*arty foods, by definition, are full of flavour and not short on fat. They crunch, they dazzle with their good looks, and they're fun to eat. But can such entertaining fare also be heart-healthy and helpful in lowering cholesterol? Yes indeed, because so many of the foods recommended for heart health are already standard party fare. Nuts to nibble, avocado in guacamole, smoked salmon with capers, and olives of all sorts are healthy foods. Making sure that they stay good for you is just a matter of how you prepare them.

In this chapter, you discover heart-healthy foods with crunch that aren't deep fried and satisfying nibbles high in the right sort of fats. We also offer up an assortment of quick and easy recipes for party food, including a vegetarian pâté and marinated olives. Presentation is part of the drill, because party food at its best is also eye-catching. Read on to find all sorts of suggestions for creating scrumptious party offerings that meet your dietary needs.

Hearty Bites to Make a Cardiologist Smile

The hors d'oeuvres and little nibbles that meet the nutritional requirements of a cholesterol-lowering, heart-healthy diet are so numerous they can fill a buffet table. These morsels feature raw vegetables, fresh herbs, healthy fats, chicken, and fish. In addition, these foods are eaten in very small amounts, but many are so tasty that you can make a meal out of them.

Popping in a party crunch

Healthy foods, perhaps because they're never deep-fried, often lack crunch, leaving you longing for the sound of crispy food and a satisfying chew. Party favourites such as potato crisps and tacos are full of crunch, whereas healthier foods, such as grains, nut butters, and vegetables, are quiet foods unless you eat them raw as crudités. The following sections give you ways to combine the best of both worlds: the cholesterol-conscious and the crispy.

Crostini

Toast is crunchy, so how about starting with that and making some crostini, which means 'little toasts' in Italian. Here's how to prepare crostini:

1. **Adjust the rack of a grill to be at least 10 centimetres from the heat source and preheat the grill.**

2. **Cut a slim baguette of French bread into thin slices and place on a large baking sheet.**

   Cut slices of bread on the diagonal for a stylish presentation.

3. **Brush the slices on one or both sides with a little olive oil and rub one or both sides with a halved and peeled clove of garlic.**

4. **Grill the bread so that one side is lightly toasted.**

5. **Turn the bread over and grill for a further minute or two, making sure that the bread doesn't toast all the way through.**

Use crostini as a platform for other foods. Here are some suggested toppings:

- A smear of tapenade – an olive paste seasoned with capers, anchovies, garlic, and lemon juice, that is sold in jars.
- Goat cheese mixed with fresh herbs, such as basil and parsley, and topped with a sliver of sun-dried tomato.
- A spoonful of garlicky, mashed cannellini or butter beans scented with oregano.

Crudité dips

Eating raw vegetables at parties became chic when they took on the name *crudité*, which is French for 'raw'. They are refreshing, crispy, and full of all the vitamins and minerals that nature gives them. But what do you do with all the bits of vegetable after you cut them? The following ideas tell you how to bring order to the chaos:

✔ Start with sticks of carrot, celery, and cucumber, and perhaps some blanched asparagus or blanched green beans, and give each vegetable a separate container, such as a glass tumbler, a colourful ceramic mug, or a small flower vase. Cluster the containers on the serving table, creating a vegetable forest.

✔ Arrange vegetables on a long, rectangular platter or a basket lined with curly lettuce or kale, and give each vegetable its own row.

✔ Tuck raw vegetables in between the leaves of a full head of lettuce, following the instructions in the later Crudité with Mango Salsa and Creamy Avocado Dip recipe.

Appetising appetisers

One of the great pleasures of party food is that it's full of hard-to-resist assertive flavours, in part because the food is also full of fat, which is a flavour carrier. Taking a holiday from diet restrictions, the most careful of eaters graciously accept the vol-au-vents and sausage rolls on offer. But there's no reason you can't enjoy the feel of fat, even if you're watching your cholesterol. You have options.

Nuts and olives

Nuts and olives are two classic cocktail nibbles that are perfectly acceptable heart-healthy foods. In numerous studies, both nuts and olives, the basis of the famed Mediterranean diet, are linked to a lower risk of heart disease. In addition, the monounsaturated and polyunsaturated fats in these foods help control cholesterol.

So which nuts have the most of these healthy fats and are low in the cholesterol-raising saturated kind? Here are a few that fit the bill:

✔ Almonds

✔ Hazels

✔ Macadamias

✔ Pecans

✔ Pistachios

✔ Walnuts

One way to include nuts in a party menu is to add walnuts to hummus, purée-ing them along with the other ingredients. The rich, mellow flavour of walnuts blends well with the other ingredients and walnuts add omega-3 fatty acids, making hummus even more nutritious. Here's how to make this dish: In a food processor, combine one tin (425 grams) chickpeas, 50 grams walnuts, 4 to 8 tablespoons tahini sesame paste (according to taste), 60 millilitres fresh lemon juice, and 1 clove of garlic, plus water or oil to reach the desired consistency. Season with cumin and black pepper.

Cheeses

You can save on fat if you eat lower-fat cheeses or soya cheese look-alikes, but you may not get great flavour or texture in all cases. You probably prefer a shaving of world-class Parmigiano-Reggiano as a garnish for slices of pear topped with a paper-thin slice of Prosciutto, than a large wedge of rubbery, low-fat mozzarella. But do sample some lower-fat cheeses and see what you think. For instance, low-fat ricotta or soft cheese spreads are usually very satisfying. If you want to cut back on fat intake and still eat cheese, modified products let you keep these creamy-tasting foods in your diet.

When shopping for cheese, check the label for content of total fat and saturated fat as well as cholesterol. The amounts present vary among producers. Cheeses such as Camembert and Brie are medium fat cheeses, whereas Roquefort, Cheddar, and processed cheese are high-fat cheeses, and contain significant amounts of saturated fat and cholesterol – even in a few bites, which isn't very much, especially for a devoted cheese eater. Best to stay away from these unless you can stop after one nibble. Feta and mozzarella, even the full-fat kind, are lower in fat and cholesterol and better options.

For the feel of fat on the tongue, use low-fat yogurt and low-fat soured cream, both very palatable, in your hors d'oeuvres.

Caviar

If any food says 'special occasion', it's caviar. Because caviar is salted fish eggs, just like chicken eggs, it's a wholefood and a balanced source of nutrition. In addition, although fat contributes 61 per cent of the calories, caviar, like fish, contains mostly the healthy monounsaturated and polyunsaturated kinds. Admittedly, caviar is high in sodium (containing 240 milligrams per tablespoon) and in cholesterol (containing 31.3 milligrams per teaspoon), but you're not likely to eat a bowlful of caviar anyway, because it's so expensive.

Here are two ways of serving caviar that give you a smidgeon of this glamorous stuff. On a budget, use black lumpfish caviar, golden whitefish caviar, or salmon red caviar, all sold in little jars in supermarkets. Otherwise, invest in some pricier imported sevruga, osetra, or beluga caviar.

1. **Boil round, red potatoes, the smallest you can find, until they're cooked through and tender.**

2. **Peel the potatoes, slice in half crosswise, and cut some potato off the base of each half, so that the potato is steady when placed on a plate.**

3. **Using the smallest end of a melon baller, cut into the flat surface of each potato half and scoop out a little bowl in the middle.**

4. **Fill the hollow of each potato with low-fat sour cream and sprinkle the sour cream with caviar.**

In this next elegant hors d'oeuvre, you display caviar on pale chartreuse coloured chicory leaves.

1. **Wash a head of chicory and cut it at the base to separate the leaves.**

2. **Using a teaspoon, place a small dollop of low-fat sour cream at the wider end of each leaf and then sprinkle caviar on the sour cream.**

3. **Garnish the caviar and sour cream with a tiny sprig of dill.**

4. **On a round serving platter, arrange the leaves like spokes, with the narrow end of the leaf pointing out.**

Impressing your guests

Not only are the following recipes attractive to the eye, but also you and your guests are likely to count them among your favourites for regular snacking. The Marinated Citrus-Scented Olives, in particular, have a reputation as highly addictive. Enjoy!

☃ *Crudités with Mango Salsa and Creamy Avocado Dip*

The combination of smooth and spicy textures and flavours in this recipe is just right. The Creamy Avocado Dip is full of healthy monounsaturated fats and high in folic acid, while the Mango Salsa is an effortless way to increase your fruit intake. For the crudités, try using only green and white vegetables, such as the suggestions here, for a designer look (see Figure 11-1).

Preparation time: *20 minutes*

Serves: *20*

1 head butter lettuce, with the outside leaves still intact (see the tip at the end of the recipe)

1 large turnip

2 dozen slim spears of asparagus, trimmed and blanched

1 head chicory, leaves separated and washed

1 cucumber, peeled, seeds removed, and sliced into spears

1 Taking the base of a head of butter lettuce in one hand, gently open the leaves of the lettuce with the other hand, wiggling your fingers down in between the leaves. (If the lettuce is sandy, submerge the opened head in a sink filled with water and briefly swish to loosen dirt. Drain upside down in an empty dish rack before proceeding. You may have to do this several times if a lot of sticky sandy dirt stays on the leaves.)

2 Meanwhile, peel the turnip and cut into thin rounds. Picture the turnip slice as the Earth and cut a small V-shaped wedge at the North Pole and South Pole. Also make two V-shaped wedges on opposite sides of the 'equator' line.

3 Bring about 2½ centimetres of water to boil in a saucepan and add the asparagus. Cook for about 2 minutes, until the asparagus is bright green and al dente. Remove with tongs, and submerge the asparagus in a bowl of cold water until they reach room temperature.

4 Tuck the turnip slices, asparagus, chicory leaves, and cucumber in between the butter lettuce leaves. Serve with the Mango Salsa and Creamy Avocado Dip (see next recipes).

Vary It! *If you decide that your crudité composition is begging for more colour, add carrot sticks.*

Per serving: *Calories 9; Fat 0g (Saturated 0g); Cholesterol 0mg; Sodium 8mg; Carbohydrate 2g; Dietary Fibre 1g; Protein 1g.*

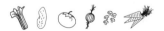

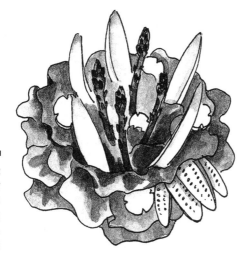

Figure 11-1:
Butter
lettuce
holding
crudités.

Mango Salsa

This recipe lives and dies on whether the mango is sweet with a smooth texture, and so chose your mango with care. When ripe, a mango yields to gentle pressure like a ripe avocado, and the stem end has a gentle aroma. Choose plump mangos, avoiding those with bruised or shrivelled skin. This fat-free mix of healing fruits and vegetables also goes well with chicken and fish.

Preparation time: 15 minutes

Serves: 12 (about 720 millilitres in total, 60 millilitres each)

1 ripe mango, peeled, pitted, and diced into small pieces

1 cup diced sweet red pepper

2 tablespoons chopped red onion

1 fresh jalapeño chilli, seeded and chopped

1 tablespoon chopped coriander

Juice of 1 lime

Black pepper

1 Put the mango, sweet red pepper, onion, chilli, coriander, and lime juice in a mixing bowl. Toss gently to combine the ingredients.

2 Season to taste with black pepper and serve immediately.

Per serving: Calories 3; Fat 0g (Saturated 0g); Cholesterol 0mg; Sodium 0mg; Carbohydrate 1g; Dietary Fibre 0g; Protein 0g.

Marinated Citrus-Scented Olives

Put one of these olives in your mouth, close your eyes, and you can taste summer in Provence! This recipe uses brine-cured olives, but if you want to cut back on salt, ordinary tinned olives work fine as well. Use pitted ones so that more of the marinade finds its way into the olives. You can also marinate these olives in olive oil, but this recipe uses water to cut back on calories and create a lighter taste.

Preparation time: *15 minutes, plus 3 days for the olives to marinate*

Marinade time: *3 days*

Servings: *24*

200 grams kalamata olives or other brine-cured olives

200 grams cracked brine-cured green olives

4 large cloves garlic, smashed

60 millilitres orange juice

60 millilitres fresh lemon juice

1 tablespoon grated orange zest

1 tablespoon grated lemon zest

2 bay leaves

2 anchovies, minced, or 2 tablespoons anchovy paste

½ teaspoon dried thyme

1 Combine the olives, garlic, orange juice, lemon juice, orange zest, lemon zest, bay leaves, anchovies, and thyme in a glass jar with a tight-fitting lid.

2 Add enough water to the citrus marinade to cover the olives.

3 Seal the jar with the lid and shake the jar several times to distribute and combine the ingredients.

4 Refrigerate the olives for 3 days, shaking the jar once each day to keep the marinade well mixed.

Go-With: *Serve the olives with goat's cheese and a baguette of French bread.*

Per serving: *Calories 40; Fat 4g (Saturated 0g); Cholesterol 0mg; Sodium 289mg; Carbohydrate 3g; Dietary Fibre 0g; Protein 0g.*

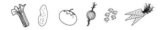

Creamy Avocado Dip

Sour cream dips have just the right tartness to complement the sweetness of fresh, raw vegetables. You can cut the saturated fat of the cream if you make the dip with low-fat soured cream, and, as in this recipe, substitute some of the soured cream with avocado to add healthier monounsaturated fats.

Special tools required: Food processor

Preparation time: 15 minutes

Servings: 30 (about 1½ cups)

1 cup non-fat sour cream

¼ teaspoon ground cumin

1 avocado, peeled, pitted, and cut into chunks

1 small clove garlic, minced

1 tablespoon chopped, fresh coriander leaves (3 sprigs), plus extra for garnish

Salt and pepper

1 Put the sour cream in a food processor fitted with a metal blade.

2 Add the cumin to the sour cream in the processor, and then add the avocado, garlic, and coriander leaves. Process until smooth, scraping down the side of the processor bowl if necessary to incorporate all the ingredients.

3 Season to taste with salt and pepper. Transfer the dip to a small serving bowl and garnish with chopped coriander leaves. Serve immediately. (You can also prepare the dip earlier on the same day you plan to serve it. Press plastic wrap onto the surface of the dip so that no air comes in contact with the avocado in the dip to keep it from turning brown. Refrigerate until ready to serve and add the coriander leaves garnish right before serving.)

Per serving: Calories 15 (From Fat 9); Fat 1 g (Saturated 0g); Cholesterol 0mg; Sodium 30mg; Carbohydrate 1g; Dietary Fibre 1g; Protein 0g.

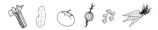

Turning Dinner into Hors d'Oeuvres

Amaze your friends with your elaborate hors d'oeuvres by cooking a main course and then serving it to them in little bites! Dinner dishes and accompaniments easily turn into fabulous party morsels, the kind that major caterers serve at gallery openings. Several of the recipes in this book are ideal for converting into hors d'oeuvres for serving to your guests on elegant platters. Experiment with the following:

- **Apple Salsa (see Chapter 16):** Enjoy as is, as a dip.

- **Sweet and Spicy Mexican Black Beans (see Chapter 19):** Warm this purée and serve it as a dip with home-baked tortilla chips.

- **Turkey Burger (see Chapter 13):** Cook 5-centimetre patties and serve on tiny biscuits.

✔ **Chicken Tandoori with Minted Yogurt Sauce (see Chapter 13):** Start with 2.5-centimetre pieces of chicken and proceed with the recipe. Thread one piece on a 15-centimetre long bamboo skewer and serve with Minted Yogurt Sauce as a dip.

✔ **Grilled Chicken with Creamy Peanut Sauce (see Chapter 13):** Start with 2½-centimetre pieces of chicken and proceed with the recipe. Thread one piece on a 15-centimetre long bamboo skewer and serve with Creamy Peanut Sauce as a dip.

Getting some help: Ready-made appetisers

Offer some of these heart-healthy, ready-made bites on their own or add them to a few of your own appetisers. You can find them in supermarkets or natural foods stores:

✔ Roasted sweet red peppers.

✔ Marinated artichoke hearts.

✔ Sun-blushed tomatoes (semi-dried).

✔ Marinated olives stuffed with almond slivers.

✔ Smoked salmon.

✔ Sliced veg from the salad bar, to serve as crudités with a dip.

✔ Stuffed tortellini (serve it on skewers).

✔ Freeze-dried vegetable crunchies, such as sweetcorn, peas, red bell peppers, carrots, and tomatoes, produced with no added fat and sold in natural food stores.

✔ Tinned stuffed vine leaves.

Doubling up: Party recipes that you can also serve as meals

All the following recipes are hearty and healthy enough to serve as main courses as well as party munchies. You can even turn the Mushroom Pâté into a pasta sauce, as the recipe introduction explains. Delicious!

Marinated Scallops with Avocado

Seviche is a popular dish from Latin America in which raw fish is marinated in citrus juice, usually lemon or lime. The acid in the fruit 'cooks' the fish. You can prepare any white-fleshed fish or scallops this way. Shellfish has a reputation as high in cholesterol, but a serving of 4 skewers of these scallops contains only 16 milligrams of cholesterol. If scallops are too expensive, try prawns or any white fish on special offer – but ensure that it's really, really fresh.

Special tools required: *36 bamboo skewers, 15 centimetres long*

Preparation time: *20 minutes, plus 4 hours marinating time*

Serves: *9 (about 4 skewers each)*

360 millilitres fresh lime juice, or enough to cover the scallops

4 sprigs coriander leaves, chopped

1 tablespoon chopped red onion

1 clove garlic, crushed and minced

36 ultra-fresh medium-sized scallops

2 avocados

225 grams cherry tomatoes, washed

Black pepper

1 In a shallow 20-centimetre square baking dish, combine the juice, coriander, onion, and garlic.

2 Rinse the scallops and remove and discard the orange roe (which has the highest cholesterol content) if present. Cut the scallops into halves to make bite-sized pieces and place in the lime juice to marinate. Cover and refrigerate for a minimum of 4 hours, or overnight. The scallops are 'cooked' when they're opaque.

3 Cut each tomato in half crosswise. Peel and remove the stone of the avocados and cut them into 2-centimetre cubes – substantial enough so that they don't fall off the skewer. Drain the seviche and season to taste with black pepper.

4 Assemble the skewers by threading the components in this order: 1 piece of scallop, 1 cube of avocado, 1 scallop, and 1 cherry tomato half. Run the skewer through the centre of the face of the tomato where it was cut and then out the top through the skin, so the tomato becomes a cap on the other foods.

5 On a round platter, arrange the skewers of seviche like spokes of a wheel, with the tomato caps at the centre. Or use a horizontal tray and place the skewers in a row with the food colours forming stripes.

Per serving: Calories 124; Fat 7g (Saturated 1g); Cholesterol 16mg; Sodium 82mg; Carbohydrate 9g; Dietary Fibre 3g; Protein 8g.

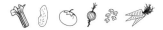

☞ Mushroom Pâté

With its hearty texture, rich brown hues, and a dash of sherry, this vegetarian mushroom pâté is much more than a passable substitute for the regular pork and liver versions. Cashews are added as a source of healthy oil. You can also thin it with a little white wine and make it into a mushroom sauce for pasta such as penne.

Special tools required: *Food processor*

Preparation time: *30 minutes, plus 4 hours chilling time*

Cooking time: *20 minutes*

Serves: *12 to 15, 2 tablespoons each*

5 tablespoons safflower oil

2 large shallots, chopped

2 cloves garlic, crushed and chopped

550 grams fresh shiitake mushrooms, stemmed and coarsely chopped (or use brown chestnut mushrooms)

140 grams roasted cashews (preferably unsalted)

1 tablespoon finely chopped fresh basil

1 tablespoon finely chopped fresh parsley, plus sprigs for garnish

2 tablespoons sherry

Black pepper

1 In a large, heavy frying pan over a medium heat, heat 4 tablespoons of the oil and add the shallots, garlic, and mushrooms. Cook for 15 to 20 minutes, stirring frequently, until the mixture begins to brown and all the liquid evaporates (timing depends on the moisture content of the mushrooms). Remove the pan from the heat.

2 In a food processor fitted with a metal blade, chop the cashews until they have a fine texture. Add the remaining 1 tablespoon of oil and continue to process to make a coarse paste.

3 Add the mushroom mixture, basil, parsley, and sherry. Pulse the processor on and off until the pâté has a coarse texture. Season to taste with black pepper.

4 Transfer the mushroom pâté to a small ceramic loaf pan, or a bowl lined with plastic wrap so you can easily pop out the pâté. Cover and chill for 4 hours. Serve in the loaf pan, or turn the pâté out of the bowl and garnish with sprigs of parsley. Enjoy on crostini.

Per serving: Calories 148; Fat 12g (Saturated 1g); Cholesterol 0mg; Sodium 4mg; Carbohydrate 11g; Dietary Fibre 1g; Protein 3g.

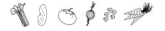

Chapter 12

Hoarding Healthy Nibbles

*P*eople used to frown upon snacking. Nowadays, however, eating between meals is perfectly acceptable, as long as you select healthy options. Succumbing to the siren call of a bag of salty crisps or a packet of salted nuts is all too easy when you're feeling a bit peckish, and so ban these items from your kitchen and make your own, more healthy snacks instead. That's where this chapter comes in.

Eating Little and Often

Grazing rather than gorging is an increasingly popular way to eat, and involves having several small meals and snacks throughout the day in place of the traditional three hearty meals. But remember that the calories you gain from snacks pile on the pounds unless you compensate and eat less at normal meal-times.

Interesting research involving macadamia nuts shows that, despite their high fat content, eating a diet that includes between 20 and 90 grams macadamias per day can significantly lower both total and LDL cholesterol without putting on weight. In fact, the study reported slight reductions in weight, despite an increase in total fat consumed. This is due to the way in which the body metabolises the monounsaturated fats, and the plentiful amount of fibre and protein macadamia nuts contain, which has a satiating effect on appetite, making you feel full.

Keeping your cupboards stocked with healthy snacks

To keep temptation at bay, avoid ready-made crisps and other types of commercial snack. Chances are they contain far too much salt and omega-6 fats and not enough vitamins, minerals, fibre, healthy omega-3, and monounsaturated fats.

To stock up on health snacks, browse through the shelves of your local health food shop and pick up packs of almonds, macadamias, walnuts, raisins, dried cranberries, prunes, apricots, acai berries, and whatever other fruits are in vogue as nutrient-rich superfoods.

Useful snacks for office life

The fact that apples, oranges, pears, and bananas are among the most popular of fruits is no coincidence. Tasty and available in snack-sized units, you can take a bag of apples to work with you and eat at least one every day. Research shows that an apple a day reduces your risk of death, from any chronic disease at any age, by one third (but especially from coronary heart disease or stroke), compared with those eating fewer apples.

Nuts are another healthy option. You're probably familiar with peanut butter but did you know that health food stores also sell nut butters made from almonds, Brazil nuts, macadamias, hazelnuts, pistachios and even pumpkin seeds? These nut and seed butters are a rich source of monounsaturated fats and antioxidants – especially vitamin E. For a really simple yet healthy snack, try thinly spreading some nut butter onto a few oatcakes. Delicious!

Store nut butters in the fridge, even when unopened, to preserve their nutritional qualities.

Avocadoes make another great snacking choice. Strictly speaking avocadoes are fruits, but their delicate colour and flavour mean that they make a great savoury snack more reminiscent of a vegetable. Avocadoes contain monounsaturated fats, beta-sitosterol, and vitamin E, which all lower LDL cholesterol. Research published in the *Archives of Medical Research* in 1996 shows that eating avocadoes on a daily basis can lower your total cholesterol by 17 per cent and increase your levels of beneficial HDL cholesterol by 11 per cent within one week.

The famous Mexican avocado spread guacamole is a great dish to take to work for snacking or for your lunch.

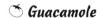 **Guacamole**

This guacamole is delicious spread over wholemeal toast, oatcakes, rice cakes, or crispbread.

Special tools required: *Avocado slicer, blender*

Preparation time: *5 minutes*

Serves: *4*

Flesh from 1 large, ripe avocado

Juice and zest from half a lemon or lime

1 tablespoon extra-virgin olive oil

1 small green chilli, deseeded and chopped

Freshly ground black pepper

Coriander, chopped

1 Place the avocado flesh, lemon or lime juice and zest, olive oil, and chilli in a blender or food processor fitted with a metal blade.

2 Season well with black pepper and blend until smooth.

3 Serve garnished with chopped coriander.

Per serving: Calories 117; Fat 11g (Saturated 2g); Cholesterol 0mg; Sodium 6mg; Carbohydrate 5g; Dietary Fibre 3g; Protein 1g.

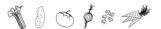

Snacking on nuts and seeds

Almonds and macadamia nuts contain monounsaturated fats and antioxidants that prevent oxidation of LDL cholesterol, which means that it clears more readily from your circulation. Eating a handful of these nuts per day (around 20 nuts) can lower LDL cholesterol by 5 per cent and increase HDL cholesterol by 6 per cent. Eating walnuts also has a beneficial effect on LDL and HDL cholesterol. So you can see why people who eat nuts frequently are between one third and a half less likely to develop coronary heart disease than those eating nuts infrequently. But be sure to buy those without added salt!

⏱ *Cinnamon and Spice Almonds*

Scent some almonds with spices, add some raisins, and you have a healthy treat. The small amount of butter in this recipe imparts its inimitable flavour without adding much saturated fat. When you toast nuts in this way, they don't absorb much of the cooking oils because they already contain a large amount of fats of the beneficial type. Serve this snack with cocktails or after-dinner coffee.

Preparation time: *5 minutes*

Cooking time: *10 minutes*

Serves: *24*

1 tablespoon butter	*1 tablespoon ground ginger*
1 tablespoon extra-virgin olive oil	*1½ teaspoons nutmeg*
400 grams whole raw almonds	*200 grams seedless raisins*
1 tablespoon cinnamon	*Salt*

1 In a frying pan over a medium heat, melt the butter and combine with the oil.

2 Add the almonds and toss to coat with the oil. Sprinkle the almonds with the cinnamon, ground ginger, and nutmeg, and toss to combine the ingredients. Cook, stirring frequently, for 5 minutes.

3 Add the raisins and continue to cook the almond mixture for an additional 2 to 3 minutes, until the nuts begin to brown. Season to taste with salt and allow the nuts to cool completely before storing.

Per serving: *Calories 133; Fat 10g (Saturated 1g); Cholesterol 1mg; Sodium 1mg; Carbohydrate 10g; Dietary Fibre 3g; Protein 4g.*

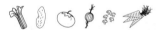

⏱ *Toasted Mixed Nuts*

This recipe for toasted mixed nuts makes an ideal between-meal or evening snack. Although 25 grams is an average serving, you can easily find yourself consuming more so keep an eye on how much you're eating!

Preparation time: *5 minutes*

Serves: *12*

50 grams shelled almonds

50 grams shelled hazelnuts

50 grams shelled cashews

50 grams shelled walnuts

50 grams shelled Brazil nuts

50 grams shelled macadamias

1 Warm a pan over a medium heat, and then pour in all the nuts.

2 Cook the nuts gently for a few minutes, moving the pan and shaking or stirring them frequently as they turn golden. Take care not to burn them.

3 Turn them out into a shallow dish and leave to cool.

Vary It: *Adding a handful of seedless raisins or dried cranberries gives this snack an additional healthy flavour.*

Per serving: Calories 161; Fat 15g (Saturated 2g); Cholesterol 0mg; Sodium 10mg; Carbohydrate 4g; Dietary Fibre 2g; Protein 4g.

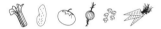

☞ Toasted Nuts and Seeds

This simple-to-make snack makes getting an extra helping of monounsaturated fat from the almonds and macadamias a cinch, while the seeds provide extra fibre to help lower your cholesterol even further.

Preparation time: *5 minutes*

Serves: *12*

100 grams almonds, shelled

100 grams macadamias, shelled

100 grams mixed seeds (for example, pumpkin, sunflower, linseed, sesame), hulled

1 Warm a pan over a medium heat, and pour in the nuts and seeds.

2 Cook the nuts and seeds gently for a few minutes, moving the pan and shaking or stirring them as they turn golden. Take care not to burn them.

3 Turn them out into a shallow dish and leave to cool before eating.

Per serving: Calories 157; Fat 14g (Saturated 1g); Cholesterol 0mg; Sodium 2mg; Carbohydrate 5g; Dietary Fibre 3g; Protein 4g.

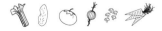

Combining Your Favourite 'Good' Foods

So now you're nutty about nuts, what else can you combine them with apart from raisins and cranberries? Chocolate, of course!

Dark chocolate containing at least 70 per cent cocoa solids contains large quantities of antioxidants and is especially rich in the super-protective variety known as procyanidin flavonoids. These help to prevent harmful LDL cholesterol from oxidising and furring up your artery walls. Although increasingly recognised as good for the heart, dark chocolate is still high in calories. White chocolate and milk chocolate don't provide the same benefits and are also high in fat and sugar; so avoid these and train your palate to prefer the dark, more bitter versions.

Chocolate goes especially well with nuts and fruit, and here are some recipes to prove it.

☞ *Chocolate Nuts and Grapes*

These chocolate-coated nuts and grapes make a deliciously healthy finish to a meal. As well as making healthy snacks, you can serve them with coffee as petit-fours.

Special tools required: *Bain marie or a simple glass bowl over a pan of simmering water*

Preparation time: *15 minutes plus one hour chill time*

Serves: *12*

100 grams dark chocolate (at least 70 per cent cocoa solids)

100 grams seedless black grapes

50 grams macadamia nuts

50 grams Brazil nuts

1 Break the chocolate into small pieces and place in a metal bain marie or glass bowl over boiling water. Stir gently until the chocolate has melted.

2 Using 2 teaspoons, dip the grapes and nuts into the chocolate to coat them – all over or just on one side, depending on your preference.

3 Lay the coated grapes and nuts on a nonstick baking sheet lined with waxed paper, and chill in the fridge for at least one hour, or until needed.

Per serving: *Calories 106; Fat 10g (Saturated 3g); Cholesterol 0mg; Sodium 1mg; Carbohydrate 7g; Dietary Fibre 1g; Protein 2g.*

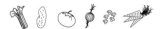

⏱ *Chocolate Florentines*

These nutty chocolate discs are so delicious you may find it hard to believe that they're good for you. You can serve them with coffee or after meals, or bag them up as gifts for friends at dinner parties.

Special tools required: *Bain marie or a simple glass bowl over a pan of simmering water*

Preparation time: *15 minutes plus 1 hour chill time*

Serves: *12*

200 grams dark chocolate (at least 70 per cent cocoa solids)

50 grams flaked almonds

50 grams sliced macadamia nuts

Zest of one lemon

1 Break the chocolate into small pieces and place in a metal bain marie or glass bowl over boiling water. Stir gently until the chocolate has melted.

2 Using a dessert spoon, drip small drops of chocolate (about the size and thickness of a pound coin) onto a sheet of grease-proof paper, to form small rounds.

3 Top the rounds with the flaked almonds, macadamias, and lemon zest and chill in the fridge for at least one hour, or until needed.

Per serving: *Calories 137; Fat 12g (Saturated 4g); Cholesterol 0mg; Sodium 0mg; Carbohydrate 10g; Dietary Fibre 2g; Protein 2g.*

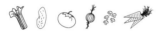

Quick recipes for warm snacks

Sometimes, only a warm snack hits the spot, especially during cold weather. Here are some ideas to keep you going:

✔ Spread some tomato purée on a wholemeal pitta bread, and top it with low-fat mozzarella cheese and other favourite toppings such as sliced mushrooms, peppers, onion rings, fresh herbs, capers, and anchovies. Place under the grill and you have a healthy snack in minutes.

✔ Wrap a small, washed, unpeeled potato in a piece of kitchen roll, and microwave for a couple of minutes. Hey presto, you have an instant jacket potato! Add some low-fat crème fraîche and chives, or some flaked tuna (canned in spring water rather than brine or sunflower oil), or even some baked beans for a quick and healthy meal.

✔ Make up a bowl of warm porridge according to the instructions on a packet of instant

(continued)

(continued)

porridge oats. Add grated apple, sliced banana, a sprinkling of cinnamon, or some fresh berries for additional health benefits.

✔ Open a tin of sardines in tomato sauce, place in a non-metal dish, warm them through in the microwave or under the grill, and serve on wholegrain toast topped with slices of fresh tomato.

✔ Cut some sweet potatoes into wedges, brush them with extra-virgin olive oil (or garlic-infused oil), and season well with freshly ground black pepper. Transfer the potatoes to a large roasting tray and bake them at 200 degrees for 30 minutes or until cooked through. Serve with low-fat fromage frais or tomato dip.

✔ Cut some unpeeled russet potatoes into chunky chips. Brush them with extra-virgin olive oil and dust with chilli powder. Bake at 200 degrees for 25 minutes or until cooked through and golden.

Perhaps the healthiest warm snack of all is a baked banana. This works well with the blackened, over-ripe bananas that so many people throw away. Simply wrap the unpeeled banana in aluminium foil and cook it for 3 minutes on barbeque coals, or for 3 minutes per side under the grill. Top with some lemon juice, a little ground cinnamon, and low-fat crème fraîche. Yum!

Part IV
Cooking with Poultry, Fish, and Meat

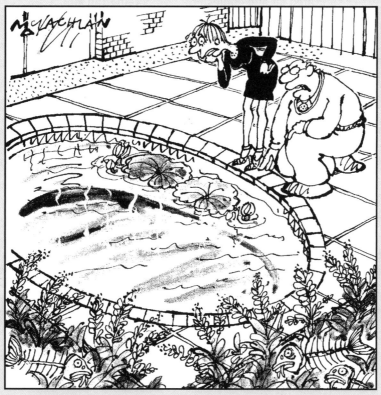

'The koi carp have gone again – that's the
<u>very</u> last time you bring your Dieting &
Nutrition Club round for afternoon tea!'

In this part . . .

Here's where you discover how to include poultry, fish, and meat on a cholesterol-balancing menu. This part gives you tips on selecting the right cuts and deciding on portion sizes so that you can limit the amount of saturated fat and cholesterol you obtain from animal foods. We also introduce you to some ways of preparing chicken that are tasty and a little different, and show you why freeing turkey from its confines as a seasonal Christmas dinner is sensible when watching your cholesterol.

Then you can dive into the subject of cooking fish, including how to select, store, and cook it in ways that enhance its succulence and flavour. The seafood chapter also includes a checklist of the healthiest fish for controlling cholesterol. The chapter on meats covers beef, pork, lamb, and a few exotic meats, while the final chapter looks at enlivening flavours with some carefully selected seasonings and sauces. To prepare sauces and salsas, you find out how to start with nutritious ingredients such as apples, onions, and chilli peppers to turn out your own special concoctions. You also discover all the good things garlic does for your heart!

Chapter 13

Flocking to Chicken and Turkey: New Ways with Old Favourites

*E*ven if you eat a million chickens during your lifetime, we can still think of good reasons to eat more. And although most people only eat turkey at Christmas, this seasonal bird is starting to show up in all sorts of dishes, and in many new forms. Experts now recognise turkey to be an undisputed health food, too. In this chapter, you find the specifics on why chicken and turkey belong in a cholesterol-lowering diet. You also find useful information and tips on selecting, storing, and cooking poultry, along with eight scrumptious recipes to experiment with.

But don't limit your avian intake to these two birds. Duck is fine to eat from time to time although its meat is swathed in all that fat under the skin. The total fat and saturated fat levels in duck meat, eaten without the fat and skin, falls somewhere between the fat in dark meat chicken and rump steak, and the cholesterol content is comparable. So, you can still enjoy lean slices of duck breast, glazed with an orange sauce, for a special occasion without feeling too guilty.

Discovering the Cholesterol-Lowering Benefits of Poultry

The popularity of chicken and turkey is due to their lower fat content; these types of poultry have less total fat and saturated fat than red meat and, as a bonus, poultry also supplies vitamins and minerals that are good for the heart.

Crowing over cutting fat

Compared with red meats, poultry has less fat overall, and contains significantly more monounsaturated and polyunsaturated fats that are better for heart health. As most of the fat is in the skin, you can easily remove it before or after cooking.

Table 13-1 gives a quick comparison of the fat and cholesterol in a single serving (100 grams) of chicken, turkey, and beef. This is equivalent to half a chicken breast or one chicken leg. We display the total fat in grams, and the type of fat as a percentage of total fat. The column for omega-3s (a type of polyunsaturated fat that lowers cholesterol) tells you the percentage of your daily requirement that a serving of these foods delivers.

Table 13-1		Comparison of Fat in Chicken, Turkey, and Beef				
Animal Protein	Total Fat	Saturated	Monounsaturated	Polyunsaturated	Omega-3s	Cholesterol
Chicken, roast light meat, skinless	3.6 grams	33%	41%	25%	10%	105 milligrams
Chicken, roast drumstick	9.1 grams	27%	47%	20%	27%	135 milligrams
Turkey, roast light meat	2.0 grams	35%	35%	25%	13%	82 milligrams

Animal Protein	Total Fat	Sat-urated	Mono-unsatu-rated	Poly-unsatu-rated	Omega-3s	Chol-esterol
Turkey, roast dark meat	6.6 grams	30%	36%	26%	24%	120 milli-grams
Beef, lean mince; stewed	8.7 grams	46%	51%	3%	2%	75 mil-ligrams

Derived from: McCance and Widdowson's The Composition of Foods, 6th Summary edition. Food Standards Agency.

For cholesterol balance, choose the light meat of chicken and turkey rather than dark meat, which is higher in fat.

The advantage of home-cooked chicken is that you control the amount of fat that you eat. Here are several ways to remove fat and calories at the same time:

- Remove the skin from chicken or turkey, before or after cooking.

- When preparing a whole bird, remove all the fat from inside the body cavity before cooking.

- Cook a whole chicken or turkey on a roasting rack set in a baking tray, so that fat drips into the bottom of the pan.

- Refrigerate chicken broth overnight, so that the fat hardens in a layer on the surface of the liquid, which you can lift off with a spatula and discard.

- Bake vegetables to serve with the chicken or turkey in a separate dish. If placed in the bottom of the baking pan, they absorb the fat that collects.

- Use a gravy separator or a baster to remove the fat.

- To remove fat floating on the top of room-temperature stock, float an absorbent kitchen towel, laid out flat, on the surface. When soaked in fat, lift the towel with a spatula and discard. Repeat if necessary.

Think twice before eating chicken liver – because cholesterol is made in the liver, cooked chicken liver contains 350 milligrams of cholesterol per 100 grams.

Pecking orders with vitamins and minerals

Chicken and turkey both contain high amounts of vitamin B6, a nutrient that helps to lower levels of homocysteine. Homcysteine is an amino acid in the blood that, when elevated, increases the risk of heart disease. (Chapter 1 has more on homocysteine.) Poultry also contains riboflavin (B2) and vitamin B12, which play a role in keeping homocysteine levels in check, plus niacin (B3), which doctors sometimes prescribe in addition to a statin drug to help lower 'bad' LDL and triglycerides.

Heat doesn't destroy B vitamins, but as poultry cooks, the meat loses juices that contain these water-soluble vitamins. To recover these nutrients, use pan drippings in your final dish. Skim the fat and add a little white wine to produce a light sauce. Serve your chicken au jus to get your B vitamins, too!

Poultry is also a source of selenium, a trace mineral your body needs for normal heart function.

Taking Out the Batteries and Going Free-Range

When shopping for chickens, knowing how to judge freshness is important, as is handling raw meat safely to prevent any bacteria it may harbour from reaching other foods in your kitchen.

Shopping for the freshest chickens

Chicken that's labelled 'fresh' hasn't just flown in from the barn. Although producers pack some chickens with ice cubes to reach nearby markets the next day, they chill and ship most mass-produced chickens in temperatures near freezing. Technically, the meat itself isn't frozen, but water in the birds does freeze, and carcasses are many days old before they are for sale in the shops.

The next time you go shopping, take a good look at the poultry, with the following in mind:

- When buying a whole chicken, look for one whose breast is full in relation to its legs.
- Chicken skin should look fresh and not broken, mottled, or transparent.
- Chicken meat should look clear and unblemished.

- The breast bone should easily bend. Flexibility shows that the bird is younger, and therefore the meat is more tender and lower in fat.

- Fresh chicken smells fresh. Before buying a package, give it a sniff.

- A package of chicken that contains water suggests it was frozen and then defrosted. If purchased and refrozen at home, it may contain bacteria that developed during the time the chicken was first thawed.

Don't judge a chicken by the colour of its skin, which has nothing to do with quality. The colour of chicken ranges from creamy white to yellow, and depends on the breed and whether the feed contains yellow pigments.

Chilling-out: Buying frozen chicken

Frozen chickens can taste good, but ensure that you buy a chicken that's handled properly after arriving in the shop. Both for flavour and safety, you need to stay fussy about its condition. Keep the following in mind when buying a frozen bird:

- The chicken should feel rock hard.

- Frozen liquid inside the package is a sign that the bird has thawed and refrozen, which can increase the likelihood of contamination with bacteria. Avoid these birds.

- Avoid those with heavy frost – a sign that they were frozen long ago.

- Avoid chickens whose skin appears powdery or has discoloured patches.

Have a chat with your butcher if you're not clear whether the chickens for sale were once frozen, or how long ago the frozen birds arrived at the store.

Handling poultry safely

The first consideration in preparing chicken is making sure that it's safe to eat. Shops sell poultry with the skin on, and more bacteria are present on an animal's skin than in the meat. Room-temperature chicken is the Promised Land to toxic bacteria such as salmonella, which thrive in the warm, moist environment found on chicken skin and on the surface of chicken cavities. Food poisoning from eating contaminated chicken is extremely common. These bacteria multiply exponentially every 20 minutes. Millions of bacteria can breed within just four hours. Your chicken has no hope of recovery.

The iron-clad rule for chicken left unrefrigerated longer than four hours is to throw it out.

Storing chicken

When shopping for chicken, bring it home immediately and place in the refrigerator. Don't rinse raw chicken – cooking it thoroughly kills any germs on it, and washing the meat can splash bacteria onto the sink and nearby worktops and dishes. Chicken and turkey have a short shelf life in your fridge. Whole birds and pieces, if raw, last two days at most. Raw chicken pieces, cut into chunks, have an even shorter time limit of 24 hours. You can refrigerate cooked chicken for 3 to 4 days, but if it has a sauce, the safe storage time is just 2 days. If you want to store a chicken dish with sauce for a longer period of time, freeze it.

Preparing chicken

To ensure that chicken is safe to eat, take these precautions during preparation:

- ✔ Wash all utensils, such as cutting boards and knives that come in contact with the chicken. Clean them thoroughly with soap and hot water to prevent cross-contamination that can occur when you use these same utensils to prepare other foods.

- ✔ Wash the kitchen table and your hands after handling chicken.

- ✔ If a recipe calls for marinating a chicken after the chicken is cooked, make sure that you don't add any uncooked marinade to the final dish. If you do want to use the marinade in a sauce, first heat it in a small pot and bring it to the boil.

Know the tell-tale signs of foul fowl – a slimy film on the surface of the bird and an unpleasant odour.

Touring the world for chicken recipes

Chicken travels well, at least in culinary terms. It's at home in all major world cuisines, featuring in traditional dishes and modern variations from the sun-drenched lands of the Mediterranean to the Indian continent and Asia.

In the following recipes, you journey to the northern shore of the Mediterranean to sample the flavours of Spain, France, and Italy – oranges, olives, rosemary, thyme, garlic, Prosciutto, and basil. Then you move on to Morocco and cook a chicken inspired by the offerings of the spice bazaar. Next you visit India for that country's special tandoori chicken, and finally you go to Thailand for chicken treated to a spicy peanut sauce.

Roast Chicken Provençal

This recipe results in a bird that's succulent and infused with the flavours of lemon and herbs. Rosemary and thyme are tucked under the skin, which holds the juices in the meat. If you happen to have a source of fresh lavender, you can also add this to the mix of herbs – a very Provençal touch! You don't need to eat the skin after the chicken is cooked, but the skin does seal in flavours while the chicken is roasting.

Preparation time: *15 minutes*

Cooking time: *About 1 hour*

Serves: *4*

1 teaspoon dried thyme, or 1 tablespoon finely chopped fresh thyme

1 teaspoon dried rosemary, or 1 tablespoon finely chopped fresh rosemary

1 teaspoon finely chopped fresh lavender (optional)

3 tablespoons extra-virgin olive oil

1 tablespoon lemon juice, plus half a lemon

1 clove garlic, minced

Black pepper

1 whole chicken, 1.1 kilograms, cut into pieces

1 Preheat the oven to 180 degrees. Combine the thyme, rosemary, lavender (if desired), 2 tablespoons of the olive oil, the 1 tablespoon lemon juice, garlic, and black pepper to taste in a small bowl.

2 Using your fingers, carefully spread the herb mixture under the skin of the chicken breasts and, if possible, the legs, keeping the skin intact.

3 Place the chicken in a medium roasting pan. Rub the skin with the remaining 1 tablespoon of olive oil and, using the lemon half, squeeze some of the juice over the chicken pieces. Season to taste with black pepper.

4 Place the chicken in the oven and roast for 60 minutes, basting once or twice. Check for doneness by making a small cut in any section, right to the bone. You should see no red whatsoever but a slight tinge of pink is acceptable, because the meat finishes cooking by the time you bring the chicken to the table.

Tip: *To reduce the fat content of this dish, remove the skin before serving the chicken pieces.*

Tip: *To save some pennies, when a recipe calls for chicken pieces as this one does, buy a whole chicken and cut it up yourself.*

Per serving: *Calories 412; Fat 29g (Saturated 7g); Cholesterol 108mg; Sodium 105mg; Carbohydrate 1g; Dietary Fibre 0g; Protein 34g.*

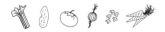

Roast Chicken with Marinated Olives, Rosemary, and Oranges

This versatile recipe uses the Marinated Citrus-Scented Olives from Chapter 11. You can also use shop-bought kalamata olives, but to ensure that the brine used for curing them doesn't overpower the flavour of the dish, soak the olives in water overnight.

Preparation time: *20 minutes*

Cooking time: *1 hour*

Serves: *4*

650 grams red potatoes with skins, washed, cut into 1-centimetre thick slices

1 medium onion, cut lengthwise in quarters

5 tablespoons extra-virgin olive oil

Black pepper

2 cloves garlic, crushed

3 tablespoons fresh orange juice

2 large navel oranges, peeled and thinly sliced (about 8 to 10 slices per orange)

4 skinless chicken breast halves (about 800 grams)

4 plum tomatoes, halved lengthwise

10 marinated, pitted black and/or green olives (see the Marinated Citrus-Scented Olives recipe in Chapter 11), sliced thin lengthwise

1 tablespoon fresh rosemary leaves

1 Preheat the oven to 190 degrees.

2 Put the sliced potatoes and onions in a large bowl. Add 2 tablespoons of the olive oil and black pepper to taste. Toss to coat. Arrange the vegetables in a 22-x-30-centimetre baking dish and place in the heated oven. Set the timer for 15 minutes.

3 In a small bowl, combine the garlic, orange juice, 2 tablespoons of the olive oil, and black pepper to taste. Put the chicken breasts in the bowl used for the vegetables. Add the marinade and turn the chicken to coat.

4 Arrange the orange slices in a second baking dish of similar size, making individual beds of overlapping slices for each of the chicken breasts. Place 1 chicken breast on each bed.

5 Arrange the tomatoes around the chicken and drizzle the tomatoes with the remaining 1 tablespoon of olive oil. Sprinkle the olives and rosemary over the chicken. Cover the baking dish with aluminium foil. When the potatoes have roasted for 15 minutes, put the chicken in the oven.

6 When the chicken has cooked for 20 minutes, remove the foil and cook the chicken uncovered for another 15 minutes. Baste the chicken with the remaining marinade and cook for an additional 10 to 15 minutes. To check the chicken breasts are done, cut into one with a thin-bladed knife – ensure that the centre of the breast is white or slightly pink.

7 Transfer the chicken and roast vegetables to an oval platter, with a bouquet of fresh rosemary set at one end of the plate, and serve immediately.

Tip: For a less sweet, spicier taste, omit the orange slices from the recipe. The dish still has a Mediterranean flavour, but of a different type.

Per serving: Calories 553; Fat 24g (Saturated 4g); Cholesterol 89mg; Sodium 251mg; Carbohydrate 47g; Dietary Fibre 6g; Protein 38g.

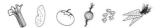

Chicken Stew with Prosciutto and White Beans

This stew is full of flavour but not fat. It has two low-fat sources of protein: chicken and beans. The small amount of saturated fat in the Prosciutto, added for its rich, smoky taste, balances with the two classic Italian seasonings, onions and garlic, which thin the blood.

Preparation time: *30 minutes*

Cooking time: *60 minutes*

Serves: *6*

60 grams (2 heaped tablespoons) plain flour

60 grams (2 heaped tablespoons) wholewheat flour

Black pepper

6 small chicken breasts (skinless and boneless), or 3 large breasts cut in half

2 tablespoons extra-virgin olive oil

1 large onion, diced

5 cloves garlic, crushed

85 grams sliced Prosciutto, chopped into small pieces

2 tins (400 grams each) diced tomatoes

2 tins (400 grams each) low-salt chicken broth

180 millilitres dry white wine

1 tin (400 grams) cannellini or white kidney beans, drained and rinsed

1 handful (20 grams) fresh basil leaves, cut into narrow strips

1 Put the plain flour and wholewheat flour in a shallow bowl. Season with black pepper. Place a chicken breast in the flour and turn to coat all sides. Set on a separate plate. Do the same with the rest of the chicken meat.

2 Put the olive oil in a heavy, large pan over a medium-high heat. Sauté the chicken in the oil for about 3 minutes per side. Using tongs, transfer the chicken to a large bowl.

3 Add the onion and garlic to the pan and sauté until the onion becomes translucent, after about 10 minutes. Add the Prosciutto, tomatoes, chicken broth, and white wine. Bring to the boil, scraping off any browned bits on the bottom of the pan.

4 Return the chicken and any accumulated juices to the pan. Cover and simmer the stew for about 30 minutes until the chicken is thoroughly cooked. Add the cannellini and basil. Simmer for an additional 10 minutes to develop flavours. Season to taste with black pepper and serve.

Per serving: Calories 343; Fat 11g (Saturated 3g); Cholesterol 88mg; Sodium 667mg; Carbohydrate 24g; Dietary Fibre 5g; Protein 37g.

Moroccan Chicken with Couscous

Seat yourself on cushions around your coffee table and pretend you're dining in the Kasbah as you savour this roast chicken filled with couscous and infused with spices. The recipe calls for a spice mix called ras el hanout, which you can make by following the recipe in Chapter 16. The extra time is worthwhile when you taste the delicious results.

Special tools required: *Food processor*

Preparation time: *30 minutes, plus 10 minutes while the couscous soaks*

Cooking time: *1½ hours*

Serves: *4*

85 grams couscous, preferably wholewheat	1 stick cinnamon
150 millilitres water, boiled	Thumb sized piece of root ginger, peeled and sliced
50 grams golden raisins	
1 tablespoon homemade ras el hanout (see the recipe in Chapter 16)	120 millilitres white wine
	Black pepper
2 tablespoons extra-virgin olive oil	1 whole chicken, 1.3 to 1.8 kilograms
Black pepper	1 teaspoon turmeric
1 medium onion, chopped	2 tablespoons honey

1 Preheat the oven to 200 degrees. Put the couscous in a bowl, add the water, and stir to combine. Set aside for 10 minutes while the couscous absorbs the water. Add the raisins, ras el hanout, 1 tablespoon of the olive oil, and black pepper to taste. Toss to combine and set aside.

2 Truss the chicken (see Figure 13-1). Rub the chicken with the remaining olive oil. Put the onion, cinnamon, ginger, wine, and black pepper to taste in a 22-x-30-centimetre roasting pan. Place the chicken on top of this mixture.

3 Roast the chicken for at least 1¼ hours depending on the size. Meanwhile, combine the turmeric and honey in a small bowl. After the chicken has cooked for 55 minutes, spread the top with the honey mixture. Cook for an additional 20 minutes to allow the honey to caramelise. At this stage, place the set-aside couscous in the oven to heat through.

4 Check chicken for doneness by making a small cut in any section, right to the bone. You should see no red whatsoever, but a slight tinge of pink is acceptable. Transfer the chicken to a platter and let it rest for about 5 minutes before carving. Meanwhile, pour the pan juices into a clear measuring cup and pour or spoon off as much fat as possible. Remove the couscous and set it aside to use as a side dish.

5 Put the pan juices in a blender or a food processor. Add the bits of onion and ginger but not the cinnamon stick. Blend until the mixture is a thick sauce. Reheat in a small pan. Serve the chicken promptly with the sauce and couscous.

Per serving: Calories 609; Fat 30g (Saturated 7g); Cholesterol 128mg; Sodium 128mg; Carbohydrate 40g; Dietary Fibre 5g; Protein 44g.

Trussing a Chicken

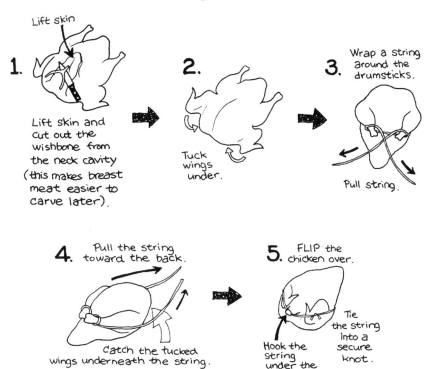

1. Lift skin

Lift skin and cut out the wishbone from the neck cavity (this makes breast meat easier to carve later).

2. Tuck wings under.

3. Wrap a string around the drumsticks.

Pull string.

4. Pull the string toward the back.

Catch the tucked wings underneath the string.

5. FLIP the chicken over.

Hook the string under the backbone.

Tie the string into a secure knot.

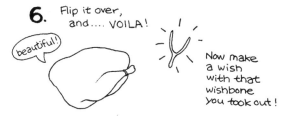

6. Flip it over, and.... VOILA!

beautiful!

Now make a wish with that wishbone you took out!

Figure 13-1:
Simple steps for trussing a chicken.

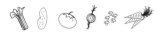

Grilled Chicken with Creamy Peanut Sauce

One of the tastiest items you can order from a Thai restaurant is Chicken Satay, which is grilled chicken served with a sweet and spicy peanut sauce. This recipe shows you how to make it at home. A large-scale study associated eating more nuts, including peanuts, with an impressive drop in heart disease – so dip into this sauce. It's lusciously creamy and full of healthy, unsaturated fats.

Special tools required: *36bamboo skewers (15 centimetres long), or 18 bamboo skewers (15 centimetres long), soaked in water for 30 minutes*

Preparation time: *20 minutes, plus 1 hour to marinate the chicken*

Cooking time: *10 minutes for one batch*

Serves: *6*

3 tablespoons fresh lime juice	240 millilitres water
2 tablespoons minced fresh root ginger	900 grams skinless, boneless chicken breasts
2 cloves garlic, crushed	Creamy Peanut Sauce (see recipe below)
1 tablespoon honey	Lime wedges for garnish

1 In a shallow baking dish, make the lime marinade by combining the lime juice, ginger, garlic, honey, and water.

2 Cut each chicken breast in half, lengthwise, to produce strips about 3 centimetres wide. Again cutting lengthwise, slice each strip in half to produce chicken strips that you can easily thread onto a skewer.

3 Place the chicken strips in the lime marinade. Spoon the marinade over the chicken to coat. Cover and refrigerate for 1 hour.

4 Thread the chicken strips on the bamboo skewers. Use 30-centimetre skewers if you plan to cook the chicken on a barbecue grill and shorter, 15-centimetre skewers if you need to fit them on a grill pan.

5 Prepare the barbecue or the grill pan by first wiping the surface with vegetable oil and setting the heat source to medium high. Cook the chicken for 3 to 4 minutes on each side or until cooked through. To ensure that the chicken is done, cut into one of the pieces with a thin-bladed knife to check the centre of the chicken is white or slightly pink.

6 Serve with the Creamy Peanut Sauce on a platter garnished with wedges of lime.

Tip: *If you have a grill pan with a lip, an easier way to cook the chicken strips is to just lay them down on the pan and use tongs or a spatula to turn them.*

Creamy Peanut Sauce

Preparation time: *15 minutes*

Cooking time: *5 minutes*

Yield: *2½ cups sauce*

250 grams smooth peanut butter (no added salt)

3 tablespoons fresh lime juice

3 tablespoons soya sauce

2 tablespoons honey

Thumb-sized piece of fresh root ginger, peeled and chopped

½ teaspoon dried crushed red pepper flakes

1 tin (400 millilitres) low-sodium chicken broth, or homemade broth

1 Put the peanut butter, lime juice, soya sauce, honey, ginger, and red pepper flakes in the bowl of a food processor fitted with a metal blade. Process until smooth.

2 Transfer the peanut mixture to a medium-sized, heavy saucepan. Gradually add the chicken broth while stirring the sauce. Warm on a medium heat, stirring as the sauce reduces, until it is the consistency of heavy cream, which takes about 5 minutes.

3 Pour the peanut sauce into a bowl and serve with the grilled chicken.

Tip: *You can make this sauce as much as 3 days ahead. Store covered in the refrigerator. Before serving, warm the sauce over medium heat until hot, stirring continuously and thinning with water if necessary.*

Per serving: *Calories 462; Fat 25g (Saturated 6g); Cholesterol 84mg; Sodium 758mg; Carbohydrate 20g; Dietary Fibre 3g; Protein 43g.*

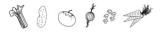

Chicken Tandoori with Minted Yogurt Sauce

This dish is one of the great classics of Indian cooking. Tandoori cooking is traditionally done in a tandoor, a small pit lined with clay, which functions as an oven. Cooks thread poultry and meats onto long skewers lowered into the tandoor pit to cook. At the same time, they slap flat breads, called naan, onto the walls of the oven where they stick, puffing and baking. With this recipe, you can simulate a version of chicken tandoori, cooked in your own oven. The cool and creamy minted yogurt sauce, which Indians call raita, is the perfect complement. Besides their wonderful flavours, the seasonings in this dish contain beneficial, active ingredients such as the garlic, onion, and turmeric that dampen inflammation. And because yogurt is full of friendly bacteria, the raita sauce aids digestion. To short-cut this recipe, buy tandoori paste, a mix of spices sold in Indian specialty stores and supermarkets. Mix this with the 240 millilitres low-fat yogurt and marinate the chicken in this mixture.

Special tools required: *Food processor*

Preparation time: *25 minutes plus 24 hours for the chicken to marinate*

Cooking time: *30 to 40 minutes*

Serves: *4*

1 medium onion, peeled and coarsely chopped	*¼ teaspoon ground mace*
6 cloves garlic, peeled and coarsely chopped	*¼ teaspoon ground nutmeg*
Thumb-sized piece of fresh root ginger, peeled and coarsely chopped	*¼ teaspoon ground cloves*
	¼ teaspoon ground cinnamon
3 tablespoons lemon juice	*¼ teaspoon black pepper*
240 millilitres low-fat plain yogurt	*¼ teaspoon cayenne pepper, or to taste*
1 tablespoon ground coriander	*4 to 6 skinless chicken pieces*
1 teaspoon ground cumin	*Minted Yogurt Sauce (see recipe below)*
1 teaspoon ground turmeric	

1 Put the onions, garlic, ginger, and lemon juice into a food processor fitted with a metal blade. Blend for about 1 minute until the mixture is a smooth paste. Transfer to a large bowl. Add the yogurt, coriander, cumin, turmeric, mace, nutmeg, cloves, cinnamon, black pepper, and cayenne. Mix thoroughly.

2 Put the chicken pieces in the marinade and turn to coat. Cover and refrigerate the chicken for 24 hours. Turn several times while the chicken is marinating.

3 One hour before cooking, take the marinated chicken pieces out of the refrigerator and bring to room temperature, ready for roasting.

4 Heat the oven to 200 degrees. Remove the chicken from the marinade. Place the pieces on a wire rack set into a shallow roasting pan lined with foil for easy cleaning. Roast the chicken, basting with marinade halfway through the cooking process. Cook for 30 to 40 minutes, or until the meat is cooked through. The chicken is done when you see clear juices if you make a small cut in the meat. Serve with the Yogurt Mint Sauce and naan or pitta bread.

Yogurt-Mint Sauce

1 medium cucumber, peeled, seeds removed, and coarsely grated

360 millilitres low-fat yogurt

¼ teaspoon ground cumin seeds, lightly toasted in a pan, stirring constantly – don't burn

1 heaped tablespoon freshly chopped fresh mint

1 Lightly toast the cumin seeds in a pan, stirring constantly. Take care not to burn them.

2 Combine the cucumber, yogurt, cumin seeds, and mint.

Per serving: Calories 199; Fat 8g (Saturated 3g); Cholesterol 56mg; Sodium 121mg; Carbohydrate 20g; Dietary Fibre 2g; Protein 20g. Based on recipe using skinless chicken.

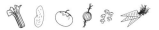

Talking Turkey All Year Round

Turkey contains much less fat than red meat and even less fat than chicken (see Table 13-1). Turkey is also a good source of vitamin B6 and supplies selenium, riboflavin, niacin, vitamin B12, zinc, and omega-3 fatty acids. (See Chapter 2 for specifics on the benefits of these nutrients.) Shopping for turkey requires a watchful eye to judge quality and a sniff to judge freshness. Careful handling is all-important because, like chicken, turkey is an ideal host for pathogens that cause food-borne illness. As a simple roast, it's delicious, but turkey is versatile enough to prepare in a variety of other, more imaginative, ways.

Plucking the right turkey

The standard supermarket turkey, often for sale at bargain prices per pound, is often as tasty as pricier versions. But if you prefer birds raised with special feed that don't contain residues of antibiotics, free-range organic turkeys are the right choice, and are now readily available.

Although chicken is a popular bird because of its handy size, which generally cooks quickly and provides 4 servings, most people think that cooking turkey is a hefty undertaking, requiring hours in the oven. To these people, turkey is best served at family gatherings such as Christmas when lots of mouths need feeding. In fact, turkey is just as easy and convenient to cook as chicken – if you select a crown, which is simply the low-fat breast meat. Roasting a whole bird involves the same procedures as chicken, but because it's a drier meat, turkey requires more basting.

Using the best turkey pieces

You can substitute turkey breast for white chicken meat in many dishes such as in the recipes for Chicken Stew with Prosciutto and White Beans and Grilled Chicken with Creamy Peanut Sauce earlier in this chapter. You can also use turkey breast, which has a rich flavour despite its low fat, to replace veal in recipes for Italian scaloppine.

You can find an assortment of turkey pieces, such as drumsticks, wings, and thighs in many butchers. You can also ask your butcher to mince lean turkey for you (or mince your own) to make the delicious Turkey Burger later in this chapter.

 When cooking turkey breast, baste the meat every 15 minutes to keep it moist. To cook a 1.3 to 2.7-kilogram turkey breast, roast it for 45 minutes and then test it for doneness every few minutes, using an instant-read thermometer. The turkey is done when the temperature reaches 70 degrees. Before carving, let the turkey rest 5 to 10 minutes.

Turkey in other forms

Look for turkey mince, sausage, and ham. These products are out there, designed for customers who want to cut fat intake. But check labels for the amount of total fat and saturated fat in a serving, and also check how large or small a serving is suggested. Some turkey products may contain as much fat as beef. And because cutting back on salt is a good move, check the sodium content, too.

Fresh versus frozen turkey

Fresh turkey is more available throughout the year these days, but you find a lot of frozen turkeys, too. Frozen birds are often very inexpensive per pound, and make a thrifty purchase if you have a large freezer.

Defrosting a rock-solid, basketball-size bird may look like a daunting task, but if you remember to start defrosting well before you need to cook the bird, it's no problem. You usually just need to check the packaging. The Food Standards Agency provides a handy, instant calculator on its website (www.eatwell.gov.uk) and suggests the following times for defrosting a turkey:

✔ In a fridge at 4 degrees: defrost for 10 to 12 hours per kilogram.

✔ In a cool room (below 17.5 degrees): defrost for 3 to 4 hours per kilogram.

✔ At room temperature (about 20 degrees): defrost for 2 hours per kilogram.

Check the turkey is fully defrosted before cooking. If you're not roasting it straight away, place the bird in the fridge until you're ready to cook it.

Roasting whole turkeys

Choose the best-sized bird to fit your family and your love of turkey leftovers. Some people are happy to eat turkey soup every day for a week, whereas others run away from home at this thought. (See the 'Winging it with leftovers' section later in this chapter for help.) Cooking a whole turkey does require your attention. The breast meat of a whole roasted turkey becomes dry if you're not careful, and so take some preventive measures.

✔ For a smaller turkey, under 4.5 kilograms, start cooking it on its breast and then flip the turkey over on its back for the final 30 to 60 minutes.

✔ For a bird over 4.5 kilograms, just tent the breast with aluminium foil for the last hour of roasting. If you try to flip a big bird, the turkey may go flying!

✔ To stuff the bird, allow 100 to 150 grams prepared stuffing per 450 grams of turkey and pack it loosely under the skin covering the breast, because it expands during cooking. If your recipe makes more stuffing than the bird can hold, wrap the remaining mixture in foil and bake alongside the bird in the pan during the last ½ hour of roasting. Remember to take the weight of the stuffing into account when calculating turkey cooking times.

Take care not to over-roast your turkey. Follow the cooking time guidelines in Table 13-2.

Table 13-2   Cooking Times for Whole Turkeys at 180 Degrees

Weight	Cooking Times
3.6 kilograms to 5.4 kilograms	4 to 4½ hours
5.4 kilograms to 7.3 kilograms	4½ to 5½ hours
7.3 kilograms to 9 kilograms	5½ to 6½ hours
9 kilograms to 10.9 kilograms	6½ to 7½ hours

Self-defeating turkeys

Self-basting turkeys are an attempt to moisten the turkey breast meat while it cooks. One of the major pluses of turkey meat is that it's relatively low in fat, especially the breast. In self-basted turkeys, fat or oil is placed under the breast skin before the bird is packed or frozen. Pop the turkey in the oven, and as the bird heats up, the fat melts and oozes over the turkey, with some added to the meat to make it moist. To avoid these added fats, which may include hydrogenated oils and added flavourings, baste the turkey yourself with the accumulating drippings in the baking pan. Remember, these contain the B vitamins present in the turkey juices.

For a great-tasting gravy, heat 250 millilitres of white wine (making sure that you don't boil it) and pour the wine over the turkey when it's half done. When the turkey finishes cooking, collect the drippings, skimming off most of the fat, and use to make the gravy, which has a more gourmet flavour thanks to the wine.

Winging it with leftovers

The beauty of cooking a whole turkey is that it gives you leftovers. Use these as inspiration to add new dishes into your usual cooking routine. Here are some examples:

- ✔ Mince your own turkey meat to make turkey burgers, such as the Turkey Burger in the next section.

- ✔ Use minced turkey meat in a chilli, such as the Hot Turkey Chilli in the next section.

- ✔ Chop and mix your turkey leftovers with low-fat mayonnaise and rocket leaves for the ultimate turkey salad sandwich filling. If available, add fresh pomegranate seeds for extra crunch and antioxidants.

- ✔ Use your turkey meat as the basis for a risotto, with added sweetcorn, mushrooms, onions, and whatever else needs using up. Use home-made turkey stock made from boiling up the bones for a rich flavour.

Recipes for gobbling up gobblers year-round

You don't have to wait until Christmas to enjoy some turkey. Why not make some scrumptious turkey burgers or a pan of turkey chilli for a change instead of using beef.

Hot Turkey Chilli

This chilli is made with turkey breast, which is naturally low in fat; healthy extra-virgin olive oil; and barley and beans, both great sources of soluble fibre. This dish is a far cry from standard beef chillies with their little lakes of fat floating on top, but it still delivers wake-up flavours. The mix of fresh chilli peppers, herbs, and spices holds its own. Feel free to turn up the volume with more chilli and Tabasco if you want more bite!

Special tools required: *Food processor*

Preparation time: *20 minutes*

Cooking time: *1 hour and 25 minutes*

Serves: *10 to 12*

5 tablespoons extra-virgin olive oil	1 teaspoon oregano
80 grams minced onion	1 teaspoon thyme
3 cloves garlic, minced	¼ teaspoon cinnamon
4 teaspoons ground cumin	1 tin (400 grams) pinto beans, drained and rinsed
600 grams minced turkey breast	1 tin (400 grams) red kidney beans, drained and rinsed
1 litre chicken broth (homemade or fat-free and low-sodium canned broth)	
60 grams pearl barley	1 tin (400 grams) chopped tomatoes
1 jalapeño chilli with seeds, chopped fine	Tabasco sauce
	Black pepper

1 In a large nonstick frying pan, heat 4 tablespoons of olive oil over a medium heat. Add the onion and garlic and cook for about 7 minutes until tender. Add the cumin and stir with a wooden spoon for about 30 seconds until fragrant.

2 To the onion mixture, add the ground turkey. Cook, stirring occasionally, for about 10 minutes, until the meat is no longer pink.

3 Add the chicken broth, barley, jalapeño, oregano, thyme, and cinnamon. Cover and simmer until the barley is almost tender, stirring occasionally, for about 45 minutes.

4 Add the pinto beans, red kidney beans, and tomatoes. Simmer, uncovered, until the barley is tender and the chilli is thick, about 20 minutes. Add more stock or water if necessary.

5 Season to taste with the Tabasco sauce and black pepper. Serve immediately. (You can also prepare the chilli a day ahead and then cover and refrigerate. Heat thoroughly before serving.)

Tip: If you prefer a milder dish, you can unseed the jalapeño chillies.

Per serving: *Calories 198; Fat 8g (Saturated 1g); Cholesterol 41mg; Sodium 252mg; Carbohydrate 11g; Dietary Fibre 3g; Protein 19g. Analysis reflects rinsed and drained beans.*

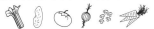

Turkey Burger

You can enjoy a hearty burger without all the fat when you use ground turkey rather than beef. However, because you need to cook your burger well done to ensure that the poultry is safe to eat, you need to add juicy ingredients to keep the burger moist. Add onion and some sort of sauce to the turkey, as in this recipe, and include a juicy condiment on the bun, such as Cranberry Sauce with Caramelised Onions and Cinnamon (see Chapter 16).

Preparation time: *15 minutes*

Cooking time: *10 minutes*

Serves: *4*

600 grams minced turkey

1 small onion, finely chopped

1 teaspoon Worcestershire sauce

¼ teaspoon dried sage

Black pepper

Cranberry Sauce with Caramelised Onions and Cinnamon (see Chapter 16)

1 In a large bowl, combine the turkey, onion, Worcestershire sauce, sage, and black pepper to taste. Form into 4 patties. For a juicier burger, handle the meat as little as possible and take care not to compact the meat.

2 Cook the burgers in a hot, well-seasoned cast-iron frying pan or ridged grill pan. Cook the burgers over a medium heat for about 5 minutes, or until brown and crispy. Flip the burgers carefully and cook for 5 minutes longer, or until golden brown and a thermometer inserted in the centre registers 75 degrees and the meat is no longer pink.

3 Serve each burger on a whole-grain hamburger bun slathered with the Cranberry Sauce with Caramelised Onions and Cinnamon.

Tip: *If the turkey meat is very lean, spray the cooking surface with oil before adding the meat, to prevent the turkey from sticking.*

Per serving (burger only): *Calories 156; Fat 7g (Saturated 2g); Cholesterol 65mg; Sodium 94mg; Carbohydrate 2g; Dietary Fibre 0g; Protein 22g.*

Chapter 14

Serving Up Soulful Seafood

Seafood is a staple of a healthy diet because it benefits heart health in a number of ways. The healthy omega-3 fats in fish improve the balance of HDL and LDL cholesterol in the bloodstream, prevent erratic heartbeats, thin the blood so that it's less likely to form artery-blocking abnormal clots, and reduce inflammation, which plays a role in the development of atherosclerosis (or hardening and furring up of the arteries).

You can divide seafood into two broad categories: fish, which are equipped with fins, and shellfish, which have shells. Both types are delectable foods that take well to all sorts of preparations and flavourful ingredients. Yet fish cooked at home is often a poor substitute for the mouth-watering flavour of fish you can order in restaurants. Dining out often sets the standard for good fish dishes.

But all this is about to change, as you make your way through the recipes in this chapter. You have the chance to experiment with different techniques and savour all sorts of fish made with complementary vegetables, spices, and herbs. Read on to find out how to handle fish so that it's safe to eat and tasty. Relax about preparing seafood in your own kitchen. The best is yet to come.

Savouring Healthy Seafood

Fish and shellfish are ideal foods for the heart because they offer a source of protein that's exceptionally low in saturated fat and contain only a moderate amount of cholesterol. The fats in seafood are the kind associated with a lower risk of heart disease and stroke. If fish is only a 'sometimes food' for you, here are some good health reasons to eat more.

Going for omega-3s and more

You want to eat fish and shellfish *because* of, not despite, the fat it contains. Isn't that a great reason to enjoy these delicious foods? Fish oils provide you with EPA (eicosapentaenoic acid) and DHA (docosahexaenoic acid), both long-chain omega-3 fatty acids that protect against coronary heart disease.

The Mediterranean diet, associated with low rates of heart disease in that part of the world, features regular consumption of fish. People who eat a lot of fish have a consistently lower risk of coronary heart disease than those following a more Western-style diet that emphasises red and processed meats. Other studies show that eating fish regularly two to four times a week nearly halves the risk of experiencing a stroke.

Fish oil benefits the heart and circulation in many ways. Here's what it does:

- Lowers triglycerides significantly (see Chapter 1).
- Cuts both total cholesterol and LDL cholesterol a little.
- Reduces abnormal blood clotting.
- Helps maintain a normal heartbeat rhythm.
- Damps down chronic inflammation in arteries (see Chapter 1).
- Lowers an elevated blood pressure.
- Reduces the progression of atherosclerosis (hardening and furring up of the arteries).

Seafood is also a great source of nutrients that function as antioxidants, maintain fluid balance, support the expansion and contraction of heart muscles, and transport oxygen in the blood. These include minerals such as selenium, potassium, magnesium, and iron. Fish is also an excellent source of B vitamins that keep homocysteine levels in check.

Counting cholesterol in fish and shellfish

Fin fish, such as salmon and cod, have a similar amount of cholesterol as white-meat chicken and turkey, foods that are routinely recommended for low-cholesterol diets. Even shellfish deserve a thumbs-up. Researchers at one time mistakenly warned against shellfish because of its supposedly high cholesterol content, but the development of more accurate testing means that we now know that clams and other crustaceans have a relatively low cholesterol content. In addition, shellfish is ridiculously low in saturated fat: 100 grams of boiled prawns contain less saturated fat than four dry-roasted peanuts.

Table 14-1 gives you a quick comparison of the amount of cholesterol in seafood with common high-cholesterol foods such as liver and red meat. Although some shellfish such as prawns are high in cholesterol, clams are relatively low, and so there's no reason not to enjoy the recipe for Anchovy and Clam Fettuccine later in this chapter.

Table 14-1	Comparing Cholesterol and Saturated Fat Content in Seafood with the Amounts in Other Foods	
Food Items (100 Grams each)	*Cholesterol (in Milligrams)*	*Saturated Fat (in Grams)*
Prawns	195	0.1
Shrimps	130	0.2
Lobster	110	0.2
Crab	72	0.7
Oysters	57	0.2
Clams	67	0.2
Scallops	47	0.4
Salmon	50	1.9
Tuna, fresh	28	1.2
Minced beef	60	7.1
Chicken white meat	70	0.3
Pork spare ribs, lean and fat	67	4.5
Calf liver	370	1.0

Note: These data are the amount in raw shellfish, fish, and meats.

Derived from: McCance & Widdowson's The Composition of Foods, Sixth Summary Edition. Food Standards Agency.

Watching for seafood catch-22

Fish is a cornerstone of healthy eating. The general recommendation is to eat fish – especially oily fish – two to four times a week. But the average adult in the UK manages to eat only a third of a portion of oily fish per week.

For all the benefits of fish, however, you do need to select your seafood wisely. Following certain guidelines to avoid the downside of eating fish is important. Seafood contains traces of toxic industrial pollutants such as PCBs, dioxins, pesticides, and heavy metals, in particular, methyl mercury. Mercury, as it accumulates, attacks nerve cells, causing loss of co-ordination and numbness, and impairs hearing and vision. Here's another problem: some of the fish highest in omega-3 fatty acids (which you *do* need) contain the most mercury. The fish that contain the highest amounts of mercury include the following: swordfish, shark, king mackerel, fresh and frozen tuna steaks, and tinned tuna.

The Food Standards Agency in the UK suggests that men, boys, and women past childbearing age (or who aren't able or intending to have further children) can eat up to four portions of oily fish a week before the possible risks from sea pollutants outweigh the known health benefits. Girls and women who may become pregnant at some point in their lives should limit their intake of oily fish to between one and two portions a week to obtain the known health benefits while limiting any possible adverse effects of pollutants on any children that they may have in the future. Pregnant and breast feeding women can also eat between one and two portions of oily fish a week, but should avoid shark, marlin, and swordfish. They can, however, eat up to four medium-sized tins or two tuna steaks a week, according to the Food Standards Agency.

Knowing which fish to favour

You can still eat plenty of fish and shellfish healthily and safely, despite concerns about polluted waters. You just need to know which fish contain the most omega-3 fatty acids, vitamins, and minerals and at the same time are the cleanest. For help in selecting fish, consult the following list for a good idea of which are good, better, and best.

Here's the A+ list, which includes seafood with high amounts of omega-3s:

- ✔ Anchovy (see the recipe for Anchovy and Clam Fettuccine later in this chapter)
- ✔ Herring
- ✔ Mackerel

- Oysters
- Pilchards
- Salmon (take a look at the Grilled Salmon with Chinese Vegetables recipe later in this chapter)
- Sardines (see the later section 'Slapping together a sardine sandwich')
- Sea bass (flip to the recipe for Baked Sea Bass with Aromatic Vegetables later in this chapter)
- Trout (see the later section 'Diving into simple fish dishes')

The A list includes seafood with moderate amounts of omega-3s:

- Flounder
- Perch
- Red snapper (see the recipe for Fish Stew with Sweet Peppers later in this chapter)
- Shellfish: scallops and clams (see the recipes for Grilled Scallops and Herby Vegetables and for Anchovy and Clam Fettuccine later in this chapter), shrimps, king crab, and crayfish
- Sole (see the Sole with Spicy Tomato Ragout recipe later in this chapter)
- Turbot

The B list includes fish with somewhat higher amounts of toxins. If you eat a fish from the B list, the next time you have fish, choose one from the A list.

- Haddock
- Halibut (see the recipe for Halibut with Coriander and Lime Salsa later in this chapter)
- Shellfish: lobster and crab

Supermarkets widely sell many of these fish and they are easy to prepare. (If you're hesitant about de-shelling – or shucking – oysters, order them in restaurants.) Make a point of eating all these various kinds of seafood every three months. That way, you're more likely to minimise your intake of toxins such as mercury, while giving yourself plenty of omega-3s and the full range of nutrients that seafood has to offer.

To reduce exposure to mercury and other toxins that accumulate in fatty tissue, trim away the skin, the fatty belly flap, and any dark meat before cooking fish. Certain cooking techniques, such as grilling and baking, also remove fat.

Salmon: The new chicken of the sea

Salmon is relatively cheap these days and is always available because it's farm-raised. Such expediency has its price: this salmon is often given doses of antibiotics, coloured artificially, and exposed to pollutants. In addition, farmed salmon are much fatter than wild salmon, and yet they're lower in the good omega-3 fatty acids. Invest in the real thing and shop for salmon labelled 'wild,' which you can find fresh, frozen, and in tins.

Tuna is a special case because different varieties contain different amounts of mercury and the healthy omega-3 fatty acids. Large tuna, which come to the table as tuna steaks, contain the most mercury but also the highest amounts of healthy oils. Albacore tuna contains moderate amounts of both mercury and omega-3s whereas tinned light tuna, from smaller fish, have the least. Opt for the tinned, light tuna packed in water (which is used in the recipe for Tinned Tuna Fish Cakes later in this chapter), and obtain fish oils by eating the A-list fish.

Bringing Home Beauties: Buying and Storing Fish

Do yourself a favour and find a fishmonger that sells really fresh, great-tasting fish, even if it costs a little more than seafood from your local supermarket. If you locate a reliable place to buy quality fish you really enjoy you're more likely to eat seafood regularly and reap the health benefits.

Considering the source

Of course, the taste of absolutely fresh fish and shellfish has no match, and really fresh offerings smell of the sea – not of fish. But such choice offerings are rare. When shopping for fish, keep the following in mind:

- Many large supermarkets and fish shops are likely to sell fresh seafood. You can find wonderful quality, but the fish may have lost texture and flavour during its hours of transport between the sea and the store.

- Look for blast-frozen fish (called IQF, standing for Individual Quick Freezing, in the trade), which is filleted or cut into steaks and then specially frozen within hours of catching. This fish can taste as fresh, or even fresher, than 'fresh' fish.

✔ Often the freshest fish is pre-cut and pre-wrapped. But do avoid fish that is sold as fresh but was previously frozen and then defrosted – this fish is definitely the worse for wear. Fish that is in a watery package and dis-coloured, with whitish edges, is a tell-tale sign.

If you're lucky enough to live by the sea, you're likely to find fishermen selling freshly caught fish from their boats along the harbour, or in local markets.

Keeping fish fresh

To ensure that you bring the freshest seafood possible to your table, give it your full attention after buying it. Refrigerate seafood quickly and correctly so that it doesn't spoil, and handle it carefully during preparation. All the attention pays off in terms of flavour and texture as well as safety. In this sec-tion, you find what to do and what not to do when handling seafood.

Storing seafood safely

After you purchase seafood, you're in charge of its care, just like when buying a plant or adopting a puppy. It soon lets you know if you haven't given it proper care. Here's the drill:

✔ After buying your fish, immediately take it home and put the fish in the refrigerator. Plan your errands so you can go right home.

Bring a cool bag filled with ice to the shop to transport your seafood home.

✔ To store fresh fish in the fridge, wrap it tightly in foil or plastic and seal it in an airtight plastic bag. Store it in the coldest part of your refrigera-tor, down towards the bottom (because heat rises).

If you buy packaged fish, remove the fish from its package, rinse under cold water, and pat dry with kitchen towels. Then wrap it in fresh foil or plastic and keep it in an airtight plastic bag near the bottom of the fridge.

✔ Fish held at normal refrigerator temperatures of 2 to 5 degrees stays fresh for only a few hours. You can double the holding time for fish by storing it at 0.5 degrees. If you can't adjust the temperature of your refrigerator to just above zero, and you don't want your lettuce to freeze, fill a lidded container with crushed ice, cover the ice with a layer of greaseproof paper, and place your fresh fish on this. Then seal the lid and store on a shelf in the fridge.

Handling seafood properly

For safety, you need to handle fish with respect when you're preparing it for cooking. Follow these steps:

✔ Cook fish the day you purchase it. If you do need to keep the fish for one day, store it on ice if possible, even if the packaging suggests a longer use-by date. Fish starts to smell 'fishy' amazingly quickly when it's not absolutely fresh and kept chilled.

✔ When making a fish dish with several ingredients that need preparing, finish the chopping and mixing of the other ingredients and then take out the fish from the refrigerator and add it to what you've prepared, such as a marinade or poaching stock.

✔ To trim a fish, place it on a brown paper bag or in the plastic bag, cut open, that the fish came in. After you've done your preparations, you can throw away the bag, which may harbour bacteria. Don't use a cutting board – wood, plastic, and acrylic can harbour bacteria.

Fishing for Compliments: Using the Right Cooking Method

You can wow family and friends with great-tasting seafood dishes if you simply observe a few basic guidelines and choose the right cooking method for the specific type and cut of fish.

Fish has little connective tissue, unlike meat, and so doesn't require long cooking to tenderise it. However, fish cooks quickly and tends to dry out. Techniques such as poaching, basting, steaming, and marinating help solve this problem. Your fish is done when it's no longer translucent, easily flakes when you break it apart with a fork, and the internal temperature is 63 degrees.

Suiting the fixing to the fish

Match seafood with the right method, and you're on your way to producing great results. The recipes in this chapter give you a chance to experiment with these techniques.

✔ Grilling is ideal for fish steaks such as halibut and thick fillets such as flounder or salmon. The high heat cooks the seafood quickly, helping to stop it drying out. Arrange the fish in a single layer on a well-greased grill rack set about 10 centimetres from the heat. Season the fish if you like and baste it during cooking. Turn thick cuts once about halfway through cooking. Try the Grilled Salmon with Chinese Vegetables or the Halibut with Coriander and Lime Salsa recipes later in this chapter. Cooked grilled prawns or scallop kebabs are delicious grilled, too.

Using a special basket that holds the fish makes it easy to turn over. Look for this utensil in gourmet kitchen shops.

✔ Baking provides a drying heat and so is good for small steaks and fillets such as flounder and sole, which cook very quickly. Place the fish in a greased dish and drizzle with lemon juice, wine, and/or stock plus a sprinkling of herbs. Cook in an oven preheated to 200 to 220 degrees. You can also bake a whole fish sitting in plenty of savoury liquid such as the Baked Sea Bass with Aromatic Vegetables described later in this chapter.

A simple guide for baking fish is to allow 10 minutes per 2½ centimetres of thawed fish at its thickest point. You can even buy little devices that measure the fish and are printed with a cooking time chart to make this extra easy.

✔ Sautéing is ideal for preparing thin fillets such as plaice, sole, sand dabs, snapper, and whiting. In this cooking method, you dry, lightly flour, and sauté the fish over a medium heat. Sautéing in butter is the classic technique, but you can use olive oil to avoid the saturated fat.

✔ Poaching works well for whole fish, but you can also cook steaks and even fillets by simmering them in liquid, whether fish stock, vegetable stock, wine, or a combination of wine and water. Poached fish is often served cold or at room temperature with an accompanying sauce, such as a dill-mayonnaise or a sweet red pepper sauce.

You can also dress up fish in a variety of ways. The most versatile fish accessory is probably fresh lemon, which provides a garnish and adds a bit of flavour. Figure 14-1 shows many ways to prepare whole lemons to make your fish more stylish while adding a flavour accent.

Of course, you can use many other foods to garnish your whole fish, including fresh vegetables, fresh herbs, and types of fruit. Figure 14-2 shows how you can garnish cooked whole fish in many different ways.

Diving into simple fish dishes

Here are some basic ways to prepare fish that are useful to have in your repertoire. They don't really require measuring, and you probably have most of the ingredients to hand.

Dredging trout in bread crumbs and more

If you're frying fish such as trout, sole, flounder, or cod and the recipe calls for bread crumbs, try dredging the fish in one of these alternatives:

✔ Fine ground cornmeal (also known as maize flour or polenta flour).

✔ Oatmeal.

✔ Ground almonds mixed with bread crumbs.

✔ A mixture of 125 grams plain wholemeal flour, 2 teaspoons toasted and ground fennel seeds, and ground black pepper.

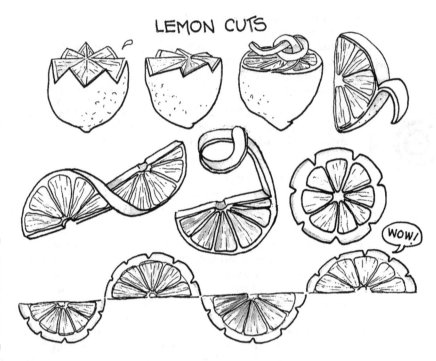

Figure 14-1:
Fancy and
easy lemon
cuts for
garnishing
fish.

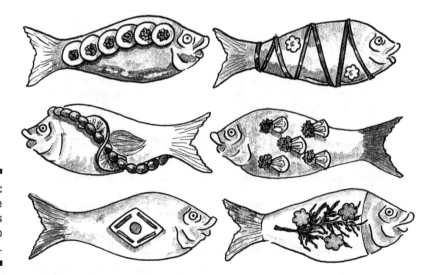

Figure 14-2:
Some of the
many ways
to dress up
a fish.

Brewing a quick fish stew

When you have little time to cook, buy some halibut or flounder and a few prawns to fix a stew, using this simple recipe:

1. Sauté some onion and garlic.

2. In a large pan, combine two 400-gram tins of tomatoes, a litre of chicken or vegetable stock, a bay leaf, some red pepper flakes, a few sprigs of parsley (or whatever fresh herbs you have), and onion and garlic. Bring to the boil over a medium-high heat and then reduce to a simmer.

3. Cut a couple of potatoes into bite-size chunks and cook them in the tomato sauce for about 15 to 20 minutes.

4. When the potatoes are almost done, add the fish and cook for 10 minutes on a medium heat.

5. Toward the end of the cooking time, add the prawns and cook for about 3 minutes, until the prawns turn opaque.

Serve with French bread and a green salad.

Slapping together a sardine sandwich

Start with a tin of sardines, bones and all, for the calcium. Add a splash of malt vinegar and black pepper. Mash together and mound on a slice of fresh bread. Add lettuce, tomato, cucumber, and so forth, if you like; close with another slice of bread; and open wide.

Feasting on Fabulous Fish Recipes

Here we go, with some lip-smacking fish dish inventions that are easy to cook and make real crowd pleasers. Start with the freshest fish possible and add a few tasty ingredients for a mid-week evening meal or a weekend dinner party. The flavours of these dishes speak of Mexico, Italy, France, and Japan, and you also have the chance to do some good old-fashioned grilling.

Halibut with Coriander and Lime Salsa

In 19th century Britain, people seasoned their halibut with freshly grated nutmeg, salt, and pepper and simply baked it in the oven. In this more modern recipe, coriander leaves and lime juice complement the firm, meaty white flesh perfectly. If this is health food, bring it on!

Special tools required: *Food processor*

Preparation time: *10 minutes*

Cooking time: *10 minutes*

Serves: *6*

8 tablespoons extra-virgin olive oil

4 tablespoons lime juice (2 limes)

3 tablespoons chopped coriander leaves

3 tablespoons chopped parsley

2 tablespoons coarsely chopped onion

1 medium-hot green chilli, sliced (optional)

6 halibut fillets (175 grams each)

Black pepper

Coriander sprigs for garnish

1 Place 6 tablespoons of the olive oil, the lime juice, coriander, parsley, onion, and chilli (if using) in a food processor.

2 Purée the ingredients until the mixture is smooth. Set aside.

3 Preheat the grill. Brush the halibut with the remaining 2 tablespoons of olive oil. Sprinkle the fish to taste with black pepper.

4 Grill the halibut for about 5 minutes per side, just until the centre of the fillet is opaque.

5 To serve, spoon a pool of the sauce on each dinner plate. Place a portion of halibut on each plate and garnish the fish with a sprig of coriander. Yummy accompaniments are oven-roasted potatoes and fresh corn on the cob.

Vary It! *Try a Basil Lemon Sauce variation. Start with 6 tablespoons extra-virgin olive oil and add 4 tablespoons freshly squeezed lemon juice. Add 3 tablespoons basil leaves, 3 tablespoons parsley, and 3 tablespoons chives, all coarsely chopped. Purée in a food processor. To serve, spoon the sauce over the grilled halibut and garnish with a dollop of low-fat sour cream and a slice of black olive.*

Per serving: *Calories 337; Fat 21g (Saturated 2g); Cholesterol 55mg; Sodium 95mg; Carbohydrate 2g; Dietary Fibre 0g; Protein 36g.*

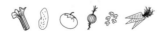

Sole with Spicy Tomato Ragout

Sole is so-named because the Greeks thought it made an ideal slipper for ocean nymphs. Small sole fillets are ideal for this recipe, which makes a great main course for a weekday dinner.

Preparation time: *15 minutes*

Cooking time: *25 minutes*

Serves: *4*

1 medium onion, peeled and sliced very thin	*1 tablespoon chopped coriander leaves*
1 teaspoon extra-virgin olive oil	*1 tablespoon chopped parsley*
2 cloves garlic, peeled and chopped	*Black pepper*
1 tin (400 grams) tomatoes, chopped	*450 grams sole fillets*
½ to 1 green chilli pepper, seeds and veins removed, chopped	*Low-fat chicken stock or tomato juice (optional)*

1 In a large, 30-centimetre frying pan, heat the onions in the olive oil on medium heat, for 7 to 10 minutes or until translucent. Stir occasionally. Toward the end of this cooking process, add the garlic.

2 Add the tinned tomatoes, chilli, coriander, and parsley to the onions and garlic. Stir the mixture and simmer, covered, for 15 minutes to combine the flavours. Season to taste with black pepper.

3 Place the sole fillets in the pan and spoon the tomato sauce over them. If you don't have enough sauce to cover the fish, add a small amount of liquid, such as water, low-fat chicken stock, or tomato juice. Cover and cook on medium-low for about 10 minutes, until the flesh of the fish is opaque. Add additional liquid if necessary while the fish is simmering to prevent it from sticking to the bottom of the pan. Serve immediately.

Tip: *If you don't have a large frying pan, put the fish in a baking dish, pour the sauce over the fish, and bake at 180 degrees for 15 to 20 minutes.*

Tip: *You can add about 4 tablespoons of liquid to give the fish a little something to steam/ poach in; white wine works well.*

Per serving: *Calories 152; Fat 5g (Saturated 1g); Cholesterol 53mg; Sodium 210mg; Carbohydrate 7g; Dietary Fibre 2g; Protein 20g.*

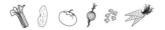

Grilled Salmon with Chinese Vegetables

Salmon used to be the fish of kings, but is now often on sale at a cheaper price than cod. This easy dish provides a gourmet treat even when you think you don't have time to cook. It boosts your intake of omega-3 fatty acids, which promote heart health in many ways, and sneaks in some green vegetables, too.

Preparation time: *20 minutes, plus 1 to 2 hours to marinate the salmon*

Cooking time: *15 minutes*

Serves: *4*

60 millilitres white miso (fermented soya bean paste)

2 tablespoons unseasoned rice vinegar

2 teaspoons soya sauce

1 tablespoon minced fresh ginger

1 spring onion, trimmed and finely chopped

450 grams wild salmon fillets, skin and bones removed

1 clove garlic, grilled

1 tablespoon unrefined sesame oil

4 shiitake mushrooms (or brown chestnut mushrooms), quartered

4 miniature pak choi, roughly chopped

125 grams mange tout

2 teaspoons toasted sesame oil (optional)

1 In a shallow baking dish, make a marinade by whisking together the miso, rice vinegar, soya sauce, ginger, and spring onion. Place the salmon in the marinade and turn to coat. Cover and chill for 1 to 2 hours.

2 In a large frying pan or wok, cook the garlic in the sesame oil for 30 seconds. Add the mushrooms and pak choi. Cook on medium-high, stirring frequently, for 5 to 7 minutes, until the vegetables begin to soften. Then add the mange tout for the last 3 minutes of cooking. If desired, finish with a splash of toasted sesame oil.

3 Meanwhile, preheat the grill. Using a rubber spatula, gently scrape any excess marinade from the salmon and discard. Oil a shallow baking pan and arrange the salmon fillets in the pan.

4 Place the salmon under the grill and cook for about 7 to 10 minutes until the edges turn golden brown. Gently turn the fillets over and grill for an additional 3 minutes. Cook the fish until it is opaque in the centre. Cooking times may vary depending upon the type of grill and the thickness of the salmon fillets. Keep an eye on them – after you flip them they cook quickly.

5 Divide the vegetable mixture among 4 large dinner plates. Place the grilled salmon on top of the vegetables. Serve immediately with steamed brown rice.

Per serving: Calories 272; Fat 12g (Saturated 2g); Cholesterol 71mg; Sodium 501mg; Carbohydrate 11g; Dietary Fibre 3g; Protein 29g.

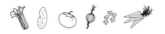

Baked Sea Bass with Aromatic Vegetables

Sea Bass has a soft, dense flesh and delicate flavour. You can use this recipe to prepare fillets or the whole fish. With miniature vegetables as a garnish, this dish dresses up for company but is also a great solution for a quick, high-protein, mid-week meal.

Preparation time: *10 minutes*

Cooking time: *20 to 25 minutes*

Serves: *4*

240 millilitres white wine

240 millilitres bottled clam juice or fish stock (see Chapter 9 for a fish stock recipe)

1 bulb fennel, stem and fronds trimmed, and sliced horizontally

350 grams baby carrots (or regular carrots with tops removed), peeled, quartered lengthwise, and cut into 5-centimetre lengths

10 grams chives, cut into 2½-centimetre lengths

1 teaspoon dried marjoram

2 tablespoons tarragon vinegar

2 tablespoons extra-virgin olive oil

Black pepper

900 grams whole sea bass (see the tip at the end of the recipe)

1 Preheat the oven to 220 degrees. Put the white wine and clam juice or stock in a medium-sized pot. Add the fennel and carrots and cook over a medium heat for 5 to 10 minutes. Remove from the heat and add the chives, marjoram, tarragon vinegar, olive oil, and black pepper to taste.

2 Place the sea bass in a shallow baking pan. Pour the vegetable and stock mixture over the fish, making sure that some vegetables are also in the fish cavity.

3 Bake the fish for 10 minutes per 2½-centimetres of thickness (measured in the thickest part of the fish) usually for about 15 to 20 minutes. To test for doneness, insert a thermometer at an angle into the thickest part of the flesh. The fish is edible at 60 degrees. Because fish tissues begin to break down at 65 degrees, allowing both juices and flavour to escape, remove the fish from the oven when it is no hotter than 63 degrees. The fish continues to cook a little after it's removed from the oven. Alternatively, stick a toothpick into the thickest part of the fish. When the fish is done, the pick meets with little resistance and comes out clean. Serve immediately on a platter, with the vegetables scattered over the whole fish for decoration. Cut serving portions at the table.

Tip: *Leaving the head on the fish while it cooks helps to seal in juices and keeps the fish moist.*

Tip: *Placing the fennel inside the fish gives the flesh a very nice flavour.*

Per serving: *Calories 227; Fat 10g (Saturated 2g); Cholesterol 50mg; Sodium 271mg; Carbohydrate 12g; Dietary Fibre 4g; Protein 23g.*

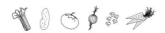

Making more Sensational Seafood Recipes

The following recipes are good ones to have for a quick meal at home or for an informal get-together with friends. This section also includes a chance to prepare scallops, shellfish that are perfectly fine to have on a cholesterol-controlling diet because they're low in saturated fat and cholesterol.

Grilled Scallops and Herby Vegetables

Scallops are one of the many shellfish that easily fit into a heart-healthy diet because they're low in cholesterol and contain only a trace of saturated fat. Their mild flavour with a hint of the sea combines well with the flavour of fresh herbs.

Grilled Scallops

Special tools required: *4 lightly oiled, 38-centimetre long metal or bamboo skewers (see the later tip under Grilled Vegetables)*

Preparation time: *15 minutes, plus 2 hours for marinating the scallops*

Cooking time: *5 minutes*

Serves: *4 (for dinner)*

2 tablespoons extra-virgin olive oil	*1 clove garlic, chopped*
2 tablespoons fresh lemon juice	*Pepper*
2 tablespoons finely chopped basil	*12 large sea scallops*
2 tablespoons finely chopped parsley	*Lemon wedges*

1 Preheat the grill. In a medium-sized, non-metallic bowl, whisk together the olive oil, lemon juice, basil, parsley, garlic, and pepper for the marinade. Divide into two portions.

2 Add one half of the herb marinade to the scallops and toss well. Cover and refrigerate to marinate for 1 to 2 hours.

3 Using 2 skewers, thread 6 scallops through the centre rather than crosswise. Repeat with the remaining scallops.

4 Lay the scallop skewers on an oiled grill or on an oiled grill rack set over the grill, keeping the skewers about 1 centimetre apart. Cook for 2 minutes per side, removing from the grill as soon as the scallops become opaque. Using the blunt side of a knife, slide the scallops onto the vegetable platter.

Grilled Vegetables

Special tools required: *4 lightly oiled, 38-centimetre long metal or bamboo skewers (see the first tip at the end of the recipe)*

Preparation time: *10 minutes*

Cooking time: *15 minutes*

Serves: *4 (for dinner)*

8 cherry tomatoes

8 slices of courgette, 1 centimetre thick

½ medium onion, peeled and cut into 8 wedges

1 Toss the vegetables with the remaining half of the marinade. Using 1 skewer, thread the onion wedges on this. Leave several centimetres of skewer free of vegetables so that the handle-end of the skewer extends beyond the edge of the grill so you can manoeuvre the skewer easily. Next, skewer the courgette slices, threading the skewer through the length of the slice. Finally, using 2 skewers, double-skewer the tomatoes to keep them from twirling.

2 Place the onion skewer on a medium-hot, oiled grill or on an oiled grill rack made for vegetables set over the grill. (See the second tip at the end of this recipe for how to test the heat of the grill.) Cook for 10 minutes, turn over, and cook for an additional 10 minutes. Transfer to a bowl some of the marinade used to marinate the vegetables, and occasionally brush the onions with the marinade.

3 When the onions have cooked for 5 minutes, put the courgette on the grill, flat side down. Grill each side for about 7 minutes. Brush frequently with the marinade as they cook.

4 When the courgette has cooked for 5 minutes and the time comes to turn the onions, add the skewer of tomatoes to the grill. Cook all the vegetables together for an additional 10 minutes or less, until they're cooked through.

5 Remove the vegetable skewers from the grill and place on a platter. Using the blunt edge of a knife, gently slide the vegetables onto the plate. Serve the scallops and vegetables on a bed of rice pilaf or Quinoa Italian-style (see the recipe in Chapter 20). Garnish with lemon wedges.

Tip: Soak bamboo skewers in water overnight before using to prevent them from burning. They're a better option than thick metal skewers for grilling small pieces of delicate foods because a thick metal skewer may split.

Tip: To check the temperature of a grill, hold your hand about 12 centimetres above the cooking surface. When you have a low heat, you can hold your hand under the grill for 5 to 6 seconds; with a medium heat, 3 to 4 seconds; and with a high heat, 1 to 2 seconds.

Per serving: *Calories 136; Fat 7g (Saturated 1g); Cholesterol 28mg; Sodium 135mg; Carbohydrate 5g; Dietary Fibre 1g; Protein 12g.*

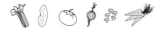

Tinned Tuna Fish Cakes

These fish cakes are coated in bread crumbs to give the crunch everyone likes, but without the fat. These cakes make great fish sandwiches or go well on top of a green salad for a light lunch. They also make a handy main course when you need dinner fast. Try them garnished with a wedge of lemon and an easy sauce you can whip together in an instant using low-fat mayonnaise and wasabi, the hot, Japanese version of horseradish.

Preparation time: *15 minutes*

Cooking time: *Approximately 35 minutes total*

Serves: *8 to 10 medium cakes*

140 grams fine, dry, unseasoned bread crumbs, preferably wholegrain	2 teaspoons dried thyme, or lemon thyme if available
1 teaspoon paprika	2 tins (175 grams each) light tuna (packed in water and no added sodium), drained of liquid
Black pepper	
450 grams potatoes, with skins, cut into equal chunks	1 level tablespoon capers
	2 tablespoons chopped fresh parsley
2 large shallots, finely chopped	2 egg whites
4 tablespoons extra-virgin olive oil	Lemon slices
2 cloves garlic, finely chopped	Low-fat mayonnaise
	A pinch of wasabi, to taste

1 In a small bowl, mix the bread crumbs, paprika, and black pepper to taste. Transfer the bread crumbs to a flat plate and set aside. Fill a large pan with water and bring to the boil.

2 Cook the potatoes in boiling water for 15 to 20 minutes until tender. Drain, mash, and set aside.

3 Use a paper towel to wipe out the frying pan used to toast the bread crumbs. Cook the shallots in 1 tablespoon of the olive oil over a medium heat for 5 minutes. Add the garlic and thyme, and cook for another minute.

4 Place the tuna in a large bowl and break it up with a fork. Add the potatoes, shallot mixture, capers, and parsley. Combine and form into cakes about 7½ centimetres in diameter.

5 Put the egg whites and 60 millilitres of water in a shallow bowl and beat together with a fork. Dredge the fish cakes in the bread crumbs. After each fish cake is covered, gently dip the cake in the egg-white solution and again in the bread crumbs. Your hands get covered with crumbs and egg whites while you do this, and so try putting the cakes directly in the heated pan or on a piece of waxed paper between dips. This double-dip procedure seals the cake and ensures a moist interior.

6 Again, wipe out the same frying pan. Add another tablespoon of oil, and heat. Add a batch of the fish cakes and cook over a medium heat, for about 5 minutes per side, until the bread crumb crust is golden brown. Transfer the cooked fish cakes to a platter and cover loosely with aluminium foil to keep warm or place in the oven and turn the oven temperature to warm. To make a second batch of fish cakes, put 1 tablespoon of oil into the pan and proceed as with the first batch. Serve with lemon slices and low-fat mayonnaise that you've seasoned with wasabi.

Per serving: Calories 241; Fat 8g (Saturated 1g); Cholesterol 13mg; Sodium 350mg; Carbohydrate 25g; Dietary Fibre 2g; Protein 16g. (Analysis doesn't include mayonnaise.)

Fish Stew with Sweet Peppers

Here's a much more fun way of giving yourself a dose of fish oils and antioxidants than swallowing pills. Take your omega-3s and lots of selenium, an important trace mineral, in the different types of fish present in this stew. It also offers plenty of cholesterol-lowering phytonutrients in the variety of vegetables it contains.

Preparation time: *30 minutes*

Cooking time: *30 minutes*

Serves: *6*

2 tablespoons olive oil

1 large onion, peeled and sliced

2 leeks, cleaned and sliced

1 baby bulb Florence fennel, trimmed and cut into strips

3 cloves garlic, chopped

2 x 400 grams tins chopped tomatoes

3 sweet red peppers (or 1 yellow, 1 orange, and 1 red), cut into thin strips

1 pinch saffron

250 millilitres dry white wine

½ teaspoon mixed Italian dried herbs

Black pepper

900 grams mixed, non-oily fish fillets such as red snapper, red bream, cod, John Dory, or gurnard

1 Heat the olive oil in a large sauté pan and add the onion, leek, Florence fennel, and garlic. Cook over a medium-high heat for 2 minutes, stirring occasionally, until starting to colour. Add the tomatoes, peppers, saffron, white wine, and herbs. Continue to cook for 15 minutes, until the vegetables soften. Season to taste with black pepper.

2 Drop in the fish fillets, larger pieces first, and simmer for 5 minutes.

3 Strain the stew and place all the fish and vegetables in a large dish. Keep warm.

4 Bring the strained liquor to the boil and whisk continuously for one minute to aid the emulsion of water and oil. When the stew has thickened, season to taste.

5 Pour the thickened liquor over the fish and serve.

Per serving: Calories 259; Fat 7g (Saturated 1g); Cholesterol 53mg; Sodium 262mg; Carbohydrate 20g; Dietary Fibre 6g; Protein 33g.

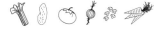

Anchovy and Clam Fettuccine

The robust flavour of this pasta is just calling for Chianti. What a lovely way to have your antioxidants (in the red wine) and meet your weekly quota of seafood. Make this dish with top-quality imported pasta, or fresh pasta, which you can find in the chill section of most supermarkets. Or use the recipe to experiment with whole-grain pastas; their rich flavours are a match for the gutsy ingredients in this sauce. Tinned clams make this dish quick and easy, but you can dress it up for company and use fresh instead.

Preparation time: *15 minutes*

Cooking time: *15 minutes*

Serves: *4*

225 grams fettuccine

2 tablespoons extra-virgin olive oil, plus extra for cooking the fettuccine

3 cloves garlic, chopped

120 millilitres white wine

1 tin (180 grams) clams, drained and juice reserved, or 900 grams fresh clams, juice reserved

1 tin (55 grams) anchovies, chopped

2 tablespoons chopped Italian parsley, plus extra for garnish

1 teaspoon mixed Italian dried herbs

Hot pepper flakes (optional)

1 Fill a large pan with water and bring to the boil. Add the fettuccine slowly enough to maintain the boil, and add a splash of olive oil. Cook the pasta for about 10 minutes, until the fettuccine is almost al dente, or a few minutes less than the instructions on the package indicate for cooking the pasta.

2 Meanwhile, heat the oil in a large 30-centimetre frying pan. Add the garlic, cooking until the garlic begins to turn golden and immediately add the wine and reserved clam juice. Add the anchovies, parsley, dried herbs, and, if desired, the pepper flakes.

3 Bring the wine mixture to the boil as the pasta finishes cooking. Drain the pasta and add to the wine mixture, tossing constantly for about 3 minutes until the pasta absorbs the liquid. Add the clams and toss with the pasta for 30 seconds. Serve garnished with more parsley.

Warning: *Adding more than a dash of pepper flakes obscures the seafood flavours.*

Vary It! *Add 2 seeded and diced tomatoes to the sauce when you add the anchovies. Finish the dish with a grinding of black pepper.*

Per serving: *Calories 365; Fat 10g (Saturated 2g); Cholesterol 42mg; Sodium 559mg; Carbohydrate 45g; Dietary Fibre 2g; Protein 23g.*

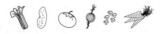

Chapter 15

Managing Meats in a Healthy Diet

....

In This Chapter

▶ Including meat in a low-saturated-fat diet

▶ Discovering the kindest cuts of beef and lamb

▶ Going wild over venison

▶ Keeping lean pork tender and juicy

....

Meat is still welcome in a diet designed to lower cholesterol. Yes, you have options beyond chicken breast in one of its many disguises! You can eat beef, pork, and lamb, as well as more exotic options such as venison or rabbit, several times a week, especially if you serve them with plenty of wholegrains, legumes, and vegetables that have virtually no saturated fat and zero cholesterol.

In this chapter, you find out which cuts of meat are the leanest and how much makes up a heart-healthy portion. We introduce you to cooking techniques that reduce fat and keep the meat juicy, together with specific times, temperatures, and guidelines to help you prepare various meats in your own kitchen. And you can experiment with the recipes, which are designed to minimise fat while maximising flavour.

Finding Healthy Ways to Eat Meat

Several strategies can help you include meats in a cholesterol-controlling diet:

✔ Choose leaner cuts that are lower in saturated fat.

✔ Reduce your usual portion sizes if you usually have large servings.

✔ Cook the meat in a way that eliminates some of the fat.

The following sections provide the important details.

Starting with the leanest cuts

Believe it or not, certain cuts of beef and pork compare well with lean chicken and fish because they have a good content of monounsaturated fats, which lower LDL cholesterol without affecting beneficial HDL levels. Take a look at Table 15-1 to see how these items compare in terms of total fat, saturated fat, and cholesterol. The numbers refer to the amount in 100 grams of cooked, trimmed meat.

Table 15-1	Fat Content of Lean Meat, Poultry, and Fish			
Item (raw, lean)	Total Fat	Saturated Fat	Monoun- saturated Fat	Cholesterol
Beef				
Fore rib	6.5 grams	2.9 grams	2.8 grams	56 milligrams
Lean rump steak	4.1 grams	1.7 grams	1.7 grams	59 milligrams
Topside	2.7 grams	1.1 grams	1.2 grams	50 milligrams
Beef sirloin	4.5 grams	2.0 grams	1.9 grams	51 milligrams
Pork				
Pork fillet steaks	3.4 grams	1.2 grams	1.3 grams	62 milligrams
Pork leg joint	2.2 grams	0.7 grams	0.9 grams	64 milligrams
Lamb				
Breast	11.2 grams	5.2 grams	4.2 grams	76 milligrams
Leg	12.3 grams	5.9 grams	4.8 grams	78 milligrams
Venison	1.6 grams	0.8 grams	0.4 grams	50 milligrams
Rabbit	5.5 grams	2.1 grams	1.3 grams	53 milligrams
Chicken				
Skinless chicken white meat	1.1 grams	0.3 grams	0.5 grams	70 milligrams
Skinless chicken dark meat	2.8 grams	0.8 grams	1.3 grams	105 milligrams
Fish				
Cod	0.7 grams	0.1 grams	0.1 grams	46 milligrams
Salmon	11.0 grams	1.9 grams	4.4 grams	50 milligrams

Consider upgrading to organic meat that's free of toxic residues from pesticides, antibiotics, and added hormones.

Practising portion control

As you alter the way you eat to lower your cholesterol, confine large steaks to a distant memory. You don't have to go short on your protein intake, just on sources of protein that contain excess saturated fat and cholesterol.

A portion size of cooked meat is 85 grams. This translates into a not-too-thick beefburger the size of the palm of your hand. (No cheating! If you have large hands, think of a serving as the size of a deck of cards.)

As an example, a recipe that calls for 450 grams of meat yields around five servings.

Tips from Asian cooking

At first glance, an 85-gram portion may seem appallingly skimpy, but you can make it stretch in several ways. The Chinese are experts at this: try the Steak Stir-Fry with Chinese Vegetables recipe later in this chapter.

You can also make a small portion of beef or pork stretch if you serve the meat on a skewer. Try the recipe for Grilled Chicken with Creamy Peanut Sauce in Chapter 13, but use red meat instead.

Meaty sauces

Small portions of meat can seem larger when mixed into sauces. For example, Spaghetti Bolognese from the north of Italy, made with a rich meat sauce, can be yours to enjoy even as you watch your cholesterol. Start with a bottled tomato sauce: you can find all sorts of delectable versions in standard markets. Cook some lean, minced beef, 60 grams to every 250 millilitres of sauce. Thoroughly drain the fat from the cooked meat. Pour the tomato sauce into a pot, and add the cooked meat. Simmer to combine flavours and serve over pasta. Pad it out by adding chopped onion plus grated carrot and celery, too.

Using pre-cooked minced beef helps to cut the fat when making meat loaf. This dish is often made with bread crumbs that soak up fat from the raw meat as it cooks.

Preparing meats in lower-fat ways

You can do several things to help cut down on the fat in meat. First trim away any visible fat. You don't need to do this with the precision of a neurosurgeon, but do take a moment to remove the most obvious bits. Eating this fat can double the amount of fat you consume.

Cutting away fat doesn't remove much cholesterol. Most of the cholesterol in meat is incorporated in the muscle tissue. Very little cholesterol is in the fat. However, trimming bits of solid fat is still important because, although this fat is made up of half monounsaturated fat (good) and half saturated fat (potentially bad for some people), it's a major source of calories that most people who are watching their weight can well do without.

Next, choose a cooking technique, such as grilling, that lets fat drain away as the meat cooks. Roasting meat set on a rack over the roasting pan works the same way. If sautéing, after the meat is cooked, transfer it to a platter while you skim some of the fat from the pan juices.

Make sure that you save some of the pan juices to serve with the meat. They contain all sorts of B vitamins, including vitamins B6, B12, thiamin (B1), riboflavin (B2), and niacin (B3). These nutrients are water-soluble and leach out as meat cooks. Minerals can also make their way into the juices. Meat is an excellent source of zinc that helps antioxidants do their job, as well as iron, which transports oxygen in the blood. Don't miss out on all these minerals. Serve your steaks and chops au jus.

Switching to soya

Substituting meat with soya protein in your recipes helps to lower total cholesterol and LDL cholesterol by around 4 per cent. However, a meta-analysis of many smaller studies, conducted by the University of Kentucky and published in the *New England Journal of Medicine* in 1995, found that to achieve this effect, you need to consume 2 to 3 servings of high-protein soya foods per day. This amount is equivalent to 31 to 47 grams of soya protein. Translating this into soya foods, 180 grams of firm tofu plus 360 millilitres of soya milk gives you 40 grams of soya protein. Studies have shown that eating just 25 grams of soya protein a day can lower cholesterol levels by 0.23 mmol/l (millimoles per litre) – enough to reduce your risk of heart disease by 10 per cent. Many vegetarians may already consume this much, but if you're accustomed to the taste of meat, switching to eating this much soya is a challenge.

One way to incorporate more soya in your diet is to eat only vegetarian meals one or two days a week and feature soya foods in these meals such as soya milk or yogurt, fresh or frozen soya beans (edamame), tofu, tempeh, TVP (textured vegetable protein), soya desserts, bread, and soya flour. You can also try using soya with other foods known to lower cholesterol, such as margarine enriched with plant sterols, and almonds and macadamia nuts. Soya-based vegetarian 'meats' are also available, such as 'bacon', 'sausages', and 'burgers', but check the packs for the amount of fat and salt they contain before buying. Soya also forms part of the so-called *Portfolio Diet*, which enhances a healthy eating diet with sterols, almonds, soluble fibre, and soya protein. Another source of vegetable protein is Quorn, made from a fungus-based mycoprotein similar to that found in mushrooms.

Rounding Up Healthy Red Meats

Sometimes, nothing else makes you feel well-fed like a piece of red meat. Perhaps it's the minerals in the meat, or, gosh, the fat. Red meat seems to satisfy a particular hunger, and you can have some occasionally, even if you're watching your cholesterol.

Lassoing lean beef

Beef in general is leaner these days as breeders meet the demand of health-conscious consumers. The leanest cuts of beef include sirloin and tenderloin.

When cooking lean beef, the challenge is to keep it tender and moist. Fat normally does the trick, but lean meat doesn't give you this break. Instead, to keep meat tender you need to choose the right cooking method, depending upon how well-done you want the meat.

✔ If you want medium-rare meat (reaching 55 to 60 degrees as measured with a meat thermometer), for the juiciest results use a dry heat method of cooking, such as grilling or broiling.

As meat cooks with dry heat to medium-rare, the tangled molecules of protein unfold, and the meat becomes tender.

✔ If you want lean meat well-done, moist heat is your best option. Make sure that the meat reaches internal temperatures above 70 degrees to produce tender meat.

Moist heat converts the connective tissue in meat to tender gelatine after a period of time. This process happens in the pot when you make the Vegetable Beef Stew described later in this chapter.

Counting on sheep

Some cuts of lamb are fine to include in a heart-healthy diet. Trimmed, lean leg of lamb favourably compares with pork and skinless chicken leg in terms of the amount of cholesterol it contains. However, it does provide more total fat, though a good proportion of that fat is the beneficial monounsaturated kind. Take a look at Table 15-2.

Table 15-2	Lamb Compared with Other Meats in 100 grams Servings			
Item (lean, raw)	Total Fat	Saturated Fat	Monoun-saturated fat	Cholesterol
Lamb breast	11 grams	5.2 grams	4.2 grams	76 milligrams
Lamb neck fillet	13.9 grams	6.4 grams	5.3 grams	75 milligrams
Pork leg joint	2.2 grams	0.7 grams	0.9 grams	64 milligrams
Skinless chicken leg (dark meat)	2.8 grams	0.8 grams	1.3 grams	105 milligrams

If you long for the flavour of lamb, fix yourself this lamb dish inspired by the flavours in Greek cooking, where lamb is a staple food:

1. **Place the following ingredients in a pot: 900 grams chopped plum tomatoes (tinned or fresh), 2 cloves crushed garlic, 1 teaspoon dried oregano, ½ teaspoon cinnamon, and 175 grams shredded, roast leg of lamb, trimmed of visible fat.**

2. **Cook over a medium-low heat for about 20 minutes, until the tomatoes soften and the flavours combine.**

3. **Pour over wholewheat pasta with a sprinkling of feta cheese to make 4 servings.**

Trying venison and other exotic meats

Many supermarkets stock more exotic fresh and frozen meats such as venison, rabbit, and even buffalo. If caught from the wild, these animals are lean and mean with little excess fat. Farmed animals, however, are often more fatty. Raw venison typically contains only 1.6 grams of fat and 50 milligrams of cholesterol per 100 grams, and raw rabbit provides 5.5 grams of fat and 53 milligrams of cholesterol per 100 grams. Talk to your butcher to see what's available and ask for the leanest cuts on offer to help you regularly vary your menu.

Preparing Pork That's Lean and Mean

Pork earns its place as a meat of choice in cholesterol-controlling cooking for flavour and fat content. This meat is a remarkably versatile ingredient, adapting well to all sorts of flavourings and preparations. But what kept the pork of yore so moist and succulent was all that fat. Nowadays, pork is bred for leanness and the leaner cuts can quickly dry out during cooking.

Keeping pork juicy

Choose a method of cooking that uses dry heat, such as grilling, barbecuing, sautéing, or roasting. Moist heat cooking, such as stewing and braising, draws juice out of the pork. Next, decide on a cooking temperature.

✔ When preparing thick chops, first brown them in a frying pan and then finish them in the oven at a moderate heat of 180 degrees to cook them through without drying the exterior. See Juicy Pork Chops with Rosemary as an example.

✔ When roasting a pork loin, start the oven at 200 to 220 degrees, roasting the meat for 15 minutes. Then lower the temperature to 160 degrees to keep the juices in the meat.

Don't buy those very thin chops that supermarkets sell in large packages. The meat toward the edge is overcooked by the time the meat next to the bone is done. Instead, start with a chop that is 3 to 4 centimetres thick. Such a chop amounts to about two 85-gram-servings. Share it with someone or have the rest in a sandwich for lunch the next day.

Knowing when pork is done

The main worry when cooking pork is that undercooking it can result in the roundworm infection called *trichinosis*. Although rare in the developed world, prevention is still of utmost importance. The good news is that trichinosis is killed off at around 60 degrees, a temperature much lower than once thought. A digital instant-read thermometer gives an accurate temperature even if you insert it only 5 millimetres. Consequently, you can use it to take the temperature of pork chops and meat patties as well as roasts. This inexpensive thermometer displays the temperature to two decimal points and is powered by a small watch battery.

Here are some tips to ensure properly cooked pork:

✔ Cook loin pork chops until they reach an internal temperature of 65 to 70 degrees. Then cover the chops loosely with aluminium foil, and let them rest 5 minutes to absorb juice and equalise the temperature, which rises another 5 degrees.

✔ Heat a loin roast until the meat thermometer reads 65 to 70 degrees. Then cover the meat and let it rest for 20 to 30 minutes, while the temperature rises another 10 degrees.

✔ When pork is sufficiently cooked, the meat may still look slightly pink.

Meeting some Meaty Recipes

Try these recipes for beef, pork, and meatballs the next time you want red meat. The beef recipes include lots of vegetables, and we've designed the pork recipes to keep the meat moist.

Roast Tenderloin of Pork with Hazelnut and Marmalade Glaze

Tenderloin of pork is remarkably simple to cook and goes with all sorts of marinades and glazes. Try this recipe before concocting your own variations, such as adding dark rum to the marmalade mixture. Baked sweet potatoes and cauliflower go well with this dish.

Preparation time: *15 minutes*

Cooking time: *Approximately 40 minutes*

Serves: *4*

160 grams orange marmalade	1½ teaspoons apple cider vinegar
2 tablespoons Dijon mustard	¼ teaspoon sage
60 grams hazelnuts, finely chopped	400 grams pork tenderloin, trimmed of visible fat
¼ teaspoon crushed black peppercorns	1 tablespoon extra-virgin olive oil

1 Preheat the oven to 200 degrees. Put the marmalade, mustard, hazelnuts, peppercorns, and vinegar in a bowl. Stir to combine and set aside.

2 Rub the sage into the pork.

3 Heat the olive oil in a frying pan over a medium-high heat. Put the tenderloin in the pan and lightly brown on all sides, turning frequently, for 6 minutes.

4 Transfer the meat to a baking dish. Spread the marmalade mixture over the meat. Roast in the oven for 30 minutes, or until the internal temperature is 65 degrees.

5 Remove the meat from the oven and loosely cover with aluminium foil. Leave to rest for 5 minutes to allow the meat to absorb the juices and equalise the temperature. Serve immediately, cut into thin slices.

Per serving: Calories 364; Fat 18g (Saturated 3g); Cholesterol 66mg; Sodium 258mg; Carbohydrate 30g; Dietary Fibre 2g; Protein 24g.

Vegetable Beef Stew

One way to enjoy red meat while watching your saturated fat and cholesterol intake is to eat small portions with lots of vegetables. This stew follows this formula, with about 85 grams of meat per serving, but is still substantial thanks to the barley, which gives you soluble fibre.

Preparation time: *15 minutes*

Cooking time: *About 2¼ hours*

Serves: *6*

600 grams lean sirloin, cut into 2 to 3-centimetre pieces (allow to reach room temperature before cooking)

1 tablespoon olive oil

1 medium onion, trimmed and chopped

1 tablespoon paprika

5 carrots, peeled and cut into 2-centimetre lengths

1 stalk celery, cut into 2-centimetre lengths

130 grams pearl barley, rinsed

1 clove garlic, minced

1 bay leaf

¼ teaspoon red pepper flakes

240 millilitres red wine

720 millilitres fat-free, low-sodium beef broth or homemade beef stock (see Chapter 9 for a method of making your own beef stock)

¼ head cabbage, sliced

1 Allow the beef to reach room temperature. In a large pot, heat the oil and then cook the beef in the oil on a medium heat for 5 to 10 minutes, stirring occasionally so all the sides brown.

2 Add the onion and paprika. On a medium heat, cook the onion until it softens and begins to brown, about 5 minutes.

3 Add the carrots, celery, barley, garlic, bay leaf, pepper flakes, red wine, and broth. Stir to combine and bring to the boil.

4 Lower the heat so that the mixture simmers and cook, covered, for 1½ hours. Add the cabbage and cook for an additional half-hour. Remove the bay leaf before serving.

5 Serve the stew in bowls and enjoy with a glass of red wine.

Tip: *The barley continues to absorb water so if you make this ahead and then reheat it, you need to add additional broth or water.*

Per serving: *Calories 279; Fat 8g (Saturated 2g); Cholesterol 56mg; Sodium 123mg; Carbohydrate 27g; Dietary Fibre 6g; Protein 25g.*

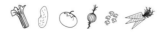

Juicy Pork Chops with Rosemary

This is an attractive and easy-to-make recipe that uses several strategies to keep the meat moist: searing, breading, and roasting with a wine reduction at a low temperature. It also requires that you start with extra-thick loin pork chops. However, one of these chops makes quite a large portion, about 225 grams. Consequently, this recipe means you forsake appearance in deference to juiciness, and carve up 2 chops to serve 3 persons. The portions may seem modest, but the point here is to retain the juiciness of the meat and cut down on total meat consumption. Enjoy it with your favourite vegetable side dishes.

Preparation time: *15 minutes, plus 15 minutes for the chops to refrigerate after breading*

Cooking time: *About 45 minutes*

Serves: *4*

40 grams wholewheat flour

80 grams wholegrain bread crumbs

2 egg whites, lightly beaten with 1 tablespoon water

2 bone-in loin pork chops (at least 225 grams each), 3 to 4 centimetres thick, trimmed of extra fat

1 clove garlic, sliced in half

Black pepper to taste

3 tablespoons extra-virgin olive oil

½ red onion, peeled and diced

2 teaspoons fresh chopped rosemary

1 bay leaf

120 millilitres dry white wine

120 millilitres water or chicken broth

1 Spread the flour out on a large plate. Cover a second plate with the bread crumbs. Put the egg whites in a shallow bowl and lightly beat until frothy. Using a paper towel, pat the chops dry. Rub the meat with the garlic half and season to taste with pepper.

2 Dredge each chop in the flour, shake off excess, and dip the chop in the egg white. Coat each side of the chops with bread crumbs, pressing the crumbs into the meat. Set the chops aside on a platter. Refrigerate the chops at least 15 minutes before cooking.

3 Preheat the oven to 180 degrees. Put 2 tablespoons of the oil in a large frying pan and fry the chops on a medium-high heat until browned, about 3 minutes per side.

4 Transfer the chops to one end of a 20-centimetre square baking dish. Reduce the heat under the pan and add the remaining 1 tablespoon oil along with the onion and rosemary. Cook until the onion pieces soften and begin to brown, about 5 minutes. Add the bay leaf and wine, reducing the liquid to 2 tablespoons. Add the water or chicken broth and simmer for an additional 5 minutes. Remove the bay leaf.

5 Place the onion mixture in the baking dish with the chops, ensuring that the chops sit on top of the onions so they remain nice and crispy. Cover tightly with foil and bake the chops in the oven for about 30 minutes. The internal temperature when done is 65 degrees. Transfer to a platter and cover loosely with aluminium foil. Let the chops rest for 5 minutes. The meat may still remain slightly pink. Cut the chops in half and serve immediately, along with assorted side dishes such as roasted sweet potatoes, broccoli, and carrots.

Tip: Wholegrain bread crumbs are sold in health food stores.

Per serving: *Calories 307; Fat 16g (Saturated 3g); Cholesterol 49mg; Sodium 162mg; Carbohydrate 19g; Dietary Fibre 3g; Protein 23g.*

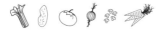

Memorable Meatballs

These meatballs are delicious, eaten as hors d'oeuvres, dipped in ketchup or barbecue sauce, or piled onto wholewheat pasta and smothered in a fragrant tomato sauce.

Preparation time: *20 minutes*

Cooking time: *15 minutes*

Serves: *24 cocktail-sized meatballs*

450 grams extra lean minced beef

1 finely chopped onion

2 egg whites

1 clove garlic, minced

1 tablespoon finely chopped fresh parsley

1 teaspoon mixed dried Italian herbs

½ teaspoon black pepper

Unrefined safflower oil to coat baking dish

2 tablespoons chopped fresh parsley

1 Preheat the oven to 200 degrees. In a large bowl, put the mince, onion, egg whites, garlic, parsley, herbs, and black pepper. Mix until thoroughly combined.

2 Line a large baking dish with foil and lightly coat with the oil.

3 Shape the mixture into meatballs about 2 centimetres in diameter, placing these in the baking dish as you finish each one. Space them out to keep the meatballs separate.

4 Place the meatballs in the oven and bake for 15 to 20 minutes, until the meat is cooked to your liking. Serve with toothpick skewers and tomato or barbecue dipping sauce.

Per meatball: *Calories 36; Fat 2g (Saturated 1g); Cholesterol 12mg; Sodium 14mg; Carbohydrate 1g; Dietary Fibre 0g; Protein 4g.*

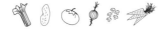

Steak Stir-Fry with Chinese Vegetables

This recipe is a great introduction to stir-frying, a useful technique for turning small amounts of meat into a satisfying meal. Stir-frying cooks food at very high temperatures, using only a small amount of fat. Constant stirring and tossing stops the ingredients burning as they cook. The shiitake mushrooms in this dish give a rich flavour, but as an alternative, use the more exotic dried wood ear mushrooms that you can find for sale in Chinese grocery stores. Wood ear mushrooms contain blood-thinning compounds also present in garlic and onions.

Preparation time: *20 minutes, plus 2 hours for the meat to marinate*

Cooking time: *8 minutes*

Serves: *4*

60 millilitres low-sodium soya sauce

2 tablespoons hoi sin sauce

1 tablespoon sherry (optional)

350 grams steak, cut across the grain in ½-centimetre slices, cut into 3-centimetre lengths (see Figure 15-1)

2 tablespoons unrefined safflower oil

1 clove garlic, crushed and minced

1 tablespoon minced fresh root ginger

1 tablespoon roasted sesame oil

225 grams pak choi (Chinese cabbage) cut crosswise in 2-centimetre pieces

60 grams fresh mushrooms, shiitake or wood ear

2 spring onions, trimmed and cut crosswise into ½-centimetre slices

225 grams mangetout washed and trimmed

1 Mix the soya sauce, hoi sin sauce, and, if desired, the sherry in a medium-sized bowl. Add the beef and turn to coat with the marinade. Cover the bowl with plastic wrap and set the beef in the refrigerator to marinate for 2 hours.

2 Remove the meat from the refrigerator and transfer it to a plate where excess marinade can drain. Turn the heat on under a wok or large frying pan. Put the olive oil in the wok, and when it's very hot, add the meat. Stir and toss continuously, cooking for no more than 2 minutes. Halfway through, add the garlic and ginger. Transfer the meat to a clean bowl and cover with a plate to keep warm. Set aside the leftover marinade to add to the stir-fry later.

3 Add the roasted sesame oil to the wok, along with the pak choi and mushrooms. Stir-fry for 2 minutes and then add the reserved marinade. After 30 seconds, add the spring onions and mangetout. Stir-fry for an additional 45 seconds, making sure that the marinade comes to the boil to cook any meat juices in the liquid. Add water if necessary.

4 Remove the wok from the heat. Add the meat and combine with the vegetables. Serve immediately with regular brown rice or aromatic brown basmati rice.

Tip: *If you want large portions, add more vegetables.*

Per serving: *Calories 253; Fat 14g (Saturated 2g); Cholesterol 50mg; Sodium 734mg; Carbohydrate 9g; Dietary Fibre 3g; Protein 23g.*

Cutting Across the Grain

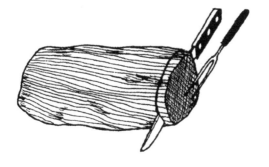

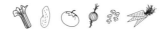

Chapter 16

Sparking Flavours with Seasonings and Sauces

. . . .

In This Chapter

▶ Replacing salt with lots of herbs and spices

▶ Savouring heart-friendly salsa

▶ Stirring up homemade sauces

. . . .

Recipes for a healthy heart are usually low in fat and salt. Sadly, this means that though your heart benefits, your taste buds can lose out. Both fat and salt help you taste the flavours of other ingredients, which is why hollandaise and steak sauce enhance the taste of meat in such a delicious way. However, this chapter proves that creating tantalising sauces and condiments using other ingredients such as fresh herbs, exotic spices, garlic, celery, and onions is perfectly possible. Reducing a sauce to intensify flavour also works, and is the secret to the Sweet Red Pepper Sauce later in this chapter.

Some of the recipes in this chapter are updated versions of old favourites, with added healthy ingredients, such as the one for Cranberry Sauce with Caramelised Onions and Cinnamon. Others, such as the recipe for Asian Cucumber Relish, provide a new condiment to add to your culinary skills. You also have the chance to experiment with herb and spice pairings and come up with your own combinations. And this chapter gives you tips on shopping for herbs and spices, too. You can turn an ordinary dish into something quite special when you serve it with one of the condiments prepared from recipes in this chapter.

Seasoning for Less Salt

Heart-friendly diets aimed at lowering cholesterol usually include a recommendation to limit sodium intake. If you have high blood pressure, your doctor has probably already advised you to cut back on salt during cooking and at the table. This advice probably sounded like being sentenced to a lifetime of eating bland food, but fear not. As you cut back on salt, your taste buds adjust to this change and soon – usually within four weeks – you start to find that even lightly-salted foods are more than salty enough for you.

You can also bring out the flavour of food with substances other than salt. Adding fresh lemon or lime juice or a dash of vinegar can enhance flavours, with lime in particular interacting with taste buds to accentuate low salt flavours. Strong herbs and spices, such as garlic, ginger, cayenne, and hot pepper sauce, also eliminate the need for salt. Or make up some herb and spice mixtures with complex flavours that keep your mind off the missing salt while your taste buds are adjusting. This chapter tells you how.

Another way to cut back on salt is to stay away from seasoned salts, pickle condiments, and salty commercial sauces. Here are some likely suspects:

- ✔ Garlic salt
- ✔ Onion salt
- ✔ Celery salt
- ✔ Lemon-pepper
- ✔ Seasoning blends
- ✔ Hot dog and burger pickles and relishes
- ✔ Soya sauce
- ✔ Barbecue sauce
- ✔ Tomato sauce
- ✔ Brown sauce

When buying seasoning blends, always check the labels for their sodium content. Some brands even include salt in spice rubs, chilli powder, and curry powder. As a guide, more than 1.5 grams of salt or 0.6 grams of sodium per 100 grams is high. Low is less than or equal to 0.3 grams of salt or 0.1 grams of sodium per 100 grams. Figures between these two levels are classed as medium.

Doing the herb shuffle

Herbs are the leaves and soft stems of plants. You can buy them fresh in the produce department of any supermarket and the range available is now much wider than just traditional parsley. You can also grow fresh herbs at home. Plant nurseries carry an assortment, which changes according to the season. Often a pot containing a living plant doesn't cost much more than a meagre pack of fresh herbs from the shops. Just set the pot in a sunny spot on your kitchen window, water regularly, and harvest a continuous supply.

When shopping for fresh herbs select those with a healthy green colour and avoid those that are limp and yellowing. And do the sniff test – check that the herbs have a clean scent.

If you don't want to look after plants, your other option is to buy dried herbs, which are widely available, easy to measure, and come whole, flaked, ground, or powdered. The main concern here is whether the dried herbs are old and stale. The flavour in dried herbs comes from their essential oils, which lose their strength and character after exposure to air, heat, and light. Discard any that smell of old hay.

Buy only dried herbs packaged in airtight jars instead of those that come in Cellophane bags, which let in air, and buy in small amounts that are less likely to go off before they are used.

To cook with herbs, try simply adding a single herb to a recipe you're preparing, such as basil in tomato sauce or sage in a chicken stew. Often one extra flavour note is all you need to elevate an ordinary dish to something special. Certain herbs are best with certain foods. Here's a list of herbs (and spices, which are usually more fragrant and aromatic) that partner well with various staples:

- **With beef:** Bay leaf, rosemary, parsley, chives, marjoram, garlic, summer savoury, and cloves.
- **With pork:** Sage, summer savoury, cumin, coriander, garlic, rosemary, and bay.
- **With poultry:** Rosemary, bay, thyme, oregano, summer savoury, garlic, and tarragon.
- **With fish:** Dill, fennel, garlic, parsley, tarragon, coriander, and parsley.
- **With grains:** Parsley, coriander, mint, summer savoury, garlic, dill, and sage.
- **With vegetables:** Basil, chives, oregano, garlic, rosemary, tarragon, and parsley.

Garlic is a bulb, and so is technically a spice, rather than a herb.

Stepping out with spices

Spices are aromatic or pungent seasonings that come from the bark (cinnamon), buds (capers), berries (vanilla), roots (ginger), flower stigmas (saffron), and seeds (coriander) of plants. They are usually for sale dried. Spices are at the heart of such culinary classics as Indian curry, Mexican sauces, Chinese Szechwan, and Thai dishes. For best results, cook with the freshest, highest quality spices. We like to use organic, Fairtrade spices, bought online – take a look at the Steenbergs website (www.steenbergs.co.uk).

Several spices are good for heart health. Ginger thins the blood and enhances circulation, and may help to lower cholesterol levels by stimulating the conversion of cholesterol to bile acids. Turmeric, thanks to a compound called curcumin, helps to dampen down inflammation that can promote hardening and furring up of the arteries (atherosclerosis). Curry powder and the Moroccan spice mixture, ras el hanout (also available from www.steenbergs.co.uk), both contain turmeric (try the curcumin-containing Moroccan Chicken with Couscous in Chapter 13).

Certain spices are best with specific foods. The following pairings guarantee a successful combination:

- ✔ **With beef:** Onion, garlic, cloves, mustard, ginger, paprika, and pepper.
- ✔ **With pork:** Ginger, garlic, onion, mustard, coriander, cardamom, and allspice.
- ✔ **With chicken:** Cumin, coriander, cinnamon, star anise, garlic, turmeric, and sesame.
- ✔ **With fish:** Fennel, capers, onion, garlic, ginger, saffron, and celery seed.
- ✔ **With grains:** Saffron, cinnamon, clove, nutmeg, turmeric, garlic, and onions.
- ✔ **With vegetables:** Onions, garlic, ginger, celery seed, nutmeg, capers, and pepper.

Both onion and garlic are roots, and so they're technically spices, not herbs.

Wanting more: A chorus line of complex herb and spice mixtures

When you combine herbs or spices, the results are often symphonic. Some mixtures are true classics, developed over many centuries:

✔ **Chinese five-spice powder** is a pungent mixture of equal parts cinnamon, cloves, fennel seed, star anise, and Szechwan peppercorns.

✔ **Herbes de Provence** is a savoury blend of basil, fennel seed, lavender, marjoram, rosemary, sage, summer savoury, and thyme.

✔ **Ras el hanout,** which comes from Morocco, means literally 'head of the shop', referring both to the spice shop owners who assemble their own blends, and to the Ethiopian king, known as the Ras. An authentic mixture may contain between 20 and 50 ingredients, including dried rose buds.

Many upscale markets sell these spice mixtures ready-made.

You can also try blending your own herbs and spices by grinding the ingredients with a mortar and pestle or in an electric spice/coffee grinder. Below, we suggest three magical formulas:

✔ **Savoury herb seasoning:** 3 teaspoons basil, 2 teaspoons summer savoury, 2 teaspoons celery seed, 2 teaspoons ground cumin seed, 2 teaspoons sage, 2 teaspoons marjoram, and 1 teaspoon thyme, or better yet, lemon thyme.

✔ **Lemon garlic seasoning:** 2 teaspoons garlic powder, 1 teaspoon dried basil, and 1 teaspoon dried lemon peel.

✔ **Spicy seasoning:** 1 teaspoon black pepper, 1 teaspoon ground ginger, 1 teaspoon ground coriander, and ½ teaspoon dried oregano.

Saffron luxury

Saffron is a rare spice that consists of the stigmas of a certain small purple crocus (*Crocus sativus*). The stigmas are the wispy parts in the centre of a flower that receive pollen during bee pollination. Obviously, harvesting and gathering a sizeable amount of these tiny bits presents a challenge. Each crocus has only three stigmas, and it takes almost 14,000 of these stigmas to produce just 28 grams of spice. This makes saffron the world's most expensive spice by weight, which is why supermarkets sell saffron in tiny glass vials holding only a few saffron strands and charge you as if it were gold. If you see large amounts for sale at an unusually cheap price, you can bet it isn't true saffron. Fortunately, a little of this precious spice goes a long way; a couple of strands are sufficient to flavour an entire dish such as a poached sea bass.

Saffron is an essential ingredient in recipes for Spanish paella, Italian risotto, and French bouillabaisse. European cooking uses saffron in stews and broths. In India, to develop the richest saffron colour, cooks briefly dry roast the spice, crush it, and then soak the saffron for an hour in a couple tablespoons of warm milk. Cooks also use saffron to impart its yellow-orange colour to dishes such as rice pilaf.

You can buy saffron in powder form, although it loses its flavour readily and is easily adulterated, and so only buy whole saffron threads if you can.

You can make your own version of ras el hanout with just 11 herbs and spices. Here's what you need:

- 2 teaspoons black pepper
- 2 teaspoons dried ginger
- 1 teaspoon ground cumin
- 1 teaspoon ground cinnamon
- 1 teaspoon ground coriander
- 1 teaspoon ground allspice
- 1 teaspoon ground cardamom
- ½ teaspoon ground nutmeg
- ½ teaspoon turmeric
- ¼ teaspoon ground cloves
- ¼ teaspoon cayenne

Put all the spices in a small bowl and thoroughly combine. The Moroccan Chicken with Couscous in Chapter 13 calls for this spice mixture.

If you own only a couple of these spices, you may feel hesitant to invest in all the others. In fact, the ingredients in ras el hanout make a great starter set for a spice cabinet, so why not stock up on all these useful seasonings.

Dancing Salsa

Salsa is rapidly taking its place next to other popular British condiments such as ketchup and mustard. Like so many time-honoured, traditional foods, salsa is naturally healthy. Standard salsa includes tomato, onion, garlic, and chillies – all good for the heart. Here's a rundown of their specific benefits.

Twirling with tomatoes

Tomatoes are a rich source of carotenoid antioxidants, such as betacarotene and lycopene, as well as vitamins C and E. These are necessary ammunition for protecting your cardiovascular system because they prevent oxidation of cholesterol in your circulation (see Chapter 2 for more on antioxidants). Fresh tomatoes are also naturally low in sodium and high in potassium, a ratio that counteracts high blood pressure. What's more, a single medium tomato adds up to only about 35 calories.

One of the main antioxidants in tomatoes is lycopene. Cooked tomatoes have more available lycopene than raw tomatoes, and fat increases its absorption into the body. Now there's a good reason to think of pizza as a healthy food!

Some supermarket tomatoes have a tendency to taste flavourless, mushy, and under-ripe. But some of the problems come from how they're handled after you get them home. Here are a few guidelines to follow:

- Store vegetables at room temperature. Cold arrests the ripening process of tomatoes, turns them mushy, and kills their flavour.

- Place tomatoes on the worktop, stem end up, not on the 'bumps', the shoulders of the tomato that are the most tender part. If you leave them on their shoulders for a few days, the weight of the tomato itself is enough to bruise them. And when bruises appear, spoilage eventually follows.

- Ripe tomatoes hold perfectly well for a few days at room temperature. Buy enough to last you only three or four days.

Stepping out with onions

Onions are also good for your heart. Research shows that adding onions to a high-fat diet helps to lower your LDL cholesterol levels. Onions also raise the 'good' HDL cholesterol. In fact, eating one medium-sized onion a day, preferably raw, raises HDL as much as 30 per cent (but may not win you many friends). Onions also act as a blood thinner, able to counteract the effects of a fatty meal and help reduce inflammation. They're even a good source of antioxidant vitamin C and provide small amounts of B vitamins and trace minerals.

When you want red meat and nothing else will do, select lean steak and top it with lots of sautéed onions. The onions contain antioxidants that help to protect LDL cholesterol from oxidation.

With all these benefits, onions are worth eating every day, which is easy to do because their flavour goes well with practically any food, from eggs and fish to vegetables, grains, and beans. But which kind of onion is best for each dish? The variety of onions you sometimes see for sale is confusing. Identifying the spring onions and leeks is easy, but what about all those white, red, yellow, and brown globes? The following list explains their differences:

- **Yellow onions:** A truly all-purpose onion, good raw or cooked. They have a medium to strong flavour that stays intact even when you cook them for hours.

- **Red onions:** Best for eating raw to add a sweet crunchy bite to salads. Cooking turns red onions watery, and they lose their royal colour.

- **White onions:** The most pungent onions in the market, with a sharp flavour and strong bite, white onions have a shorter shelf life because of their higher water content.

- ✔ **Green onions:** Most of the onion, including the white base and the green leaves, is edible except for the white roots. The bottom has a rounded base, indicating the beginning of a bulb. Select those with the most white up the stem. Eat raw or prepare them like leeks, braised in stock.

- ✔ **Spring onions:** Similar to green onions but with a flat base. You can use spring onions interchangeably with green onions although spring onions are milder.

- ✔ **Spanish onions:** Large, spherical onions with a golden brown skin. Their sweet taste suits all types of cooking.

- ✔ **Pearl onions:** This very small onion is best for peeling and simmering whole in casseroles and stews, and dishes such as coq au vin (chicken in wine).

- ✔ **Shallots:** Crisp, with a refined, delicate flavour, more intense than onions but not as hot. You can eat shallots raw and use them to add sophistication to oil-and-vinegar dressings. You can also roast or grill shallots for an elegant onion topping on chops and steaks.

Gambolling with garlic

For garlic lovers, you can never have too much. If you like the taste, you're in luck because garlic is one of the most medicinal of foods. Garlic helps to protect against heart disease and stroke because it lowers blood pressure, makes the arteries more elastic, and inhibits unwanted clotting to thin the blood.

Some scientific evidence exists that garlic lowers cholesterol. In one combined analysis of 12 well-designed studies from various countries, published in 1994 in the *Journal of the Royal College of Physicians*, supplementation of garlic in many forms was associated with a 12 per cent reduction in total cholesterol after only 4 weeks of treatment. In another meta-analysis, garlic was shown to reduce cholesterol levels by around 6 per cent. Although the benefits of taking garlic supplements to reduce cholesterol is still under debate, research does suggest that regular consumption of garlic in the diet can lower total cholesterol. Indeed, garlic belongs in a cholesterol-lowering diet as part of an overall strategy. Aiming for one or two average-sized cloves of garlic a day isn't difficult to do if you like Italian food.

Allicin, a sulphur compound in garlic, is responsible for garlic's health benefits. Heat destroys allicin, and so eating garlic raw or lightly cooked is best.

The medicinal properties of garlic develop when you crush or chop a bulb and the garlic juices begin to flow, releasing two substances that react with each other to form allicin. When cooking with garlic, first crush the bulbs and let them sit for 10 minutes while this alchemy proceeds, and add garlic only towards the end of cooking so that the heat doesn't destroy it. The fresh minced garlic that you can buy in jars from supermarkets retains these active compounds, but don't expect benefits from garlic powder or garlic salt.

Chomping on chilli peppers

Chillies get your attention; they are a fiery addition that can enliven mild ingredients. The heat comes from *capsaicin*, the medicinal compound in chillies that is concentrated in the soft core of the pepper, in the white membranes that support the seeds. By carefully removing these seeds, you can temper the heat of a chilli. You can also avoid the capsaicin altogether by using sweet bell peppers instead. Figure 16-1 shows you how to deseed a pepper and cut it into strips – a technique known as *julienning*.

HOW TO SEED AND JULIENNE A CHILLI PEPPER

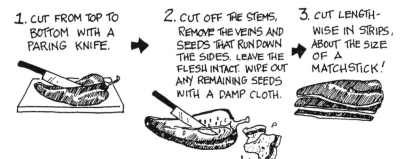

Figure 16-1: Coring a chilli pepper and removing the seeds and membranes.

1. CUT FROM TOP TO BOTTOM WITH A PARING KNIFE.

2. CUT OFF THE STEMS, REMOVE THE VEINS AND SEEDS THAT RUN DOWN THE SIDES. LEAVE THE FLESH INTACT. WIPE OUT ANY REMAINING SEEDS WITH A DAMP CLOTH.

3. CUT LENGTH-WISE IN STRIPS, ABOUT THE SIZE OF A MATCHSTICK!

If you chomp down on a fiery chilli and can't take the heat, put out the fire with a swig of milk. Milk contains *casein*, a protein that's particularly effective at washing away capsaicin. When you're handling chillies without gloves, dipping your fingers in milk also helps cool fiery hands.

Chillies stimulate circulation and thin the blood. Some evidence also suggests that capsaicin can lower blood pressure. Chillies are also loaded with antioxidant carotenoids and vitamin C. The hotter the pepper, the more capsaicin it contains. Here's how some various chillies rank:

- **Hottest:** Dorset Naga, Habanero, and Scotch bonnet
- **Medium hot:** Cayenne, jalapeño, and Tabasco sauce
- **Mildest:** Anaheim, Pimento, and Pepperoncini

Beating Better Sauces

We're not suggesting that you should never buy a bottle of ketchup or hot dog mustard, but we do hope you remember that bottled sauces and condiments are loaded with salt, and often sugar. Ketchup contains table sugar (sucrose) and salt – each tablespoon gives you 210 milligrams of sodium. So don't load them on your food like there's no tomorrow. In addition, some condiments, such as mayonnaise, may contain partially hydrogenated oil, a source of trans fatty acids, and so check labels.

But you can sidestep the search for a healthy condiment or sauce by making your own. Heart-healthy condiments and sauces are very easy to make at home, and you're likely to find that they taste even better than those you usually buy. Try the following condiment and sauce recipes to add a healthy little zing to your meals.

Saucing things up

Sample the three condiments that follow. The first is a gourmet version of cranberry sauce with sautéed onions to update a turkey dinner.

The second is a version of salsa that replaces the tomato with fruit. Although mango salsa is a winner, you're more likely to have an apple on hand than a mango, and so this recipe shows you how to cook up some Apple Salsa. It tastes so good that this salsa may miss the dinner table altogether, because it's often eaten straight from the bowl!

The third recipe uses many of the standard salsa ingredients but with the addition of rice wine vinegar it becomes an Asian relish, creating a relish that complements Asian food.

☉ Cranberry Sauce with Caramelised Onions and Cinnamon

Even though fresh cranberries are naturally very tart, this relish proves that you don't always have to add cupfuls of sugar to make them tolerable, thus saving you empty calories and carbs. The caramelised onions in this dish, and even the salt and pepper, distract the palate. The result is a relish that offers a bright balance of flavours, savoury and fruity. Try this cranberry relish on the Turkey Burger in Chapter 14.

Preparation time: *10 minutes*

Cooking time: *20 minutes*

Servings: *25 (about 500 millilitres in total, 20 millilitres each)*

200 grams fresh or frozen cranberries, rinsed

250 millilitres unsweetened apple juice

1 cinnamon stick, or ½ teaspoon cinnamon, ground

1 tablespoon extra-virgin olive oil

1 medium yellow onion, cut in half vertically and each half cut crosswise into ½-centimetre slices

2 teaspoons honey

Black pepper, crushed

1 Put the cranberries, apple juice, and cinnamon in a saucepan. Bring to the boil over a medium-high heat.

2 Reduce the heat and simmer gently for about 5 minutes, cooking until the cranberries soften and begin to pop. If using frozen berries, cook them for 10 minutes. Remove from the heat and set aside.

3 Meanwhile, in a large, heavy-bottomed frying pan, heat the oil over a medium heat. Add the onion and honey. Cook for about 12 minutes, stirring occasionally, until the onion turns golden brown. Season to taste with black pepper.

4 Add the onions to the cranberry mixture and combine. Season to taste with additional pepper, and honey.

Tip: *This is a really tasty recipe, but if you find it too tart, try sweetening with a little more honey or a splash of orange juice.*

Per serving: Calories 16; Fat 1g (Saturated 0g); Cholesterol 0mg; Sodium 1mg; Carbohydrate 3g; Fibre 0g; Protein 0g.

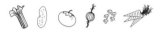

Apple Salsa

The classic ingredients in this salsa – onions and chillies – stimulate circulation and counteract inflammation. Adding to the flavour and texture, the apple also provides a source of soluble fibre that lowers cholesterol.

Special tools required: *Food processor*

Preparation time: *15 minutes, plus 1 hour refrigeration time*

Servings: *25 (500 millilitres in total, 20 millilitres each)*

1 red apple, cored and coarsely chopped	*1 clove garlic, peeled*
1 medium onion, coarsely chopped	*1 tablespoon apple cider vinegar*
Handful coriander leaves, stems removed	*2 teaspoons chilli powder*

1 Place the apples, onion, coriander, garlic, vinegar, and chilli powder in a food processor fitted with a metal blade.

2 Process the ingredients, pulsing on and off 2 or 3 times, until the pieces of apple and onion are cut into ½-centimetre pieces.

3 Transfer mixture to a bowl. To combine the flavours, refrigerate for 1 hour before serving.

Go-With: *Serve with the Tinned Tuna Fish Cakes in Chapter 14 or as a substitute for the Cranberry Sauce with Caramelised Onions and Cinnamon on the Turkey Burger in Chapter 13.*

Per serving: Calories 6; Fat 0g (Saturated 0g); Cholesterol 0mg; Sodium 3mg; Carbohydrate 1g; Dietary Fibre 0g; Protein 0g.

☞ Asian Cucumber Relish

This relish tastes just like those delicious relishes you find in Thai restaurants, only prettier because of the red pepper and red onion. It's a truly mouth-watering way to ensure that you eat heart-healthy onions, red peppers, and ginger. Enjoy this relish with the Grilled Chicken with Creamy Peanut Sauce in Chapter 13.

Preparation time: 15 minutes, plus 1 or 2 hours refrigeration time

Servings: 40 (720 millilitres in total, 18 millilitres each)

1 cucumber	½ red onion
½ sweet red pepper, prepared as in Figure 16-1	1 tablespoon chopped coriander leaves
	60 millilitres rice wine vinegar
1 tablespoon ginger root, minced as in Figure 9-2 in Chapter 9	Black pepper, crushed

1 Peel the cucumber and cut it in half lengthwise. Cut each length crosswise in very thin slices, using a knife or a mandolin slicer. Place in a medium-sized bowl.

2 Place the prepared pepper and ginger root in the bowl with the cucumbers.

3 Cut the ½ onion in half vertically. Cut each quarter horizontally into very thin slices.

4 Place the onion, along with the coriander and rice wine vinegar in the bowl with the cucumbers and red pepper.

5 Mix all the ingredients well. Season to taste with black pepper.

6 Refrigerate, covered, for an hour or two before serving to allow the flavours to mingle.

Per serving: Calories 2; Fat 0g (Saturated 0g); Cholesterol 0mg; Sodium 1mg; Carbohydrate 1g; Dietary Fibre 0g; Protein 0g.

Savouring sauce and spread recipes

The two recipes that follow give you alternatives to mayo and ketchup in the forms of a tofu-based sandwich spread and a spicy purée of sweet red peppers. Both recipes are full of flavour, without loads of added salt or sugar.

⊙ Creamy Sandwich Spread

This pleasantly light tofu-yogurt mixture provides an eggless spread with the look and feel of mayonnaise. For best results, use mild-flavoured tofu to act as a background for the more assertive flavours of mustard and garlic. This keeps for around a week in the fridge.

Special tools required: *Food processor*

Preparation time: *15 minutes*

Serves: *8*

115 grams firm tofu, drained and pressed dry

4 tablespoons low-fat, plain yogurt

2 tablespoons white wine vinegar

1 clove garlic, peeled and chopped

1 teaspoon Dijon mustard, preferably wholegrain

Pinch of salt (optional)

Black pepper, crushed

1 Place all the ingredients in a food processor. Process for about 1 minute until very smooth.

2 Transfer the tofu mixture to a bowl. Season with salt and pepper to taste. Store this spread in an airtight container in the refrigerator.

Per serving: Calories 17; Fat 1g (Saturated 0g); Cholesterol 1mg; Sodium 23mg; Carbohydrate 1g; Dietary Fibre 0g; Protein 2g.

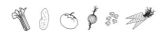

○ Sweet Red Pepper Sauce

This mouth-watering sauce is welcome just about anywhere you put it: on fish, steaks, and sandwiches, and as a garnish in soups. It's even good as a dip. All the ingredients are praiseworthy, from the garlic and onions with all their healing properties, to the sweet red peppers, which are high in the antioxidant betacarotene.

Special tools required: *Food processor*

Preparation time: *20 minutes*

Cooking time: *35 minutes*

Servings: *30 (360 millilitres in total, 12 millilitres each)*

6 medium, sweet red peppers, with skins, and coarsely chopped	*3 green chillies, seeds and veins removed, and minced*
2 cloves garlic, peeled and chopped	*240 millilitres water*
6 spring onions, trimmed and coarsely chopped	*Black pepper, crushed*

1 Put the red peppers, garlic, spring onions, chillies, and water in a large pan. Bring to the boil over a medium-high heat. Reduce the heat to medium and simmer for about 25 minutes until the vegetables are tender.

2 Season with black pepper. Set aside for 5 minutes to allow the red pepper mixture to cool slightly.

3 Using a food processor, purée the red pepper mixture in batches. Have a bowl nearby so that, as you purée each batch, you can transfer it to this bowl.

4 Strain the red pepper purée through a strainer, using a wooden spoon to rub the purée through the mesh. Discard the bits of pepper skin left behind in the sieve.

5 Return the purée to the pan and simmer over a medium heat, for 10 to 15 minutes, stirring occasionally, until the sauce is thick enough to coat the back of a spoon. Season to taste with black pepper.

Tip: Use the sauce as a sandwich spread, a garnish for soups, a sauce for chops, and a condiment for the Tinned Tuna Fish Cakes in Chapter 14.

Per serving: Calories 8; Fat 0g (Saturated 0g); Cholesterol 0mg; Sodium 1mg; Carbohydrate 2g; Dietary Fibre 1g; Protein 0g.

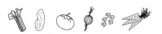

Part V
Cooking with Cholesterol-Controlling Vegetables, Beans, and Grains

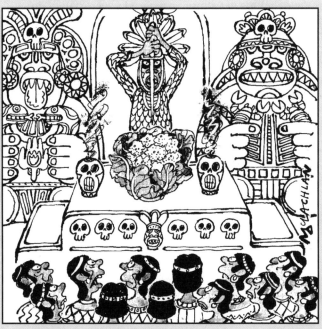

'Sacrifices are just not the same since the tribe went vegetarian.'

In this part . . .

*Y*es, you really can get excited about eating vegetables, legumes (such as beans and lentils), and
wholegrains. The four chapters in this part show you how
to prepare these foods and explain why they belong in a
cholesterol-balancing diet so that you're inspired to eat
lots of them.

This part points out which vegetables are best for your
heart and circulation, and outlines how to store and cook
them to retain the most nutrients. We lead you through
some delicious yet simply prepared vegetarian main
courses. Chapter 19 gives you insider information on preparing beans, from soaking to simmering and cooking
them, and you also discover a few bean recipes that are
destined to join your favourites list. Finally, we make a big
to-do over eating wholegrains, which do so much more for
your heart than refined products. We introduce you to the
large variety of grains available, as well as explaining how
to keep them fresh and cook them.

Chapter 17

Welcoming Heart-Friendly Veg into Your Kitchen

*V*egetables are often forgotten when talking about lowering cholesterol. In fact, they play a significant role in cholesterol balance, because of the nutrients, antioxidants, and soluble fibre they contain. Vegetables are actually more important than fruit. The only thing is, you do have to eat them!

The UK Department of Health recommends that you eat at least five or more servings (or around 450 grams) a day of fruit and vegetables, not including potatoes. However, the average Brit manages only between two and two and a half servings – half the ideal amount. Of course, if you're vegetarian, you're probably already ahead of the pack.

Whether eating vegetables is a sometimes event or you're already devoted to plant foods and just want to fine-tune your eating habits, this chapter is for you. It shows which vegetables are especially good for heart health and which are especially good to include on your shopping list. Information about the nutrients they contain follows, along with cooking tips and some suggestions for salt-free seasonings.

The chapter concludes with recipes that call for each of the vegetables we discuss. Some are treated to full-flavoured, gutsy seasonings such as the Spinach with Onions, Garlic, and Greek Olives and the Roasted Carrots with Walnuts, baked with a dusting of nutmeg and allspice. Such combinations are certain to convince the most reluctant of vegetable eaters that these plant foods are for lions and tigers and not just for rabbits.

Getting to know the Veg VIPs

Studies confirm that vegetables, along with fruit, are essential for cardiovascular health. One such study, involving over 84,000 men and 42,000 women, found that those eating the most fruit and vegetables a day were 20 per cent less likely to experience a heart attack, over the follow-up period of 8–14 years, than those with the lowest intakes. Each serving of fruit or vegetables eaten per day reduced the risk of coronary heart disease by 4 per cent. The greatest protection came from green leafy vegetables, each daily serving of which reduced the relative risk of a heart attack by an incredible 23 per cent.

Another study looking at 75,000 women and over 38,000 men found that each additional serving per day of fruit and vegetables lowers the risk of a stroke by 7 per cent in women and 4 per cent in men. *Cruciferous vegetables* (those that belong to the Cruciferae or cabbage family), such as broccoli, cabbage, cauliflower, and Brussels sprouts, are most protective, but green leafy vegetables and vitamin C-rich fruits and vegetables are also beneficial. So eat your spinach and broccoli! This chapter, and the next, give you several tasty recipes to help you to eat more heart-healthy vegetables.

Aim to have a vegetarian day one or two days a week.

Writing your vegetable shopping list

The produce section is the prettiest part of the supermarket – full of colour, and even the air feels full of life. But walk down the aisle where canned vegetables are on display, and you don't get the same buzz.

When you desire a vegetable that's out of season and not on display, go ahead and buy it frozen. First, eating vegetables that are frozen is better than eating none at all, and frozen ones are quite nutritious. The produce is flash frozen within 24 hours of harvesting and is likely to contain good amounts of nutrients at least equal to a 'fresh' vegetable that travels long distances to market and sits around in storage for a few days. The heating process used in tinned vegetables, however, can damage vitamins and phytonutrients – and some have salt and sugar added, too. Some items such as tinned beans and tomatoes, though, do seem to hold up well.

Farmers' markets offer an array of fresh produce, usually picked just the day before. You can tell how extra fresh the fruits and vegetables are when you bring them home and are pleasantly surprised at how long they stay fresh and edible in your kitchen, often much longer than shop-bought produce.

Certain vegetables are essentials for your cholesterol-lowering shopping list. They contain more of the nutrients that have beneficial effects on your heart and arteries, and many are good sources of soluble fibre that lower cholesterol, just like oat bran does. A wide variety of veg is available throughout the year, and so try to eat something different most days of the week rather than buying the same old, same old. Here are some suggestions to help get your juices flowing:

- Artichokes (both globe and Jerusalem types)
- Asparagus
- Broccoli
- Carrots
- Celeriac
- Courgettes
- Dark green cabbages (such as spinach, curly kale, and spring greens)
- French beans
- Green peas
- Leeks
- Mangetout
- Onions
- Pumpkin
- Spinach
- Swede
- Sweet potatoes

So, you have no excuse to ever get bored with veg!

Starchy versus non-starchy veg

Vegetables are basically of two main types – starchy and non-starchy. Sweetcorn, potatoes, and root vegetables such as potatoes and parsnips are starchy because they're a more concentrated source of carbohydrates and calories than other vegetables. The non-starchy veg includes leafy greens, celery, mushrooms, peppers, and tomatoes (okay, so these last two items are really fruits!). A healthy diet includes both kinds of veg, with an emphasis on the non-starchy type because they are lower in calories and supply several phytonutrients that control cholesterol and protect arteries. Another reason to opt for non-starchy is that these vegetables digest slowly and have a lower glycaemic index, causing less of a rise in blood sugar levels.

Loading up on vitamins and minerals

Think over the vegetables you eat regularly – maybe carrots, peas, sweet-corn, and some potatoes (no chips don't count!). For many people, variety means adding green beans once or twice in the summer, and yet so many other types are out there waiting for you, including important ones for heart health. The ten vegetables we feature in this chapter provide a wide range of nutrients that play a role in controlling cholesterol and are good for the heart (see Chapter 2). These nutrients include antioxidants such as betacarotene, vitamins C and E, several B vitamins such as vitamin B6 and folic acid, and important minerals such as magnesium and potassium.

Asparagus, broccoli, spinach, and sweet potatoes supply all these nutrients, with spinach having the highest amounts. And both carrots and sweet potatoes provide loads of betacarotene. You don't know how to tackle artichokes or asparagus? Don't worry! The recipes in this chapter guide you through the steps, in case cooking these vegetables is new to you.

Stocking up on plant power: The potent phytonutrients

The ten vegetables we feature in this chapter contain phytonutrients, which we explain in Chapter 2. Besides fighting cancer, these compounds also protect the heart. For example:

- Asparagus is a source of rutin, a flavonoid that strengthens capillary walls, working in combination with vitamin C.

- Globe artichoke contains cynarin, which lowers 'bad' LDL, improving the ratio of LDL to HDL cholesterol. Cynarin also increases the liver's production of bile, which requires cholesterol to produce. Bile is then excreted from the body, taking some of your cholesterol with it. Hooray!

- Broccoli and other green (and orange-yellow) vegetables contain lutein, a carotenoid that prevents the progression of atherosclerosis.

- Spinach contains lutein plus alpha-lipoic acid and glutathione – extra-powerful antioxidants that guard against stroke and heart attack, too.

The top ten includes cruciferous vegetables – broccoli, cabbage, and kale – but other cruciferous veg such as cauliflower and Brussels sprouts are also good for the heart. They contain sulforaphane, a compound that boosts antioxidant activity in several ways.

Dishing potatoes

Potatoes contain readily digested starch that quickly raises your blood glucose levels, and if you pile on the butter and sour cream, you're likely to add kilos to your weight as well as raise your cholesterol. Sweet potatoes are a better option because they have less impact on blood glucose levels and contain sky-high amounts of antioxidant betacarotene.

Chips, crisps, and other forms of processed spuds may be cooked in oils that contain trans fatty acids, and so reserve them for occasional treats. However, you can enjoy a freshly baked potato, steaming and hot, with a topping of reduced-fat yogurt and chives or non-fat sour cream and freshly ground black pepper. Baked potatoes are delightful drizzled with healthy olive oil and sprinkled with rosemary, before baking in the oven. Or try the Vegetarian Potato and Bacon Wedges in Chapter 7 and the recipe for Sweet Potato and Parsnip Purée with Toasted Pecans later in this chapter. Delish!

Supping on soluble fibre

Vegetables also provide soluble fibre, the kind that lowers cholesterol. Around 2 grams of soluble fibre is present in every 100 grams of vegetables. Admittedly, the amount of soluble fibre in veg is significantly less than in oats, but every little helps!

Here's how vegetables rank in terms of soluble fibre content, with the best sources at the top:

- ✔ Green beans and baked potatoes with the skin on.
- ✔ Brussels sprouts and pumpkin.
- ✔ Asparagus, beetroot, broccoli, and sweet potato.
- ✔ Cauliflower and boiled potato without the skin.
- ✔ Carrots, green peppers, and mushrooms.

Okra, cabbage, aubergines, and mushrooms – albeit the latter is a fungus and not a vegetable – are also good sources of soluble fibre.

Readying Vegetables for the Table

Cooking vegetables is easy because they take well to all sorts of preparation, from steaming, roasting, and stir-frying to stewing and puréeing. You can even cook them in a microwave. Whichever method you choose, the important thing is not to over-cook them, and not to pile on the salt or melted butter.

Pampering veg in the pot

Cook vegetables using a method that preserves the nutrients. When a vegetable is subjected to heat, the cell walls eventually break down, releasing juices and the nutrients inside. When you boil a vegetable to death, the good stuff ends up in the water, and you eat the depleted vegetable, a shadow of its former self. Instead, lightly steam or bake your vegetables, so that many more nutrients reach your plate.

If you do boil vegetables, use the water to make gravy, sauces, or a vegetable soup such as the Leek and Mixed Vegetable Soup recipe in Chapter 9.

Steaming basics

To steam vegetables, use a collapsible steamer insert set inside a large pan with a tight-fitting lid. Steaming is cooking over, not in, liquid, so you don't want to use so much water that it rises above the bottom of the steamer to where the vegetables sit. If you don't own a steamer, please buy one!

If you see steam escaping from the pan and you no longer hear the water moving, check to see if enough water is present. If necessary, add more boiling water to the pan from a freshly-boiled kettle.

Smartening up steamed vegetables with healthy toppings

Although steamed vegetables are very healthy, their simplicity is sometimes boring. Make them more interesting by adding some of these toppings, which all enhance the flavour without adding salt:

- ✔ A squeeze of lemon juice, plus freshly ground black pepper.
- ✔ A drizzle of healthy oil, such as extra-virgin olive oil or walnut or hazelnut oil, perhaps mixed with chopped herbs or garlic.
- ✔ A scattering of seasoned bread crumbs, along with a drizzle of oil.
- ✔ A sprinkling of gourmet vinegar, such as aged balsamic or tarragon, perhaps combined with oil to make a vinaigrette.
- ✔ A splash of hot sesame oil or pepper flakes to add some punch.
- ✔ A toss of toasted nuts – whole, slivered, or ground – to add some crunch.
- ✔ A dash of a salt-substitute or herbal seasoning.

Don't assume that a dish is low in calories or saturated fat just because it is labelled vegetarian. Sometimes, vegetarian main courses served in restaurants or included in vegetarian cookbooks have slatherings of melted cheese on top. If you can't resist eating such a dish, increase your intake of nuts and seeds and cook with healthy vegetable oils.

Because steamed vegetables have no camouflage, use only top-quality, very fresh produce.

A Diversity of Delicious Vegetarian Recipes

After you try these dishes, you'll never again have reason to assume that a vegetable meal is tasteless and boring. These recipes are packed with exuberant flavours, such as toasted nut toppings or caramelised onions. And some are so substantial – such as the Broccoli and Shiitake Mushroom Stir-Fry – that you can use them as a vegetarian main course.

⊙ *Antipasto Artichoke*

The steaming broth that cooks and scents the artichoke contains the best of Italian flavours – garlic, onion, wine, and basil. It's too good to throw away after the artichokes are cooked, so strain it and use as a dipping sauce for the artichoke leaves. When you remove all the leaves, you come to the fuzzy inner choke. Remove this with a spoon and discard, before enjoying the artichoke heart, which you eat with a knife and a fork.

Preparation time: *15 minutes*

Cooking time: *45 to 60 minutes*

Serves: *4 (as a first course)*

4 large artichokes

1 litre water

250 millilitres white wine

60 millilitres extra-virgin olive oil

1 onion, minced

4 cloves garlic, chopped

3 sprigs flat-leaf parsley, stems removed and chopped

2 sprigs fresh basil, stems removed and chopped

1 Using a serrated knife and kitchen shears, prepare your artichokes as shown in Figure 17-1. (The V-shaped cuts add a decorative touch.)

2 Put the water, wine, oil, onion, garlic, parsley, and basil in a large pot. Stir to mix. Place the artichokes, stem side down, on the bottom of the pot and cover with a tight-fitting lid.

3 Steam the artichokes on a medium heat for 30 minutes to 1 hour, depending on the size of the artichokes. Add additional water if necessary while the artichokes cook. An artichoke is done when the bottom leaves come off easily as you pull them and the flesh is tender.

Per serving: Calories 197; Fat 14g (Saturated 2g); Cholesterol 0mg; Sodium 152mg; Carbohydrate 17g; Dietary Fibre 9g; Protein 5g.

PREPARING AN ARTICHOKE

Figure 17-1: Cutting an artichoke before cooking it.

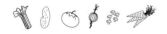

🍅 Asparagus with Mustard Vinaigrette

The flavour of fresh asparagus is so fine that fancy preparation is unnecessary. Poaching in a little water is all you need to do. Preparing the asparagus for cooking is the only thing that takes some time. First remove the tough base of each spear by holding it in one hand. Next, take the stem end in the other hand. Gently bend the asparagus until it snaps, leaving you with a tender spear and a woody portion to discard. If thick skin still remains at the base of the spear, pare this away with a vegetable peeler. To clean sand from the asparagus, set the vegetable in a large pan filled with cool water for at least 10 minutes. Repeat if necessary.

Preparation time: *15 minutes*

Cooking time: *6 minutes*

Serves: *4*

2 tablespoons extra-virgin olive oil	*½ teaspoon Dijon-style mustard*
1 tablespoon balsamic vinegar	*Black pepper*
1 tablespoon chopped shallots or more if desired	*1 large bunch asparagus, about 450 grams trimmed and cleaned*
1 clove garlic, chopped	

1 To make the vinaigrette, put the olive oil, vinegar, shallots, garlic, and mustard in a small bowl. Whisk to combine the ingredients. Season to taste with black pepper. Set aside.

2 Fill a large, wide frying pan with 2 centimetres of water. Bring the water to the boil.

3 Add the asparagus. Cover and cook the asparagus on a medium heat until just tender, about 3 to 6 minutes.

4 Drain the asparagus. Using a wide spatula, transfer the asparagus to a platter. Drizzle with the mustard vinaigrette.

Tip: *You can eat asparagus daintily by hand, picking each spear up and dipping it into a sauce, such as this vinaigrette. Arrange the asparagus tips so that they point towards the diner, making it easier to reach across the plate to pick up the thicker end of the asparagus and dip the asparagus point.*

Per serving: *Calories 80; Fat 7g (Saturated 1g); Cholesterol 0mg; Sodium 23mg; Carbohydrate 4g; Dietary Fibre 1g; Protein 2g.*

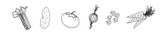

☽ *Broccoli and Shiitake Mushroom Stir-Fry*

The succulent texture of this buttery mushroom isn't the only reason to eat shiitakes: a Japanese study showed that shiitakes lower cholesterol, possibly because of a protein they contain. This is a stir-fry dish, which means that you briskly 'stir' the food by lifting up portions with a spatula and flipping these over so all the ingredients, at various times, are directly exposed to the hot surface of the wok or frying pan.

Preparation time: *15 minutes*

Cooking time: *15 minutes*

Serves: *6*

3 tablespoons hoi sin sauce

1 teaspoon hot sesame oil, or 1 teaspoon sesame oil plus 3 or 4 drops chilli oil or to taste

180 millilitres water

2 tablespoons extra-virgin olive oil

6 fresh shiitake mushrooms, stems removed, quartered

450 grams pak choi, stems cut crosswise in ¼-centimetre slices and leaves cut into strips (reserve separately)

225 grams broccoli florets, cut into 3-centimetre pieces

1 In a small bowl, whisk together the hoi sin sauce, sesame oil, and water. Set aside.

2 Heat the olive oil in a wok or a large, deep frying pan, over a medium-high heat.

3 Add the shiitake mushrooms and pak choi stems and raise the heat to high. Cook, stir-frying with a spatula for 2 minutes, and then add the broccoli. Cook the vegetables for an additional 3 minutes, until the broccoli is bright green and begins to soften. Add the pak choi leaves and continue to stir-fry for 3 minutes.

4 Add the hoi sin sauce mixture. Stir-fry and continue to cook the vegetables for about 5 minutes more, until almost all the liquid evaporates and the broccoli is tender. Serve immediately.

Per serving: Calories 94; Fat 6g (Saturated 1g); Cholesterol 0mg; Sodium 188mg; Carbohydrate 10g; Dietary Fibre 3g; Protein 3g.

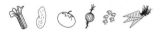

✎ Roast Carrots with Walnuts

This recipe is a great, savoury accompaniment for meats and poultry. Baking is a useful method for cooking vegetables because it takes little effort and preserves nutrients. The addition of walnuts and walnut oil adds cholesterol-lowering essential fatty acids.

Preparation time: *15 minutes*

Cooking time: *45 to 55 minutes*

Serves: *6*

2 celery sticks	*8 garlic cloves, peeled*
8 medium carrots	*1 teaspoon ground nutmeg*
4 parsnips	*½ teaspoon allspice*
80 millilitres walnut oil	*30 grams walnut pieces*
10 shallots, skinned	*½ teaspoon ground black pepper*

1 Preheat the oven to 200 degrees.

2 Trim the celery and peel the carrots and parsnips, leaving a little of any green tops. Wash in cold water and dry thoroughly.

3 Pour the walnut oil into a large roasting pan. Add the vegetables as you cut them. Slice the carrots and parsnips lengthwise in quarters.

4 Add the shallots and garlic cloves.

5 In a small bowl, combine the nutmeg, allspice, walnuts, and pepper. Sprinkle this mixture evenly over the vegetables. Mix well until the vegetables are well coated with the seasonings and oil.

6 Cover the baking pan with foil. Roast the vegetables until they're tender and browned, around 45 to 55 minutes. Stir occasionally so that the vegetables brown more evenly.

Per serving: Calories 310; Fat 16g (Saturated 2g); Cholesterol 0mg; Sodium 86mg; Carbohydrate 40g; Dietary Fibre 8g; Protein 5g.

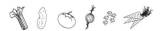

⏱ Spinach with Onions, Garlic, and Greek Olives

These greens are so dressed up with mouth-watering ingredients that even the most timid will dare to sample them. Spinach gives you a lot of carotenoids such as betacarotene and lutein, which protect your arteries. Alternatively, you can also use other leafy greens such as kale and spring greens for this dish.

Preparation time: *10 minutes*

Cooking time: *10 minutes (20 if using kale)*

Serves: *4*

3 tablespoons extra-virgin olive oil

1 onion, halved vertically and each half cut crosswise into ½-centimetre slices

1 teaspoon dried oregano

1 teaspoon dried thyme

4 cloves of garlic, skins removed and chopped

450 grams roughly-chopped green leafy vegetables (spinach, kale) thoroughly washed with any woody stems trimmed off

70 grams marinated Greek olives, pitted

Juice of 1 lemon

1 Heat a heavy-bottomed sauté pan with 2 tablespoons of the olive oil. Add the onion, oregano, and thyme. Cook, stirring occasionally, for 3 minutes. Add the garlic and cook the seasonings for an additional minute.

2 Add the spinach or kale. Cover the pan and bring to the boil over a medium-high heat. Reduce the heat and continue to cook for about 5 minutes until the greens wilt (15 minutes for kale).

3 Transfer the greens to a serving bowl. Add the remaining 1 tablespoon of olive oil, the olives, and the lemon juice. Serve hot or at room temperature.

Vary It! *For even more flavour, add a pinch of red pepper flakes to the onion and garlic when cooking this dish.*

Tip: *Store-bought marinated Greek olives sometimes have an overpowering taste. To tame them, store them in water to leach out the flavours. If the olives are still too strong-tasting after a day or two, change the water and repeat. Store marinated olives in the refrigerator.*

Tip: *Thoroughly wash your spinach to remove sand and grit. Dry in a salad spinner or on paper towels.*

Per serving: *Calories 184; Fat 15g (Saturated 2g); Cholesterol 0mg; Sodium 376mg; Carbohydrate 11g; Dietary Fibre 4g; Protein 4g.*

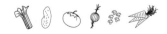

☙ *Ratatouille*

When you eat a range of colours, you consume a variety of nutrients because many phytonutrients are also pigments. A bonus of such colourful foods is that, when combined, they make a gorgeous dish. Cook this ratatouille recipe for a look at its artful shapes and hues. Serve this mixture as a side dish with chicken or fish, or as a topping for pasta to create a vegetarian meal.

Special tools required: *Collapsible metal steamer*

Preparation time: *20 minutes*

Cooking time: *40 minutes*

Serves: *6*

1 tablespoon extra-virgin olive oil

2 cloves garlic, peeled and minced

1 large Spanish onion, chopped

1 large aubergine, trimmed and chopped

1 large, sweet red pepper, trimmed and chopped

1 tablespoon coriander seeds, crushed

4 beef tomatoes, chopped

1 large courgette, trimmed and chopped

1 tablespoon fresh parsley, chopped

1 teaspoon fresh thyme, chopped

1 tablespoon fresh basil, chopped

150 millilitres dry white wine

150 millimetres water

Black pepper

1 In a large saucepan, heat the olive oil over a medium-low heat. Add the garlic and onions and cook, stirring occasionally with a wooden spoon, for about 7 minutes until the onions are translucent and the garlic is golden.

2 Add the aubergines, red pepper, and coriander seeds, and stir fry for five minutes.

3 Add the tomatoes, courgette, herbs, wine, and water. Bring nearly to the boil on a medium-high heat. Cover, reduce to a medium heat, and cook for 30 minutes, stirring occasionally with a wooden spoon, until the vegetables have softened.

4 Season to taste with black pepper and serve.

Tip: *For the vegetables in this recipe, trim tough stems and any damaged parts, but keep as much of the skins, membranes, and seeds as possible. The more complete a food is, the more health giving.*

Per serving: Calories 109; Fat 3g (Saturated 0g); Cholesterol 0mg; Sodium 18mg; Carbohydrate 20g; Dietary Fibre 6g; Protein 3g.

◌ Red Cabbage Braised in Red Wine

Red cabbage, but not green, contains red anthocyanin pigments. Anthocyanins are anti-oxidants that have a positive effect on cholesterol, preventing the build-up of arterial plaque. This benefit aside, the dish tastes great, too. The recipe uses a cooking technique called braising, in which you first brown a food (usually meat or veg) in fat and then cook it, tightly covered, in a small amount of liquid for a lengthy period of time. Braising is an easy yet handy cooking skill to have for many different recipes.

Preparation time: *15 minutes*

Cooking time: *1 hour and 45 minutes*

Serves: *6*

1 tablespoon extra-virgin olive oil	*2 whole cloves*
2 medium onions, 1 thinly sliced and 1 halved	*60 millilitres red wine vinegar*
1 red cabbage, shredded	*480 millilitres dry red wine*
2 green Granny Smith apples, peeled, cored, and thinly sliced	

1 In a large frying pan, heat the olive oil over a medium-high heat. When the oil is hot, add the sliced onion and cook over a medium heat for about 7 minutes until translucent.

2 Add the cabbage and apples. Stir to mix the ingredients.

3 Stick 1 clove in each of the onion halves. Add the onion halves, vinegar, and wine to the cabbage mixture.

4 Cover and braise the cabbage over a very low heat, stirring occasionally, until the cabbage is soft, the flavours combine, and most of the liquid has been absorbed, about 45 minutes to 1 hour. Remove the onion halves. Serve warm.

Per serving: *Calories 90 (From Fat 25); Fat 3g (Saturated 0g); Cholesterol 0mg; Sodium 17mg; Carbohydrate 17g; Dietary Fibre 4g; Protein 2g.*

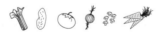

⏲ *Spinach with Peanuts and Ginger*

Even for people who don't eat their vegetables, this spinach is so full of lip-smacking flavours that it's easy to swallow. The spinach is cooked quickly to preserve nutrients. Consider chopping the spinach after it's cooked to make it even easier for your body to get at the nutrients.

Preparation time: *10 minutes*

Cooking time: *5 minutes*

Serves: *4*

1 tablespoon extra-virgin olive oil

2 cloves garlic, minced

1 tablespoon peeled and grated fresh root ginger

450 grams fresh spinach, trimmed, well rinsed, and with some of the water still clinging to the leaves

1 tablespoon plus 1 teaspoon rice wine vinegar

1 tablespoon plus 1 teaspoon reduced salt soya sauce

35 grams chopped roasted peanuts, unsalted

1 In a heavy pan, heat the olive oil over a medium heat until hot but not smoking.

2 Add the garlic and root ginger and cook for about 15 seconds, stirring, until golden.

3 Add the spinach by handfuls, stirring continuously, and cook for about 3 minutes until the spinach leaves soften. Depending upon the size of the pan, you may need to add the spinach in batches, although it cooks down quickly.

4 Add the rice wine vinegar and soya sauce. Toss the ingredients together and serve warm or at room temperature, topped with roasted peanuts.

Tip: *Thoroughly wash your spinach to remove sand and grit. Dry in a salad spinner or on paper towels.*

Per serving: *Calories 109; Fat 8g (Saturated 1g); Cholesterol 0mg; Sodium 403mg; Carbohydrate 7g; Dietary Fibre 3g; Protein 5g.*

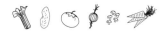

☺ Sweet Potato and Parsnip Purée with Toasted Pecans

Sweet potatoes are healthier than the name sounds, and are so loaded with beneficial antioxidant carotenoids such as betacarotene that their flesh is a lovely orange red colour. Sweet potatoes are also good sources of potassium and soluble fibre. This dish is just sweet enough and the pecans add just the right crunch.

Special tools required: *Food processor, vegetable steamer*

Preparation time: *15 minutes*

Cooking time: *45 minutes*

Serves: *8*

450 grams sweet potatoes (about 2 medium), peeled

1 Golden Delicious apple, peeled, cored, and seeds removed

450 grams parsnips (about 3 small or 2 medium)

120 millilitres semi-skimmed milk

¼ teaspoon allspice

1 teaspoon unrefined safflower oil

50 grams pecan halves (about 20)

1 Slice the sweet potatoes and apple into 1-centimetre slices. Slice the parsnip into ¹/₂-centimetre slices. Put the sweet potatoes, apple, and parsnips in a vegetable steamer over simmering water. Cover and cook for 15 minutes. Drain and cool.

2 Preheat the oven to 160 degrees. Combine the steamed ingredients with the milk and allspice in a large bowl. Purée in batches in a food processor fitted with a metal blade.

3 Transfer the purée to a 2-litre casserole. Bake until thoroughly heated, for about 30 minutes.

4 Meanwhile, heat the safflower oil in a small frying pan. Add the pecans and cook on a medium-high heat for about 2 minutes until you can smell them toasting.

5 Serve the heated sweet potato mixture topped with the toasted pecans.

Per serving: *Calories 145; Fat 6g (Saturated 1g); Cholesterol 1mg; Sodium 17mg; Carbohydrate 23g; Dietary Fibre 4g; Protein 2g.*

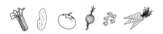

Chapter 18

Cooking Vegetarian Main Courses

In This Chapter

▶ Going without meat to keep cholesterol levels low

▶ Cooking the veggie way

More and more people are cutting back on their intake of red meat as some researchers link excess amounts with an increased risk of coronary heart disease and certain intestinal cancers. The World Cancer Research Fund recommends that we eat no more than 500 grams of red meat, such as beef, lamb, and pork, each week. Many people in the UK eat more than this.

Although you can include good quality, lean red meat in your diet (see Chapter 15), cutting back on your general intake, and excluding processed meats altogether, is a good idea for helping to improve your cholesterol balance, even if you're not a vegetarian.

If you're a vegetarian already, you have a head start in knowing how good veggie food can be. If you're a dedicated meat eater, though, aim to eat meat no more than once a day, and vary the type that you eat. For example, eat red meat one day, white meat on another day, and fish on another three days. This leaves room for two vegetarian days per week.

Tuck into the recipes in this chapter, and discover how tasty – and how healthy – vegetarian food is.

Having More Veggie Days

The vegetarian world contains so many delicious and nutritious recipes that you can be forgiven for forgetting that they're free of meat. Having one or two vegetarian days each week is a great way to explore and enjoy the variety of recipes available in cook books such as this! It's also a great strategy for lowering your intake of saturated fat and improving your cholesterol balance – as long as you don't over-indulge in butter, cream, eggs, cheese, and fried foods. Even if you don't want a full-on vegetarian day, think about having a vegetarian main meal if you eat meat for breakfast or lunch.

Going totally veggie

Some people choose to follow a 'pescatarian' or 'fishitarian' diet and follow a diet of fresh fish, fruit, vegetables, and wholegrains – a regime that can significantly improve your cholesterol balance. Other people go further and opt to become a vegetarian. Going 'veggie' is one of the healthiest ways to eat, and is associated with lower blood cholesterol levels, lower blood pressure, less obesity and, as a result, less heart disease, stroke, diabetes, and even cancer. This is partly due to its high fibre content. It's important that you don't simply cut meat out of your diet, however. New vegetarians who don't replace meat with other protein sources such as pulses, legumes, nuts, seeds, grains, and cereals are at risk of nutritional deficiencies.

Meat is a source of a number of important nutrients including protein, iron, zinc, vitamin D, and vitamin B12. Although you can get these from other food sources, a vegetarian diet can lead to low intakes of iron, zinc, vitamin B12, and if you don't get enough sunlight exposure, vitamin D. Consider taking multivitamin and mineral supplements to safeguard your intake of these nutrients.

Plant foods don't individually contain all the essential amino acids you need within one source, and so you need to eat a varied diet. For example, the essential amino acid missing from beans is present in cereals – hence, beans on toast! Combining any cereals with pulses or seeds and nuts within a meal provides a balanced protein intake, as in the Cheese and Lentil Herb Loaf recipe later in this chapter, which contains both lentils and walnuts. Other good combos include rice and bean salad, chilli beans with tortilla wraps, rice with lentil dhal, and good old bread and cheese!

Dining out on delicious veggie recipes

Vegetarian options on offer in restaurants often sound (and taste!) more delicious than the meat dishes. Try a caramelised onion and goat's cheese tart, for example, or a starter of mozzarella cheese, avocado, and tomatoes drizzled in walnut oil, or even a carrot and orange soup. Some restaurants serve nothing but vegetarian foods and are worth trying for something different. Their meals are usually low in cholesterol but remember to keep an eye on the amount of eggs, cheese, and pastry you consume.

A good restaurant that cooks food to order is always happy to fit in with your dietary needs, leaving out fatty sauces, or serving them separately on the side so you can limit the amount you consume.

Vegging Out with Vegetarian Recipes

Gone are the days when vegetarians invited for a meal resigned themselves to a cheese salad or herb omelette. The following recipes are good enough to serve to discerning guests, let alone eat yourself on your two vegetarian days per week. Pasta is a particularly good dinner option, because you can make a quick sauce using just about any vegetable and herb or spice combination you can think of. Tomato and basil, pumpkin and rosemary, spinach and nutmeg, sage and onion . . . the variations are endless.

Here are some vegetarian main meals to whet your appetite for more. When you've tried these recipes, check out Suzanne Havala's *Vegetarian Cooking For Dummies* (Wiley).

⌒ Roasted Red Pepper Devils

These devils are delicious with a simple rocket salad and some couscous or brown rice. The red peppers, tomatoes, garlic, and lemon juice in this recipe provide plenty of anti-oxidant carotenoids and vitamin C.

Preparation time: *55 minutes*

Serves: *4*

4 medium red peppers

2 tablespoons extra-virgin olive oil

4 tomatoes, diced

2 cloves garlic, crushed

2 tablespoons fresh basil, chopped

8 anchovy fillets, rinsed and drained (optional)

2 tablespoons of capers, rinsed and drained (optional)

1 red chilli pepper, deseeded and chopped

Freshly squeezed juice of one lemon

Cayenne pepper

Freshly ground black pepper

1 Preheat the oven to 180 degrees.

2 Cut the red peppers and stalks in half lengthways, and remove the seeds. Lightly brush each pepper half, inside and out, with olive oil.

3 Place the pepper halves in a nonstick, shallow baking tray. Spoon the diced tomato inside each pepper half, dividing it equally between them. Divide the garlic, basil, and chilli pepper (and the anchovies and capers, if you include them) between the pepper halves. Sprinkle with lemon juice and cayenne, and season well with black pepper.

4 Roast the stuffed peppers in the oven for 45 minutes or until the skins start to char.

Vary It! *If you prefer something less devilish, leave the chilli pepper and cayenne out of this recipe. Similarly, the anchovies and capers are optional. Have a play and invent your own combination of flavours.*

Per serving: *Calories 151; Fat 8g (Saturated 1g); Cholesterol 0mg; Sodium 318mg; Carbohydrate 18g; Dietary Fibre 5g; Protein 5g. (Analysis includes anchovies and capers.)*

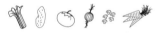

☼ Stuffed Cinnamon Aubergines

This recipe comes from Turkey and, according to legend, was so delicious that the sultan swooned on tasting it. More importantly, aubergines have a reasonably high anti-oxidant score and they provide a meaty texture to the dish.

Preparation time: *50 minutes*

Serves: *4*

2 medium aubergines, trimmed

3 tablespoons extra-virgin olive oil

2 onions, chopped

2 cloves garlic, crushed

4 tomatoes, chopped

½ teaspoon runny honey

½ teaspoon coriander seed, ground

2 tablespoons fresh parsley, chopped

½ teaspoon cinnamon, ground

1 tablespoon walnuts, chopped

Freshly ground black pepper

1 Preheat the oven to 180 degrees.

2 Cover the aubergines with boiling water and boil them for 10 minutes. Drain, and then plunge the aubergines into cold water until they are cool enough to handle. Cut the aubergines in half, lengthways. Scoop out most of the flesh, and put to one side, leaving a 1-centimetre-thick shell.

3 Lightly oil the insides of the hollowed aubergine shells and season well. Place on a greased oven tray and bake for 30 minutes.

4 Fry the onion and garlic in olive oil for five minutes or until they start to colour.

5 Add the chopped tomatoes, honey, herbs, and spices. Simmer the mixture for 15 minutes.

6 Chop the reserved scooped out aubergine flesh into small cubes, and add to the onion and tomato mixture with the walnuts and continue cooking for 10 minutes. Season to taste with black pepper.

7 Remove the aubergine shells from the oven. Stuff them with the spiced tomato and aubergine mixture. Sprinkle over the parsley, and serve immediately.

Per serving: Calories 231; Fat 13g (Saturated 2g); Cholesterol 0mg; Sodium 24mg; Carbohydrate 30g; Dietary Fibre 9g; Protein 5g.

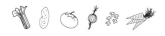

⌒ Cheese and Lentil Herb Loaf

This classic vegetarian dish combines lentils and walnuts for a balanced protein intake. You can add more or fewer nuts depending on your preference.

Preparation time: *1 hour plus 10 minutes standing time*

Serves: *4*

175 grams red lentils, rinsed

350 millilitres water

100 grams low-fat cheddar, grated

4 tablespoons walnuts, chopped

1 onion, chopped

1 tablespoon fresh parsley, chopped

1 tablespoon fresh chives, chopped

1 tablespoon fresh basil, chopped

½ teaspoon cayenne pepper

1 large, omega-3 enriched egg

3 tablespoons low-fat, natural yogurt

Juice of one lemon

1 tablespoon tomato purée

Freshly ground black pepper

A little extra-virgin olive oil for greasing the loaf tin

4 tomatoes, thinly sliced

1 Pre-heat the oven to 190 degrees.

2 Place the lentils in a tightly covered pan with the water and simmer gently for 15 minutes or until reduced to a stiff purée. Whisk the lentils to thicken them as they cook. Moisten with more water if necessary. Remove from the heat.

3 Add the grated low-fat cheese, walnuts, onion, chopped herbs, and cayenne pepper and combine well.

4 Beat the egg lightly and stir in the yogurt, lemon juice, and tomato purée. Add the egg mixture to the lentil mix and combine thoroughly. Season with black pepper.

5 Brush the inside of a 500-gram loaf tin with the olive oil. Line the loaf tin with one half of the sliced tomatoes, overlapping them to make a lining. Add one half of the lentil mixture and press down well with the back of a spoon. Top with half of the remaining tomato slices.

6 Add the remaining lentil mix and press down well with the back of a spoon. Top with the remaining tomato slices, overlapping them slightly.

7 Bake for 45 minutes or until the top is golden brown. Leave the loaf to stand in the tin for 10 minutes before turning out.

Vary It! *You can vary the herb mix and try making it with orange, yellow, green or brown lentils, or a combination.*

Tip: By arranging some nuts and chives in a pattern in the bottom of the loaf tin you can make the loaf look even more decorous when you turn it out.

Per serving: *Calories 319; Fat 9g (Saturated 2g); Cholesterol 59mg; Sodium 223mg; Carbohydrate 41g; Dietary Fibre 10g; Protein 22g.*

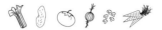

☞ *Walnut and Mushroom Nut Roast*

Mushrooms contain a form of fibre called *chitin* that helps to lower LDL cholesterol, and walnuts are an excellent source of healthy omega-3 fatty acids. Regular consumption of walnuts can also lower LDL cholesterol. So what are you waiting for? Dive in!

Preparation time: *1 hour plus 10 minutes standing time*

Serves: *6*

1 onion, chopped

120 grams chestnut or brown cap mushrooms, chopped

2 cloves garlic, crushed

1 tablespoon extra-virgin olive oil

3 medium parsnips, peeled and boiled

3 tablespoons low-fat natural yogurt

1 teaspoon fresh rosemary, chopped

1 teaspoon fresh thyme, chopped

1 tablespoon fresh parsley, chopped

1 large omega-3 enriched egg

225 grams walnuts, ground

120 grams fresh wholemeal bread crumbs

150 millilitres vegetable stock (see Chapter 9 for a home-made recipe)

A little extra-virgin olive oil for greasing the loaf tin

Freshly ground black pepper

1 Pre-heat the oven to 180 degrees.

2 Fry the onion, mushrooms, and garlic in olive oil until they start to brown.

3 Mash the boiled parsnips together with the yogurt, rosemary, thyme, and parsley, and season well with black pepper.

4 Beat the egg and add to the ground walnuts and bread crumbs. Fold them into the parsnip mix with the fried onion, mushrooms, and garlic.

5 Add the stock to the nut roast mix. Combine well and season to taste with black pepper.

6 Lightly brush a 1-kilogram loaf tin with extra-virgin olive oil. Add the nut roast mix and press down well with the back of a spoon.

7 Cover with foil and bake for 50 minutes. Leave to stand for 10 minutes before turning out.

Per serving: *Calories 425; Fat 29g (Saturated 3g); Cholesterol 36mg; Sodium 148mg; Carbohydrate 36g; Dietary Fibre 8g; Protein 11g.*

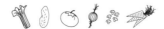

☉ Pasta with Pesto and Sun-Blushed Tomatoes

Pasta is ready to eat when it's *al dente*, which means 'sticky to the teeth'. The traditional way of checking when spaghetti is ready involves throwing a strand at a wall. If it sticks, the pasta is ready to eat!

Sun-blushed tomatoes are a good source of the antioxidant lycopene, and are a form of sun-dried tomato that is only partially dried and which therefore retains more sweetness and colour. You can buy them from good delicatessens, preserved in olive oil.

Special tools required: *Pestle and mortar, or a small food processor or blender*

Preparation time: *15 minutes*

Serves: *4*

3 tablespoons extra-virgin olive oil

3 tablespoons walnut oil (or more extra-virgin olive oil)

4 tablespoons walnuts, chopped

2 cloves garlic, crushed

50 grams fresh basil leaves, chopped

60 grams Parmesan cheese, freshly grated

60 grams sun-blushed tomatoes, chopped

Freshly ground black pepper

450 grams fresh spinach tagliatelle (or 350 grams dried pasta)

1 Pound the olive oil, walnut oil, walnuts, garlic, and basil into a smooth paste with a pestle and mortar, or use a small food processor or blender to do the same job. Stir in the Parmesan cheese and chopped sun-blushed tomatoes. Season well with black pepper.

2 Meanwhile, cook the tagliatelle or pasta in plenty of boiling water according to the packet instructions. Drain but leave moist so that the pesto sauce can coat the pasta more easily.

3 Add the pasta and pesto sauce together. Toss well and serve with a green salad.

Vary It! *Although this recipe calls for spinach tagliatelle, you can make it with any type of pasta – try wholemeal or those infused with tomato or saffron for a change. You can also get black pasta made with squid ink but, although delicious, this isn't a vegetarian option!*

Per serving: *Calories 60; Fat 34g (Saturated 7g); Cholesterol 94mg; Sodium 351mg; Carbohydrate 69g; Dietary Fibre 6g; Protein 21g.*

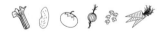

Chapter 19

Betting on Beans for Lower Cholesterol

*B*eans, lentils, and peas, otherwise known as *legumes*, are ideal foods for controlling cholesterol and supporting heart health. Legumes are very low in fat, a good source of protein, and full of the right vitamins and minerals. In addition, their high fibre content means that they have minimal effect on blood sugar levels, and reduce cholesterol absorption, too.

The only problem with beans is that most people don't eat enough. Rather than two or three portions a day, the average intake is only around one third of a serving per person per day – mostly in the form of tinned baked beans!

Let the recipes in this chapter entice you into eating more beans, and pick up a wealth of cooking tips that apply to peas and lentils as well.

Learning to Love Legumes

Plenty of evidence shows that beans and other legumes are good for your heart. A study that tracked the health of over 9,000 men and women for 19 years showed that people who eat legumes four times a week or more have a 22 per cent lower risk of coronary heart disease than people who eat legumes less than once a week. No wonder, given the many ways that legumes protect the heart. Consuming just 200 grams of beans a day can lower the 'bad' LDL cholesterol by 15 to 20 per cent in a month or so and, over a couple of years, also raises the 'good' HDL cholesterol about 10 per cent, thereby improving the important HDL:LDL ratio. Considering the dozens of ways that beans can fit into a meal, many of which we suggest in this chapter, eating the right quantity of beans regularly isn't hard to do.

Looking inside legumes

Raw legumes contain as much protein as raw steak, but with much less fat. A 200-gram serving of cooked kidney beans provides as much as 14 grams of protein, and only 1 gram of fat, almost none of it saturated. Combine legumes with a grain and you get all the amino acids your body needs to build and repair tissue. Although grains are a good source of many amino acids, they're low in, or missing, others, which are present in legumes. Because these two foods provide complementary proteins, eating them together helps you to obtain high quality protein equivalent to that found in meat. For example, you can spoon Red Lentil Dahl with Caramelised Onions (the recipe is later in this chapter) over brown basmati rice for a protein-rich main course.

Legumes are also excellent sources of folate, the B vitamin that helps keep homocysteine levels low. Homocysteine is an amino acid in the blood that needs certain B vitamins, especially folate, to break it down. Rising homocysteine levels hasten hardening and furring up of the arteries and increase your risk of coronary heart disease. One serving of lentils gives you around a third of your daily requirement of folate. Legumes also provide good amounts of magnesium, potassium, thiamin, riboflavin, and zinc. Chapter 2 outlines the benefits of these vitamins and minerals for heart health.

When you eat a variety of legumes, you're far more likely to consume good amounts of all the needed vitamins and minerals that these foods contain. Different nutrients are high in some legumes but lower in others.

Serving up soluble fibre

Legumes are a great source of soluble fibre, which lowers LDL cholesterol. In fact, a serving of kidney beans has significantly more soluble fibre than a serving of cooked oatmeal. Butter beans, black-eyed peas, and green peas also provide good amounts.

Soluble fibre forms a gel when mixed with liquid. In the intestine, it acts as a sponge, soaking up cholesterol, which the body then excretes along with the fibre. In contrast, insoluble fibre, present in the skins of fruits and vegetables, and often referred to as roughage, promotes healthy bowel movements. It doesn't seem to affect cholesterol levels.

So what, exactly, is a legume?

Legume is the species of plant on which beans, peas, and lentils grow. Beans, peas, and lentils are the mature seeds found inside the pods of the legume plants. A dried pod is called a *pulse*. So this is why a dried bean, for instance, is sometimes called a legume or a pulse. In addition, some peas are called beans, and some beans are called peas. And the chickpea is both a bean and a pea, and of course, a legume. Got all that?

Naming Names

More than 70 different varieties of legumes – beans, peas, and lentils – exist. The following list helps you sort through them:

- ✔ **Black-eyed peas:** These small, beige beans, also known as cowpeas, are easy to spot, with their deep black dot on the inner curve.

- ✔ **Black kidney beans:** The flavour of these beans is sweet, making them a perfect complement to spicy dishes. Try the Sweet and Spicy Refried Black Beans recipe later in this chapter.

- ✔ **Broad beans:** Resembling large butter beans, these tan, rather fat legumes have a pea-like flavour and a tender texture that's not starchy.

- ✔ **Butter beans:** This bean has a rich, butter flavour, and comes in two distinct varieties: the large, traditional, butter bean and the smaller baby butter bean.

- ✔ **Cannellini:** These white kidney beans are delicious in salads and soups but don't substitute them for dishes such as chilli con carne that need full-flavoured red kidney beans. Try the Cannellini and Tomato-Parmesan Ragout later in this chapter.

- ✔ **Chickpeas:** These buff-coloured, round, irregular-shape legumes have a firm texture and a mild, nutlike flavour. This bean is the primary ingredient in hummus and is used in minestrone soup.

- ✔ **Great Northerns:** Similar to butter beans in appearance, the Great Northern is a large white bean often used in baked bean dishes. Its flavour is distinctive but delicate.

- ✔ **Green beans:** Also known as string or runner beans although the fibrous string running down the pod's seam is now bred out of the bean. Both the pod and seeds are edible. Another name is snap bean, and the yellow version is wax bean.

- **Kidney beans:** This bean, curved like a kidney, is a firm, medium-sized legume with a cream-coloured flesh and a skin that is dark red, light red, or pink. Its gutsy flavour makes it a top choice for chilli con carne. Cannellini are white kidney beans, and French kidney beans are a tiny, tender version known as flageolets.

- **Lentils:** These tiny, oval pulses come in a variety of colours – green, brown, greyish-brown, red, orange, and yellow.

- **Navy beans:** These small, white legumes – also known as haricot beans – require lengthy, slow cooking.

- **Pinto beans:** This medium-sized bean is painted with reddish-brown streaks on a pale pink background. They're also known as red Mexican beans.

- **Soya beans:** Soya beans are available in many forms: whole, in custard-like cakes called tofu, as fermented tempeh, as liquid soya milk and soya yogurt, and frozen. Soya beans lower cholesterol and, thanks to the powerful iso-flavones they contain, also improve cholesterol balance. Sweet, immature green soya beans, called *edamame*, are often available in supermarkets these days, too. Try the recipe for Soya Beans with Sweetcorn and Chives later in this chapter. (See Chapter 15 for more on soya's benefits.)

Shopping for Beans and Storing Them at Home

Supermarkets stock a good assortment of beans and peas these days, whether fresh, dried, tinned, or frozen. You find an even greater variety in health food stores and farmers' markets. Ethnic stores such as Middle Eastern and Indian food shops are also great resources for the lentils and chickpeas you find in these cuisines.

When shopping for beans, shop only in stores where the turnover is high so that you're sure to bring home the freshest dried legumes.

Picking the freshest (it's okay if they're dry!)

Dried doesn't mean stale, but here's how to spot dried beans that are fresh:

- Fresh dried beans have a consistent, deep, and somewhat glossy colour.

- Beans shouldn't look faded or dry. Nor should they have wrinkles, a lot of cracks, or tiny pinholes, which are a sign of insect damage.

✓ Don't buy beans from a batch that contains a lot of broken beans.

Buy beans that have a uniform size so that all the beans finish cooking at about the same time.

Buying fresh legumes is another matter. For these, head to the produce section of the market. Look for slender beans that are brightly coloured, crisp, and free of blemishes. Fresh green peas and broad beans are usually sold in their pods, which aren't edible. The only exceptions are mangetout or sugar snap peas, which soften quickly when cooked.

A sign that bean pods are no longer fresh is that they look lumpy, the beans beneath having grown large, producing the bulges.

Fresh broad beans require special handling because they have a tough skin. To loosen the skin, cook the beans briefly in boiling water and then plunge them into cold water to stop the cooking process. Manually remove the skins before cooking the beans further.

Storing beans after bringing them home

Dried legumes keep for 12 months if you store them in tightly-sealed containers in a cool, dry place. Put them in glass jars to decorate the kitchen and so you can find them easily. Or keep legumes in re-sealable plastic bags closed with a paper-wrapped wire twist. For tidiness, you can store several of these in an airtight plastic storage box.

Fresh green beans keep for up to 5 days. Store them tightly wrapped in a plastic bag in the fridge. You can refrigerate fresh beans in their pods for up to a week if you store them in a plastic bag. Shell pod beans, such as broad beans, just before using.

Keep newly-purchased and older legumes separate. Store fresh dried beans in their own container instead of adding them to beans that are much older.

Just because beans are tinned doesn't mean that they stay edible forever. The limit of freshness for tinned beans is 12 months; that is, if the can hasn't been opened!

Doing the prep work

If you haven't cooked beans in ages, don't start thriftily and use up beans that have sat around in your kitchen for as long as you can remember. Older dried beans have less flavour and nutrients and take forever to cook. To get a better meal, you're best off buying fresh.

After buying your beans, the next step is to ready them for cooking. The prep stage is a bit involved, but after you know the drill, you can whiz through the stages quickly:

1. **Scatter the beans on a large white plate and sort through them for pebbles and stray matter to discard. Remove any broken, discoloured, or shrivelled beans.**

2. **Put the beans in a saucepan filled with water and swish them around.**

3. **Dump the beans in a colander and rinse for a minute or two.**

4. **Return the beans to the pan, which you've first rinsed out.**

5. **Add cold water, 1200 millilitres for each 100 grams of beans.**

6. **Soak the beans, refrigerated, overnight or for at least 8 hours. (You don't need to soak lentils, black-eyed peas, and split peas.)**

7. **After soaking, empty the beans into a colander and rinse them under cold, running water while moving them around with your hands.**

Now the beans are ready to cook!

Always drain and thoroughly rinse tinned beans before adding them to a recipe to remove the salt brine they're processed with.

Taking a shortcut

Yes, an alternative does exist to the overnight soaking procedure for beans:

1. **Scatter the beans on a large white plate and sort through these for pebbles and stray matter to discard. Remove any broken, discoloured, or shrivelled beans.**

2. **Put the beans in a saucepan filled with water and swish them around,**

3. **Dump the beans in a colander and rinse for a minute or two.**

4. **Return the beans to the pan, which you've first rinsed out.**

5. **Add 2400 millilitres of HOT water for each 450 grams of beans.**

6. **Heat to boiling and let boil for 2 to 3 minutes.**

7. **Remove from the heat, cover, and set aside for at least 1 hour.**

   This tenderises the beans as if they had soaked while you slept. However, at this point, the beans still need cooking.

Skipping the soak

Soaking dried beans in advance shortens cooking time by about half an hour. If you'd rather cook the beans a little longer, all you need to do is sort them, rinse them, plunk them into a pan of water, and cook them. When they're done, drain the beans in a colander. This method produces beans with more flavour but with more, er, windy side effects. (See the sidebar 'Taming beans by various means' later in this chapter.)

 Don't get surprised if you read about other ways to prepare beans that contradicts the advice in this book. You can find a range of bean truths out there, including different cooking procedures developed over hundreds, even thousands, of years. Give other methods a try and see what works for you. The way of preparing beans that you find easiest is the best way to prepare them, especially if doing it your way means that you eat heart-healthy beans more often.

Boning up on bean-cooking basics

The easiest part about preparing beans is cooking them. They go into the pan, you turn on the heat, and then you wait. Simple!

 Don't stir beans while they're cooking, especially toward the end of their cooking time: stirring breaks them up. If you must stir, use a wooden spoon, scooping the beans from the bottom of the pot as gently as if you're folding egg whites.

For guidelines on how long to cook your beans, consult Table 19-1. The cooking times are only estimates for beans that are pre-soaked; times vary depending on the age of the beans and how you prep them.

Table 19-1	Cooking Times for Soaked Legumes	
Type of Legume	*Top of Stove*	*Pressure Cooker*
Black beans	1 to 1½ hours	30 minutes
Black-eyed peas	45 minutes to 1 hour	20 minutes
Butter beans (large)	1 to 1½ hours	Not recommended
Cannellini	1 hour	30 minutes
Chickpeas	2 to 3 hours	40 minutes
Great Northern beans	1½ to 2 hours	30 minutes
Green lentils	45 minutes	20 minutes
Green split peas	1 to 1¼ hours	25 minutes
Navy beans	2½ to 3 hours	35 to 40 minutes
Pinto beans	1½ to 2 hours	30 minutes
Red lentils	20 to 25 minutes	Not recommended
Yellow split peas	1 to 1¼ hours	25 minutes

The shorter cooking times for using a pressure cooker may inspire you to buy this handy piece of cooking equipment. However, when using a pressure cooker, keep the following points in mind:

- ✔ Certain legumes, such as broad beans and chickpeas, generate a lot of foam when you cook them. To prevent this foam from jamming the valves, fill the pressure cooker only half way up.

- ✔ Legumes such as lentils and split peas are so quick cooking that they are likely to overcook in a pressure cooker. You can use a pressure cooker, but cooking them in a pan on a stove is preferable.

- ✔ Check the progress of legumes two or three times as they cook to decide if they're done. Overcooked beans in the pressure cooker may disintegrate.

- ✔ A basic formula for pressure cooking beans is to use 300 grams dried beans, 1500 millilitres water, and 1 tablespoon of oil.

Cooking kidney and soya beans

Dried kidney beans contain lectin – a natural toxin that can cause abdominal pain and vomiting. But don't worry – you can easily detoxify them by soaking them for at least 12 hours overnight, draining and rinsing them thoroughly, and then covering them with fresh water. Bring them to the boil and boil vigorously for at least 10 minutes, lower the heat, and simmer them for 1 hour until tender.

Dried soya beans contain another type of toxin that may affect the digestion of protein foods. To overcome this problem, soak dried soya beans for at least 12 hours overnight, drain and rinse them thoroughly, and cover with fresh water. Bring them to the boil and boil vigorously for 1 hour, and then lower the heat and simmer them for 2 to 3 hours until they are tender.

Tinned kidney and soya beans are fine, though, because the manufacturer has already done all this for you!

Using your bean when it comes to freezing

You can plan ahead and always have cooked beans to hand because, fortunately, beans freeze! They keep their superior flavour and texture beautifully.

Make a large batch to freeze in small portions. To use the beans in vegetable soups, meat stews, and mixed vegetable salads, put aside portions of 100 to 200 grams, an amount you can easily add to such dishes without upsetting the balance of ingredients. Freeze larger portions to have beans available for salads, starters, and side dishes. You'll thank yourself for the effort and save cooking time later.

Taming beans by various means

We all know the problem: beans are difficult to digest and can cause wind. They contain certain sugars that require a special enzyme for digestion – one that humans don't possess. To reduce this unwanted side effect of eating beans, try these tactics:

✔ Eat beans more often. Start with a small amount and increase gradually.

✔ Choose beans that are easier to digest such as lentils, butter beans, white beans, chickpeas, and black-eyed peas.

✔ Soak beans and then discard the soaking water, which is full of those hard-to-digest sugars.

✔ Add one of the many herbs that traditionally go with beans to reduce wind. Experiment with thyme, bay leaf, summer savoury, fennel seeds, or caraway seeds.

Counting beans

A few handfuls of dried beans can multiply into bowls of the finished product. Keep track of the quantity of cooked legumes you end up with by using these handy bean formulas:

✔ 200 grams of dried beans = 550 to 650 grams of cooked beans.

✔ 450 grams of dried beans = 4 to 6 servings.

✔ 1 tin (400 grams) of beans = 300 to 350 grams of cooked beans, drained.

Simmering legumes with seasonings

While your legumes are cooking, take advantage of this opportunity to let them soak up flavours. Choose seasonings that complement the recipe for a dish with deep, full flavour. Add a clove of crushed garlic, a wedge of onion, or ½ teaspoon or more of dried herbs, such as oregano, sage, or thyme. Cook the legumes in vegetable or meat broth, full strength or mixed with water, but ensure that the broth contains no salt, which toughens the beans.

Acidic ingredients such as tomatoes, lemon juice, vinegar, and wine slow down the cooking process. Don't add acidic ingredients until the beans are tender.

Drain and rinse tinned beans before using them. You remove some of the hard-to-digest sugars and about 40 per cent of the added salt as well.

Handling cooked legumes with great care

After cooking legumes, you must handle them with care. Like grains, they provide an ideal environment for bacteria to thrive. Follow these guidelines strictly:

✔ If you cook beans for later use, cool them to room temperature and then immediately refrigerate. Never leave legumes unrefrigerated for longer than 4 hours. If you do, throw them out.

✔ Store cooked beans, refrigerated, in a covered container, for up to 5 days. To make sure that they don't turn sour, bring the beans to the boil for a few minutes each day.

✔ Discard frozen beans after six months.

Loving Luscious Legume Recipes

The following recipes for preparing savoury bean dishes are accented with the flavours of piquant spices, appetising vegetables, and agreeable herbs. They give you a good mix of nutritious vegetables, legumes rich in protein and fibre, and healthy fats to satisfy your hunger and balance your cholesterol.

⌒ Garlic Butter Beans

This fierce, Greek version of butter beans is just what grilled swordfish or a chicken kebab is waiting for! Both garlic and butter beans have a positive impact on cholesterol balance, so dig in. This medicine is not hard to take!

Preparation time: *5 minutes*

Cooking time: *20 minutes*

Serves: *4*

450 grams tinned baby butter beans, drained

3 cloves garlic, crushed and chopped

2 tablespoons chopped fresh parsley

2 tablespoons extra-virgin olive oil

240 millilitres water

Black pepper, freshly ground

1 Place the butter beans, garlic, parsley, olive oil, and water in a medium-sized, heavy saucepan. Bring to the boil and cover the pan tightly.

2 Cook the butter beans on a medium heat, stirring occasionally, for about 20 minutes, until tender.

3 Season the butter beans with black pepper to taste and enjoy!

Per serving: *Calories 177; Fat 7g (Saturated 1g); Cholesterol 0mg; Sodium 121mg; Carbohydrate 22g; Dietary Fibre 7g; Protein 7g.*

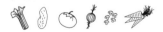

Great Northern Tuna Salad Provençal

This recipe takes its inspiration from Salade Niçoise, the speciality of southern France, and features tuna and potatoes, accented with green beans, tomatoes, sweet peppers, and hard-boiled eggs. In this version, white beans provide the starch (plus protein), and the egg garnish is omitted. For a low-sodium diet, omit the capers.

Special tools required: *Steamer or collapsible metal steamer*

Preparation time: *30 minutes*

Cooking time: *1½ hours*

Serves: *6 as a side dish, 4 as a main dish*

180 grams dried Great Northern beans (or other white beans such as navy beans or cannellini beans), soaked overnight

½ medium onion, peeled and cut into 2½-centimetre chunks

½ teaspoon Herbes de Provence

1 small bay leaf

1200 millilitres water

220 grams French green beans

1 tablespoon chopped fresh parsley

1 clove garlic, peeled, crushed, and chopped

1 teaspoon Dijon mustard

1 teaspoon capers

1 tablespoon extra-virgin olive oil

1 tin (175 grams) tuna, packed in water (not brine)

Cherry tomatoes, for garnish (optional)

Black olives, for garnish (optional)

Fresh basil leaves, for garnish (optional)

1 Place the Great Northern beans, onion, Herbes de Provence, bay leaf, and water in a medium-sized pan. Bring to the boil, partially cover, reduce the heat to low, and simmer the beans for about 1½ hours until tender. When cooked, cool and drain the beans.

2 Meanwhile, put the green beans in a steamer (or a pan fitted with a collapsible metal steamer set over water). Steam the beans, covered, on a medium heat for 4 or 5 minutes, until they are somewhat tender. Cool and cut into 5-centimetre lengths. Set aside.

3 To make the salad dressing put the parsley, garlic, Dijon mustard, capers, and olive oil in a small bowl and stir with a fork to combine.

4 Put the tuna, along with the water from the tin, in a large bowl. Add the green beans and dressing. Mix well, breaking the tuna into small pieces. Add the Great Northern beans. Toss the tuna-bean mixture together gently to mix all the ingredients.

5 Serve the salad garnished with one or more of the following: cherry tomatoes, black olives, and fresh basil leaves. Or scoop the salad into wholegrain pita pockets and eat as a sandwich.

Per serving: *Calories 160; Fat 3g (Saturated 1g); Cholesterol 9mg; Sodium 137mg; Carbohydrate 20g; Dietary Fibre 7g; Protein 15g.*

☉ Sweet and Spicy Refried Black Beans

These refried black beans offer a complexity of flavours plus a kick from the chilli pepper. The black beans also deliver lots of folate, magnesium, and fibre, and this version features only a small amount of oil.

Special tools required: *Food processor*

Preparation time: *15 minutes*

Cooking time: *30 minutes*

Serves: *6*

2 tablespoons extra-virgin olive oil	*2 tablespoons cider vinegar*
1 medium onion, peeled and chopped	*2 tablespoons honey*
1 green bell pepper, seeds and core removed, chopped	*2 teaspoons chilli powder*
	2 teaspoons ground cumin
1 green chilli, seeds and veins removed, finely chopped	*2 tins black beans (400 grams each) rinsed and well-drained*
6 cloves garlic, peeled, crushed, and chopped	*Black pepper, freshly ground*

1 Put the olive oil in a large frying pan set over a medium heat. Add the onion, bell pepper, and chilli pepper. Cook for about 10 minutes until the ingredients begin to soften.

2 To the onion mixture, add the garlic, cider vinegar, honey, chilli powder, and cumin. Using a wooden spoon, stir to combine. Then add the beans to the pan and stir until all ingredients are combined.

3 Working in batches, spoon the bean mixture into a food processor and process for about 30 seconds to purée.

4 Return the bean mixture to the pan and cook over a medium-high heat, stirring frequently, for 10 to 15 minutes until the mixture looks dry. Season to taste with black pepper.

5 Serve with a dish inspired by Mexican cuisine, such as Halibut with Coriander and Lime Salsa or Fish Stew with Sweet Peppers (see both recipes in Chapter 14). Or use the beans to top brown rice for a vegetarian main course. So delicious!

Per serving: Calories 150; Fat 5g (Saturated 1g); Cholesterol 0mg; Sodium 194mg; Carbohydrate 32g; Dietary Fibre 6g; Protein 6g.

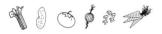

ʘ *Red Lentil Dahl with Caramelised Onions*

Dahl is a lentil dish that forms the basis of many meals in southern Asia, and is a staple food along with rice. The crowning glory of these lentils is the onions – caramelised ambrosia. Traditionally, cooking these onions requires faithful stirring for about 20 minutes while they cook. Do the best you can and make sure that you attend to the onions for at least the last 10 minutes of cooking. The lentils, onion, garlic, and seasonings in this dish are all health-enhancing ingredients.

Preparation time: *25 minutes*

Cooking time: *40 minutes*

Serves: *4*

1 tablespoon extra-virgin olive oil

1 large onion, peeled and cut vertically into very thin slices

1 clove garlic, crushed and chopped

200 grams red lentils, sorted and washed

½ teaspoon turmeric

½ teaspoon ground ginger

½ teaspoon ground cardamom

600 millilitres water

1 In a medium-sized saucepan, heat the olive oil over a medium heat for 1 minute and add the onions. Stir so that the onions cook evenly and don't burn. After about 10 minutes, the onions become limp and yellow as they lose moisture.

2 Continue to stir the onions as you cook them for another 10 minutes. The oil begins to separate from the onions, a sign that they're ready to clump together and turn light brown. Continue frying as they caramelise and start to look shrivelled up. If the onions start sticking to the pan, add a little cold water, 1 tablespoon at a time, but don't lower the heat. In the last 5 minutes of cooking the onions, add the garlic.

3 After the onions are done, add 1 tablespoon of cold water to stop the cooking. Transfer to a small bowl and set aside.

4 In the saucepan used to cook the onions, put the lentils, turmeric, ginger, cardamom, and the water. Bring to the boil. Reduce the heat, cover, and simmer until the lentils are tender, about 15 minutes.

5 Serve the red lentil dahl, topped with the fried onions, over rice for a vegetarian dish that provides high-quality protein, or as a side dish to a curry or Chicken Tandoori with Minted Yogurt Sauce (see the recipe in Chapter 13). The spiced lentils, without the onions, are also perfumed and appealing on their own.

Per serving: *Calories 211; Fat 4g (Saturated 0g); Cholesterol 0mg; Sodium 18mg; Carbohydrate 33g; Dietary Fibre 9g; Protein 13g.*

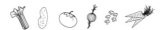

✆ Soya Beans with Sweetcorn and Chives

If you wonder just how much the flavour of butter, even a little smidgeon, can permeate a dish, try this one! One teaspoon (5 grams) of butter is a match for around a kilogram of beans and vegetables! This amount contains 4 grams of fat, including 2½ grams of saturated fat. Divide 1 teaspoon of butter into 6 servings of these nutritious beans with veg, and butter gets the green light, used as a seasoning accent. This recipe uses whole soya beans called edamame, which you can find fresh, frozen, or tinned in health food and ethnic stores. But if you can't get hold of them, just use butter beans (or any other kind of beans, for that matter) instead.

Preparation time: *15 minutes*

Cooking time: *35 minutes*

Serves: *6 (generous servings)*

1750 millilitres water	*¼ teaspoon paprika*
450 grams shelled edamame soya beans	*120 millilitres semi-skimmed milk*
1 tablespoon extra-virgin olive oil	*1 teaspoon butter*
1 onion, peeled and diced	*2 tablespoons chives, cut into 1-centimetre lengths*
1 green bell pepper, seeds and core removed, cut in 1-centimetre pieces	*Black pepper, freshly ground*
300 grams frozen sweetcorn kernels	

1 Bring 1½ litres of water to the boil over a high heat in a large pan. Add the soya beans and boil for about 8 minutes, until the beans soften. Drain in a colander.

2 Using the same pan, heat the olive oil and add the onion and bell pepper. Cook over a moderate heat, stirring frequently, for around 7 minutes until the vegetables soften.

3 Add the cooked soya beans, sweetcorn, paprika, and the remaining 250 millilitres water. Simmer, covered, for around 10 minutes, until the vegetables are tender.

4 Increase the heat to high and add the milk and butter. Boil, uncovered, for about 3 minutes until the liquid reduces by half. Stir in the chives and season to taste with black pepper.

Per serving: *Calories 197; Fat 7g (Saturated 1g); Cholesterol 3mg; Sodium 44mg; Carbohydrate 25g; Dietary Fibre 6g; Protein 11g.*

☉ Cannellini and Tomato-Parmesan Ragout

Start adding beans to your meals with this quick and easy recipe that relies on a few simple ingredients. It consists of half beans and half tomatoes, giving you a good helping of folate in the beans and the powerful antioxidant, lutein, in the tomatoes. The onions in this dish thin the blood. Scatter some Parmesan cheese over the top, and you have a high protein/low-fat dish that eats like a bowl of pasta.

Preparation time: *5 minutes*

Cooking time: *25 minutes*

Serves: *4 as a side dish, 2 servings as a lunch entrée*

400 grams diced fresh tomatoes, or 1 tin (400 grams) diced tomatoes, undrained	Black pepper, freshly ground
½ onion, diced	350 grams cooked cannellini beans (150 grams dried), or 1 tin (400 grams) cannellini beans
1 clove garlic, chopped	1 tablespoon parsley, finely chopped
½ teaspoon summer savoury or thyme	25 grams Parmesan cheese

1 Put the tomatoes, onion, garlic, savoury/thyme, and ground black pepper in a medium-sized pan. Bring to the boil and cook, uncovered, on a medium heat, for 5 minutes, to reduce some of the liquid.

2 Meanwhile, if using tinned beans, pour off the liquid and put the beans in a colander. Rinse the beans under cold water.

3 Add the drained beans and parsley to the tomato mixture. Simmer for 20 minutes. Season to taste with additional black pepper if desired. Serve with grated Parmesan on the side.

Per serving (for four as a side dish): Calories 181; Fat 3g (Saturated 1g); Cholesterol 5mg; Sodium 132mg; Carbohydrate 29g; Dietary Fibre 7g; Protein 12g.

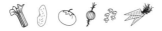

Chapter 20

Going With the Grains

*E*ating meals that include nutritious, quality grains is one way to control your cholesterol. That's why this chapter focuses on wholegrains, which are high in fibre and supply generous amounts of vitamins, minerals, and phytonutrients important for heart health. Refined grains – the standard white wheat flour and white rice of the Western diet – supply paltry amounts in comparison. This chapter compares the nutritional values of wholegrains with refined and shows you why choosing wholegrains can pay off in terms of your health.

In this chapter, you find out how easily you can add wholegrains, such as brown rice, wild rice, buckwheat, and hulled barley, to everyday meals. Wholegrains have a reputation for chewiness and looking very brown. Yet most wholegrains can fit in just fine with soups, stews, salads, and vegetables, lending a richness that's very pleasing. The pasta section is also up-to-date, featuring pasta made with wholegrains rather than refined wheat flour.

Defining the Refining Problem

Refined grains contain little to keep you healthy. Wholegrains, however, are a rich source of antioxidants such as vitamin E and selenium. The outer layer of these grains, usually lost in refining, contains the important trace minerals copper, zinc, and manganese. The grains featured in the recipes in this chapter, such as cornmeal (polenta), brown rice, wild rice, quinoa, and buckwheat provide a good dose of these nutrients, which you need for heart health.

Losing nutrients through refining

During refining, the bran and germ are removed from each kernel (see Figure 20-1), leaving only the large core of the grain, the endosperm. Unfortunately, although only a little of the bulk is removed, much of the nutrition goes with it.

Figure 20-1: Cross-section of a grain of wheat. The bran and germ contain the most nutrients, but are removed in the refining process.

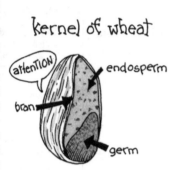

Within a kernel of grain, the nutrients are unevenly distributed. In wheat, the bran has the lion's share of fibre plus many nutrients, including 80 per cent of the kernel's entire store of vitamin B3 (niacin). The tiny germ contains over 60 per cent of the vitamin B1 (thiamin), vitamin E, and unsaturated fat. In contrast, the endosperm is mostly carbohydrate and protein, and contains only relatively small amounts of other nutrients. When wheat and other grains are refined, many nutrients for heart health are greatly reduced.

When flour is enriched, manufacturers add several nutrients back in equal or greater amounts – iron, thiamin, niacin, riboflavin, folic acid, and sometimes calcium. But even enriched, refined flour contains only 20 to 30 per cent of some 20 nutrients naturally present in wheat, and has no extra fibre added. In addition, the bleaching process that makes flour snowy white harms nutrients such as vitamin E.

Looking at what's left

Only a small percentage of the original amount of nutrients remains in refined wheat and rice. Table 20-1 shows how you're short-changed by the low level of nutrients left after refining. All these lost nutrients play a role in supporting heart health, and nutrients such as vitamin E, selenium, and zinc specifically help to control cholesterol.

Table 20-1	Nutritional Content of White Flour and White Rice	
Nutrients	*Percentage Left in Enriched White Flour*	*Percentage Left in White Rice*
Fibre	13%	22%
Vitamin B6	17%	60%
Magnesium	18%	28%
Potassium	22%	81%
Selenium	75%	77%
Zinc	20%	78%

Giving high marks to wholegrains

Scientists have put wholegrains to the test in recent years and concluded that they offer strong protection against heart disease. Researchers analysed data from 75,000 women and found that eating two and a half servings a day of wholegrain products lowered the risk of coronary heart disease by 30 per cent compared with women who consumed only 0.13 servings per day. (One serving of wholegrain is equivalent to a slice of wholegrain bread.) Another analysis of the same data found that consuming just 1.3 servings a day of wholegrains significantly reduces the risk of a stroke.

Wholegrains are beneficial for several possible reasons, including the following:

✔ They lower total cholesterol and LDL cholesterol, thanks to soluble fibre. Wheat bran in particular is beneficial.

✔ They provide antioxidants that slow the accumulation of cholesterol on artery walls.

✔ They decrease the tendency for blood to clot.

Selecting low glycaemic grains

The glycaemic index (GI) is a measure of a food's immediate effect on blood glucose levels. Eating foods with a low to moderate glycaemic index is healthier for the heart and circulation than eating those with a high GI rating. High levels of blood sugar can lead to insulin resistance (see Chapter 1) and associated high cholesterol. Eating wholegrains can help prevent this condition and, according to a recent study, even protect against Type 2 diabetes, which can raise the risk of heart disease. The benefits at least in part are due to the fibre and magnesium that wholegrains provide.

When the glycaemic index was first developed, refined wheat flour, such as that used to produce commercial white bread, was assigned a glycaemic index of 100. Based on this standard, grains such as barley, oatmeal, and wholegrain rye, which elevate blood sugar much less, rate glycaemic indexes in the range of 30 to 50.

The foods you eat along with the grain also affect its impact. A breakfast of white toast and jam is starch plus sugar and, metabolically speaking, behaves like a sweet dessert, whereas eating grains with a little meat or fish, which contain protein and fat, moderates the effect of the carbohydrates in the grains.

Growing Your Grain Choices

Consider the following easy-to-like wholegrains as you write your next food shopping list. Each has its own distinctive character. Some grains, such as basmati rice, are sweet and fragrant, whereas the flavour of buckwheat is nutlike and robust. If you want a satisfying chew, try hulled barley. Or sample quinoa, which is light on the tongue. Cook these grains for novel additions to your everyday meals, and significantly increase your intake of heart-healthy vitamins and minerals. (See Chapter 2 for their specific benefits.)

- **Barley:** Hulled barley is a wholegrain that has had only the outer husk removed. Whole barley has four times the amount of fibre present in pearl barley, which has had the hull and bran removed, and is a good source of soluble fibre, which lowers cholesterol. You can find barley and barley flakes for sale in health food shops. Barley supplies good amounts of copper, phosphorus, and zinc, as well as some vitamin B6.

- **Brown rice:** A wholegrain with a nutlike flavour, brown rice retains the germ and high-fibre bran, with only the inedible outer husk removed. Brown basmati rice is an especially fragrant variety. Brown rice supplies magnesium, vitamin B6, manganese, and selenium.

- **Buckwheat:** These triangular seeds are from a herb related to rhubarb. Buckwheat groats are hulled, crushed kernels, which cook in a manner similar to rice. *Kasha* is buckwheat groats that are toasted, and has a richer nutlike flavour compared with the milder, earthier flavour of unroasted buckwheat groats. Buckwheat groats are available in health food shops and supply magnesium, niacin, copper, manganese, riboflavin, and zinc.

- **Bulgur wheat:** These wholegrain wheat kernels are steamed, dried, and cracked before selling. This traditional grain of the Middle East has a tender, chewy texture and is used in wheat pilaf, salads, and vegetable and meat dishes. Bulgur supplies magnesium, manganese, and thiamin.

✔ **Corn:** Not a vegetable but a cereal grain, corn is a member of the grass family, along with barley and oats. The Italians use corn to make their gourmet classic, polenta. Corn supplies thiamin, pantothenic acid, niacin, folate, vitamin C, magnesium, and potassium.

✔ **Millet:** Millet is a small, high-protein grain that is a staple in human diets throughout Africa and Asia. We eat millet hulled, but pet shops sell the unhulled version as birdseed. Treat yourself to this light, nutty grain in hot cereal and pilaf, and buy a little extra for your parakeet. Millet supplies calcium, riboflavin, and niacin.

✔ **Oats:** This grain is an excellent source of soluble fibre. Whole oats, which are the grain form fed to horses, are cleaned, toasted, hulled, and cleaned again, and then steamed and flattened with huge rollers to make it ready for human consumption. (See Chapter 6 for more information on this staple grain.)

✔ **Quinoa:** One of the newly rediscovered ancient grains, quinoa (pronounced *keen-wa*) was a staple of the Inca civilisation. This tiny grain is light and fluffy when cooked and has a grassy, likable flavour. Use it just like rice in a variety of dishes. Quinoa is a quality source of protein, and is higher in unsaturated fat and lower in carbohydrates than most grains. Quinoa also supplies vitamin E, calcium, phosphorus, iron, assorted B vitamins, and fibre.

✔ **Wholewheat couscous:** A pasta made with wholegrain wheat that includes the germ and the bran, wholegrain couscous provides manganese, selenium, magnesium, thiamin, and niacin.

✔ **Wild rice:** A long-grain marsh grass, wild rice supplies magnesium, phosphorous, copper, manganese, zinc, vitamin B6, niacin, and riboflavin.

Buying wholegrain products

In a standard supermarket, you're likely to find boxed wholegrains, such as rolled oats, kasha, cornmeal (polenta), and brown rice. For greater variety, and to buy grains in bulk, which works out cheaper, visit a health food shop where millet, quinoa, and hulled barley are usually available. You can also buy just a recipe's worth to sample a grain that is new to you.

Figure 20-2 shows you some of the many types of foods you can make using a variety of grains.

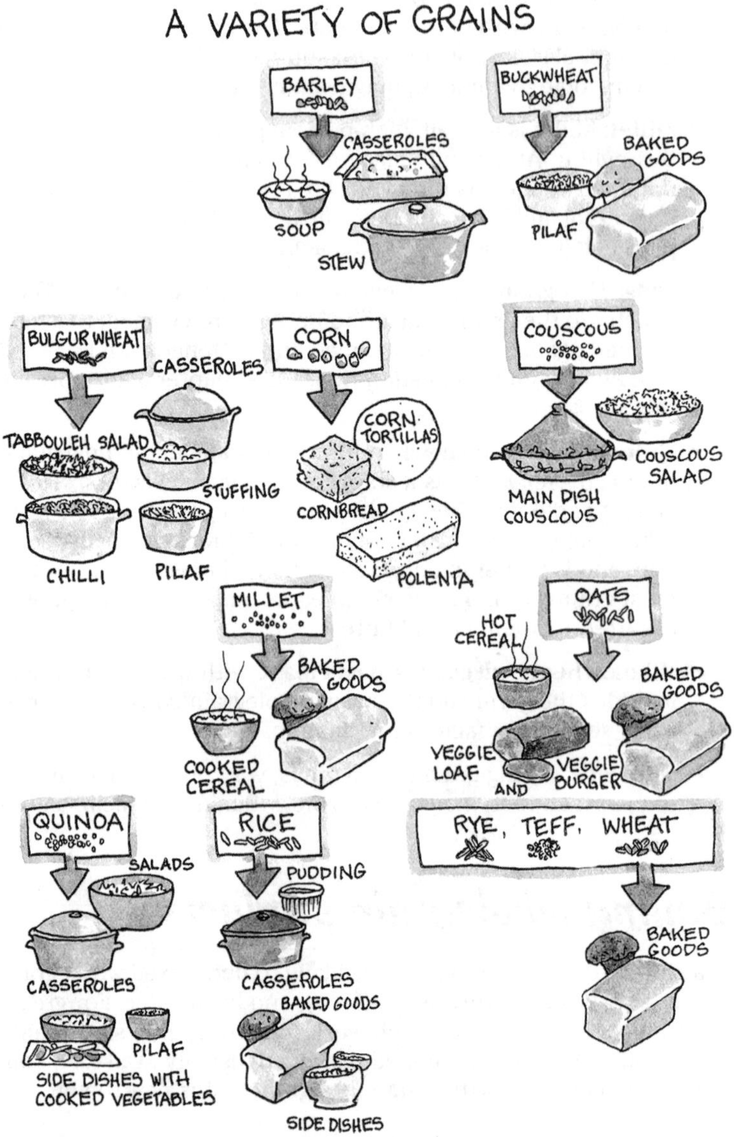

Figure 20-2: Foods made with different types of grains.

Wholegrains have a shorter shelf life than refined grains because wholegrains retain the germ, which contains oils that can go rancid. A good bet is to shop for grain in a store with a high turnover of these foods. Visit a health food store or an ethnic food shop where customers regularly go for staples such as Middle Eastern bulgur wheat or Indian basmati rice. Sniff the grain to judge freshness.

While you're at the market, also check out all the wholegrain baked goods and other products now available. Look for breads and muffins but also pitta pockets, bagels, tortillas, breakfast cereals, bread mixes, and even bread crumbs.

Look for the small loaves of thin-sliced, dense wholegrain rye and pumpernickel breads sold in the deli section of most supermarkets. The moist, rich slices are perfect with smoked salmon or toasted in the morning for a wake-up crunch.

Discovering the 'whole' truth

When it comes to wholegrain bread, the word *whole* on a label tells you that it's 100 per cent wholegrains. *Brown bread* on the other hand is a mix of white flour and wholegrain, a compromise but still a better option nutritionally than white bread. Many brands of brown bread look like wholegrain loaves, but beware; the enticing brown colour comes from caramel or molasses!

A good general rule to follow when shopping for store-bought bread is to buy a product that contains at least 3 grams of fibre per slice (or 5 to 8 grams per 100 grams) to ensure that the loaf contains a good amount of wholegrain flour. Check the label.

Reading the fine print

Shopping for wholegrain crackers, cereal, and pasta is another matter. In this case, you need to read the ingredient list to find out what's really in the product. White flour of some sort is usually the first ingredient. 'Enriched flour', 'unbleached flour', 'wheat flour', and just 'flour' also mean refined white flour. Phrases such as 'made with wholegrains' and 'all natural' are no guarantee that the items on the ingredient list are wholewheat.

Wholegrain can also mean a grain that is intact or ground, cracked, or flaked as long as all parts of the grain are present in a similar proportion to that found in the whole seed and aren't discarded during milling. A 'wholegrain food', however, is one where 51 percent or more of the ingredients (according to weight) consist of wholegrain cereal.

Easing Into Wholegrain Cookery

Cooking wholegrains isn't difficult. They only need more liquid and some extra time to cook than for refined grains. You can even cook them like pasta, without measuring the water. And preparing bulgur wheat requires no actual cooking at all! You just pour hot water over the grain and let it sit until done.

Using a sure-fire cooking technique

To prepare a grain like pasta, simply drop it into a pan of boiling water and cook until tender. This technique is easy, with no need for precise measuring or timing, and because you're cooking with plenty of water, you don't burn the grain.

Here's how to cook enough grain to yield about six servings, depending upon the grain:

1. **Fill a large pot with at least 1.5 litres of water, add ¼ teaspoon salt, and over high heat, bring the water to the boil.**

2. **Stir in 300 grams of grain, adjust the heat so that the water gently boils, and cook the grain uncovered.**

3. **If necessary, add additional hot water to keep the grains covered while cooking.**

4. **Keep testing the grain for doneness, and when it's to your taste, pour the grain into a strainer and drain. If not eating immediately, or if using in salads, place the strainer in a bowl of cold water to stop the grain from continuing to cook.**

   With wholegrains such as brown rice and unhulled barley, the cooking time is sometimes an hour or longer, although 'easy-cook' versions of brown rice are available. These versions are partially cooked and then dried – so that they can quickly reabsorb water – or are a type of Italian rice that cooks more quickly than normal brown rice.

Use boiled grain cold in a salad or as an ingredient in a cooked dish. Or eat the grain as a dish in itself. Just reheat in a frying pan with a tablespoon or two of extra-virgin olive oil plus seasonings if desired. Cook over a medium heat for about 10 minutes, stirring occasionally, until the grain is thoroughly heated.

A can't-miss grain

Bulgur wheat doesn't even require cooking. Just cover it with boiling water and let the grain soak for 15 to 30 minutes and – hey presto – it's done. Add 100 grams of fine or medium ground bulgur wheat and 200 millilitres of boiling water per person to a bowl and cover with cling film. Leave to steam. Now you have the prime ingredients in that famous Middle Eastern salad, *tabbouleh.* To the cooked grain, add equal amounts of chopped fresh parsley leaves and tomato, plus half as much again of mint, 1 chopped onion, and the juice and grated zest of 1 lemon. Serve with grilled chicken or meats, or keep your meal vegetarian and add a cucumber salad and chickpea hummus.

Cooking grain basics

Although the boiling water approach to cooking grains has its advantages, using a precise amount of water in a ratio to the amount of grain gives you a way of controlling doneness that doesn't require supervision. Just follow the recommended amounts and cooking times in Table 20-2. You may have to make small adjustments to suit the pans in which you're cooking the grain, but after you work out the right formula, you can rely on it time and again. Although the risk in boiling grains is that they become water logged, this technique gives you fluffy grains with all the liquid evaporated. And the grains are hot and ready to eat right from the pan.

Although you can cook many grains, such as brown rice and barley, using either method, buckwheat, millet, and quinoa require the measured technique. What you don't do is as important as what you do.

Here's the drill:

1. **To remove dust and pesticides, put the grain in a large bowl, add water, swish the grain around, and pour off the liquid.**

2. **Repeat Step 1 until the rinse water is clear.**

3. **Using the ratios in Table 20-2, put the grain of your choice and water, homemade stock, or tinned broth in a small saucepan; bring the liquid to the boil; and then cover with a tight-fitting lid.**

    If the lid doesn't fit properly, cover the lid with a piece of aluminium foil, tucking the foil under the lip of the lid to prevent steam from escaping from the pot.

4. Reduce the heat to low and cook for the times in Table 20-2.

If you see steam escaping, briefly remove the pan to a work surface and carefully seal the top with a square of aluminium foil wrapped over the lid and tucked under the lid's lip (take care not to burn yourself with the steam). Then place the pan back on the stove to continue cooking. This avoids ending up with undercooked or scorched grain.

Don't increase the heat to help the grains cook. They need heat, but they also simply need time in the warm liquid – think of each grain as a little sponge – to soak up moisture.

Resist the temptation to lift the lid and peek at the grains to see how they're doing during the cooking time. You lose some of the liquid as steam.

5. When the cooking time is up, turn off the heat and let the saucepan stand for 5 to 10 minutes before serving.

6. Raise the lid and fluff the grain with a fork to separate the kernels.

7. Test for doneness by taking out a few grains, allowing to cool slightly, and tasting.

If the only grain you're accustomed to eating is white rice, which is quite soft when cooked, remember that most wholegrains are slightly chewy when adequately cooked. The chew comes from all that beneficial fibre in the bran.

Wholegrains take somewhat longer to cook than their refined versions because they still retain the fibrous bran, which takes time to break down. If you plan to eat wholegrains as part of a dinner, start them when you would start fixing baked potatoes, about an hour before you expect to serve the meal, so that they're done on time.

Grain is easy to cook if you add the right amount of water for the quantity of grain, and, with a measure of patience, cook them long enough. Table 20-2 gives you guidelines to follow.

Table 20-2	Grain Cooking Times	
Grain	*Grain:Liquid Ratio (by volume measured with a teacup or mug)*	*Cooking Time*
Long-grain brown rice	1:2½	40 to 50 minutes
Hulled barley	1:3	1¼ to 1½ hours
Pearl barley	1:3	50 to 60 minutes

Grain	Grain:Liquid Ratio (by volume measured with a teacup or mug)	Cooking Time
Wild rice	1:4	50 minutes
Buckwheat and kasha	1:2	20 minutes
Bulgur wheat	1:2½	Cover with boiling water and let sit for 15 to 30 minutes
Quinoa	1:2	15 minutes
Millet	1:2	35 minutes
Wholegrain couscous	1:1½	Add liquid and turn off heat; let sit for 10 minutes

Adding grains to all sorts of dishes

Besides the grain recipes in this chapter, we've scattered many other ways of adding wholegrains to your meals throughout this book. Bake a wholewheat muffin that also includes oat flour using the recipe in Chapter 8. Turn to Chapter 6 for a basic recipe to prepare a hot porridge using assorted wholegrains starting with millet and inventing your own variations. Follow the directions in Chapter 22 and bake a cracker with rye flour or make a cake with spelt flour.

Wholegrains also show up in lunch and dinner dishes. Barley is added to soups in Chapter 9, salads in Chapter 10, and to beef stew in Chapter 15. Or stuff a chicken with wholewheat couscous in Chapter 13.

Filling grain in real meals

The following recipe gives you the chance to experiment with a very different grain – unhulled barley – which you leave alone to absorb its liquid in private.

☙ Sage-Scented Barley with Mushrooms

Made with unhulled barley, this gutsy side dish seems just right with roast pork, game birds, or beef. If you decide to cook the recipe with more tender pearl barley, you miss out on much of the barley's nutrients.

Preparation time: 30 minutes, plus 2 to 3 hours to soak the barley

Cooking time: 1 hour and 15 minutes

Serves: 6

180 grams unhulled barley, rinsed

4 tablespoons extra-virgin olive oil

170 grams sliced mushrooms, cleaned and cut into 2-centimetre pieces

1 medium onion, coarsely chopped

1 tablespoon chopped fresh sage leaves

½ teaspoon ground allspice

120 millilitres white wine

1 litre vegetable or chicken stock (see the Basic Chicken Stock recipe in Chapter 9 or use tinned, low-sodium fat-free chicken broth)

2 tablespoons chopped parsley

Black pepper, freshly ground

1 To shorten the cooking time of the barley, soak it in water for 2 to 3 hours, and then drain.

2 After the barley is soaked, heat 2 tablespoons of the olive oil in a heavy pan over a medium-high heat. Add the mushroom pieces and cook for about 7 minutes, stirring frequently. Transfer the mushrooms to a bowl.

3 Add the remaining 2 tablespoons of the oil to the pan, along with the onion. Reduce the heat to medium and cook for about 10 minutes until the onion is soft and translucent.

4 Add the barley, sage, and allspice to the onions and cook for 1 minute, stirring to coat the barley with the oil. Add the wine and cook for 5 minutes, until nearly evaporated.

5 Add the stock to the barley mixture, bring to the boil, lower the heat to low, and cover the pan tightly so that steam doesn't escape. Try to use a glass lid or peek after 40 to 50 minutes to make sure that you have enough broth in the pan. When the barley has cooked for 1¼ hours, check for doneness by taking out a spoonful, allowing to cool slightly, and tasting. Add additional broth if necessary and cook for an additional 15 minutes.

6 Stir in the mushrooms. Cook, covered, for an additional few minutes to combine the flavours. Add the parsley and season to taste with black pepper. Serve immediately.

Vary It! To prepare the barley with homemade vegetable broth, begin by cooking 2 carrots, 1 stalk celery, 1 onion, 1 bay leaf, and 1 clove in 1.4 litres of water for 30 minutes. Meanwhile, assemble the ingredients and prepare the vegetables for the barley recipe. If you choose to prepare this recipe with pearl barley, reduce the broth to 720 millilitres and cook the barley for 45 minutes.

Per serving: Calories 221; Fat 11g (Saturated 2g); Cholesterol 0mg; Sodium 82mg; Carbohydrate 26g; Dietary Fibre 6g; Protein 7g.

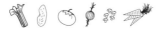

Treasuring Grains with a History

Grains are an integral part of the history of many cultures, such as rice in Asia, kamut in Egypt, and quinoa in Peru. In this section, you have the chance to add some delicious rice pilafs and risottos, and a recipe for the ancient grain quinoa, to your cooking repertoire.

Picking pilaf recipes

Rice pilaf, a mixture that is primarily grain with the addition of some other ingredients, such as chopped and cooked vegetables, poultry, meats, and seafood, originates from the Near East. Traditionally, a pilaf always begins with first browning the rice in butter or oil before cooking it in stock. A variation of this procedure is used in the following Stuffed Peppers with Turkish Pilaf recipe. In the second pilaf recipe, Herbed Wild Rice with Currants and Pecans, the grain is added directly to stock or broth, cooked, and seasoned, and then other ingredients are incorporated.

Use these pilaf recipes as a starting point to flavour your own grain mixtures. These recipes feature citrus, toasted nuts, dusky spices such as allspice and cinnamon, and refreshing mint.

We also include a traditional risotto from closer to home – Italy. Risotto is a rich and creamy dish made with Arborio rice – a sticky rice with a wonderful, creamy texture.

↺ Stuffed Bell Peppers with Turkish Pilaf

When you eat a grain with some sort of bean or pea, you give yourself a complete protein – the equivalent of that found in meats and poultry, but without the saturated fat and cholesterol. For instance, if you start with these peppers, filled with sweet raisins and spices, and have some chickpea hummus, you have a meal with high-quality protein, all from the plant kingdom. The recipe calls for long-grain, Indian basmati rice, which is aged, giving the rice a delectable nutlike flavour.

Preparation time: *30 minutes*

Cooking time: *1½ hours*

Serves: *6*

900 millilitres water

275 grams brown basmati rice (which yields 975 grams cooked rice)

3 tablespoons extra-virgin olive oil

1 onion, chopped into ½ centimetre pieces

2 tablespoons pine nuts

1½ teaspoons ground cinnamon

1 teaspoon allspice

¼ teaspoon ground nutmeg

1 large tomato, diced

2 tablespoons golden raisins

2 tablespoons fresh dill, finely chopped

2 teaspoons lemon juice

6 medium-sized green bell peppers

1 Preheat the oven to 180 degrees. Put the water in a heavy saucepan with a tight-fitting lid. Add the brown rice and bring to the boil. Cover, reduce the heat to low, and cook undisturbed for about 40 minutes, until the rice is tender. Drain.

2 Meanwhile, put the olive oil in a large frying pan. Add the onions and pine nuts and cook on a medium heat for 7 minutes, until the onions are translucent. Stir occasionally.

3 To the onions, add the cinnamon, allspice, nutmeg, tomato, raisins, dill, and lemon juice. Mix together. Add the cooked rice and combine with the other ingredients.

4 Fill a large pan with water and bring to the boil. Meanwhile, cut the tops and stems off the peppers and scoop out the seeds. Add the pepper tops and bottoms to the pot and parboil for 1 minute. With tongs, remove the peppers, drain, and arrange in a large baking dish.

5 Spoon the pilaf mixture into the pepper bottoms until they're full and cap with the pepper tops. Add 1 centimetre of water to the baking dish holding the stuffed peppers to prevent them burning on the bottom. Bake for 45 minutes, until the peppers are tender, and serve.

Per serving: Calories 296; Fat 10g (Saturated 2g); Cholesterol 0mg; Sodium 11mg; Carbohydrate 49g; Dietary Fibre 6g; Protein 6g.

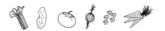

☛ Herbed Wild Rice with Currants and Pecans

This pilaf has it all – texture from the grain, sweetness from the currants and orange, a little bite from the onions, and the richness of the pecans. Made with brown rice, this recipe provides plenty of nutrients important for heart health, including magnesium, selenium, zinc, vitamin B6, and niacin. Serve as a side dish with roast turkey or chicken. The pilaf is also great at room temperature for a lunch buffet.

Preparation time: *25 minutes*

Cooking time: *1 hour and 15 minutes*

Serves: *6*

1 unwaxed orange (see the Warning at the end of this recipe)

480 millilitres chicken stock (see the Basic Chicken Stock recipe in Chapter 9 or use tinned, low sodium fat-free chicken broth)

80 grams wild rice, well rinsed

600 millilitres water

200 grams brown rice

2 spring onions, cut crosswise into thin rings

4 tablespoons chopped flat-leaf parsley

4 tablespoons chopped mint leaves

60 grams currants

50 grams pecan halves, toasted

2 tablespoons extra-virgin olive oil

Black pepper, freshly ground

1 Grate the rind of the orange to yield 1 heaped teaspoon of zest. Cut the orange in half, squeeze to yield 2 tablespoons juice, and set aside.

2 Put the chicken stock in a medium saucepan with a tight-fitting lid. Bring the stock to the boil.

3 Add the wild rice and bring back to the boil. Reduce the heat to low, cover the pot, and cook, undisturbed, until the rice is puffed up and tender, about 40 minutes. The rice is done when the grains are puffed up and are quite tender, regardless of whether the liquid is absorbed. Drain if necessary.

4 Meanwhile, in a second heavy saucepan, put the 600 millilitres water and bring to the boil. Add the brown rice and bring back to the boil. Cover, reduce the heat to low, and cook, undisturbed, for about 50 minutes until the rice is tender and the water absorbed.

5 Add the brown rice to the wild rice. Add the spring onions, parsley, mint, currants, pecans, orange zest, olive oil, orange juice, and black pepper to taste.

Warning: *Because the rind is an ingredient, use an organic orange to avoid possible chemicals used in growing the fruit and bringing it to market.*

Per serving: *Calories 328; Fat 12g (Saturated 2g); Cholesterol 0mg; Sodium 48mg; Carbohydrate 50g; Dietary Fibre 6g; Protein 8g.*

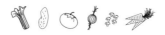

☺ *Wild Mushroom Risotto*

This classic risotto is easy to prepare, makes a great savoury lunch or supper on its own, and is also a good accompaniment for meat or fish. Although you can add the liquid left from soaking the porcini mushrooms to the risotto for extra flavour, it's often gritty, and so check before using if you want to do this. Adding hot stock to the rice a little at a time while stirring ensures that the rice is really plump and tender.

Preparation time: *25 minutes*

Cooking time: *30 minutes*

Servings: *6 (for lunch)*

50 grams dried porcini mushrooms

2 tablespoon extra-virgin olive oil

1 onion, chopped

2 cloves garlic, chopped

225 grams chestnut mushrooms, sliced

350 grams Arborio rice

150 millilitres dry white wine

1.2 litres hot chicken or vegetable stock (see the stock recipes in Chapter 9, or use tinned, low sodium fat-free chicken broth)

2 tablespoons chopped flat leaf parsley

25 grams butter

Black pepper, freshly ground

60 grams Parmesan cheese, freshly grated

1 Soak the dried porcini mushrooms in hot water for at least 10 minutes, and then drain and set aside (reserve soaking liquid).

2 Heat the olive oil in a large, heavy-based frying pan. Add the onion and garlic and fry for 3 minutes until soft. Add the sliced chestnut mushrooms and fry for a further 3 minutes, until starting to brown.

3 Stir in the rice and cook, still stirring, for a couple of minutes. Add the wine and simmer, stirring, until all the liquid is absorbed.

4 Add the hot stock, a ladleful at a time, stirring until the liquid is absorbed before adding another ladleful. Chop the drained porcini mushrooms and stir into the risotto, along with the reserved soaking water half way through this process. Continue until all the liquid is absorbed and the rice is plump, creamy, and tender.

5 Add the parsley and butter. Season well with black pepper and serve with freshly grated Parmesan cheese.

Tip: *For an even creamier risotto, stir in some low-fat mascarpone cheese or crème fraîche.*

Per serving: *Calories 404; Fat 14g (Saturated 6g); Cholesterol 20mg; Sodium 287mg; Carbohydrate 55g; Dietary Fibre 3g; Protein 17g.*

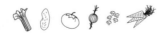

Using grains from the distant past in recipes today

Ancient grains are making their way back into the modern diet. Quinoa was a staple of the Inca civilisation, and amaranth sustained life in ancient Mexico and Peru for good reason. Both grains are an excellent source of high-quality protein. You, too, can use these as a protein source in a varied vegetarian diet to part-replace the protein from red meat. Shop for these grains in health food stores. You're likely to find amaranth as both a flour and as seeds, and quinoa in grain form. A recipe for quinoa with basil and tomato follows.

Try popping amaranth seeds just like corn. Heat a dry frying pan on the hob and sprinkle on amaranth seeds using a spoon. Cover immediately with a lid and the seeds pop in just a few seconds. Add to muesli, yogurt, and desserts.

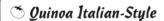

☙ Quinoa Italian-Style

The texture of quinoa is nicely soft and light but with intermittent grains that pop. The delicate taste is fine on its own but also welcomes herbs and vegetables. This version uses Italian flavourings and is especially tasty with a dusting of grated Parmesan cheese. Serve quinoa as a side dish, just as you serve rice.

Preparation time: *10 minutes*

Cooking time: *20 minutes*

Serves: *6*

250 grams quinoa	*4 tablespoons basil leaves, cut into thin ribbons*
480 millilitres water	*Black pepper, freshly ground*
2 medium tomatoes, deseeded and chopped	*Parmesan cheese, grated*

1 If the quinoa you buy is not pre-washed, rinse the quinoa in five changes of water in a bowl, sifting through the grains and moving them around. Let the grains settle before pouring off the water. If the quinoa doesn't settle, drain in a large, fine sieve after each rinse.

2 Put the quinoa in a heavy medium saucepan filled with the water. Bring to the boil and reduce the heat. Cover and simmer for about 20 minutes until the quinoa is tender and the water has been absorbed.

3 When the quinoa is tender, toss with a fork to separate the grains. Add the tomatoes and basil and combine. Add black pepper to taste. Serve with grated Parmesan cheese.

Per serving: Calories 167; Fat 3g (Saturated 1g); Cholesterol 0mg; Sodium 13mg; Carbohydrate 31g; Dietary Fibre 3g; Protein 6g. (Cheese not included in the analysis.)

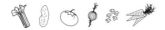

Plating Up Healthy Pasta

Pasta is a health food, but if your aim is to give yourself a serving of nutrients that help to lower cholesterol, don't turn to standard spaghetti. You can see on the labels that it's made from semolina, which sounds nutritious but is actually just a type of wheat. In addition, most pasta on supermarket shelves is made of refined white wheat flour, just like white bread.

Instead, visit a health food shop or one of the larger supermarkets and explore the impressive variety of intriguing wholegrain pastas made from wholegrain spelt (an ancient cereal grain with a mellow, nutty flavour), corn, and even Jerusalem artichoke (a tuber related to the sunflower). These are wholefood pastas, complete with fibre and all their original nutrients.

Wholegrain pastas have a stronger, more nutlike taste than white-flour spaghetti, and call for sauces that can compete in flavour. Adding meaty mushrooms, roast vegetables, and piquant chillies boosts the flavour of homemade sauces.

Allow 60 grams uncooked, dried pasta per serving. This quantity is enough to fill a pasta bowl, along with the sauce, but still keep calories in check.

Splitting the difference: Pasta that's a mix of refined flour and wholefood

If wholegrain pastas are too overbearing for you, try spinach pasta made with white flour plus a dose of green vegetable. Or, try soba noodles, a staple of Japanese cooking, which are a combination of refined wheat flour and wholegrain buckwheat. Pastas that include spinach, tomato, beetroot and even squid ink are out there, too.

You can also start with the refined durum wheat pasta and beef up your sauces with the missing bits by adding wheat bran and wheat germ, which health food shops sell, as follows:

- ✔ For each 240 grams of pasta (enough for 4 servings) add 1½ teaspoons of wheat germ and a similar amount of bran to replace around half of that lost in refining.

- ✔ Because you're adding more bulk to the sauce, add a few more tablespoons of water to retain its original consistency.

Wheat germ goes rancid quickly. Store in vacuum-sealed jars in the refrigerator or freezer. Use within 2 to 3 months.

Pasta recipes for getting your grains

These recipes are terrific on their own without any embellishments, but a fine flavoured cheese is also welcome. Even when watching your fat intake, you can afford a sprinkling of cheese on your pasta. Treat yourself to the best you can find and enjoy the superior flavour. Hunt out imported Parmesan and Pecorino Romano or some mild goat cheese produced on a local farm.

Buckwheat Noodles in Asian Sesame Sauce

These noodles, resplendent in a honeyed sesame-soya sauce, are good hot or cold. They supply magnesium, which helps the heart muscle contract, and folic acid, which keeps homocysteine levels in check (see Chapter 1 for more on homocysteine).

Preparation time: 20 minutes

Cooking time: 30 minutes

Serves: 4

2 litres water

225 grams soba noodles

2 tablespoons sesame tahini

3 tablespoons soya sauce

2 tablespoons rice vinegar

2 tablespoons honey

1 tablespoon sherry

10 grams coriander leaves

2 cloves garlic, peeled and chopped

2 teaspoons hot chilli sauce

2 spring onions, chopped

1 In a large pan, bring the water to the boil. Add the noodles and cook, uncovered, according to package instructions. Drain in a colander. Place the noodles in a large bowl of cold water to cool for 10 minutes and then drain again in the colander.

2 In a medium bowl, whisk together the tahini, soya sauce, and vinegar until smooth. Add the honey and sherry and stir again.

3 Add a few tablespoons of water to the tahini mixture, stirring well after each addition, until the mixture is of sauce consistency.

4 Stir in the coriander, garlic, and hot chilli sauce.

5 Place the noodles in a serving bowl and drizzle with the sauce. Toss and then garnish with the spring onions. Serve immediately at room temperature.

Per serving: Calories 297; Fat 4g (Saturated 1g); Cholesterol 0mg; Sodium 884mg; Carbohydrate 56g; Dietary Fibre 3g; Protein 14g.

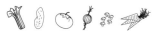

☙ Spinach Pasta with Walnut and Basil Sauce

This colourful dish in green, red, and yellow provides heaps of special nutrients for the heart. This spinach pasta sneaks leafy greens into your meal, but the recipe works just as well with wholegrain pastas because the walnut basil sauce is a match for their more robust flavours. If squash or asparagus aren't available, use other vegetables such as courgette instead.

Special tools required: *Food processor fitted with metal blades*

Preparation time: *15 minutes*

Cooking time: *40 minutes*

Serves: *4*

120 grams walnut pieces

85 grams basil leaves

2 cloves garlic, skin removed

80 millilitres plus 2 tablespoons extra-virgin olive oil

350 grams sweet red bell peppers, seeds removed and quartered

350 grams yellow squash or pumpkin

350 grams asparagus

175 grams button mushrooms, washed

225 grams spinach spaghetti

1 Put the walnuts, basil, garlic, and 80 millilitres of olive oil in a food processor fitted with a metal blade. Blend until smooth. Pour into a small bowl and set aside.

2 Slice the red peppers and squash crosswise into ½-centimetre-wide slices. Cut the asparagus into 4-centimetre lengths. Cut each mushroom vertically into 4 slices.

3 In a large frying pan filled with 2 centimetres of water, parboil the asparagus for about 4 minutes until almost tender. Drain the cooking liquid. Remove the asparagus to a bowl and set aside. Thoroughly dry the frying pan with a paper towel.

4 In the same pan, cook the peppers, squash, and mushrooms in the remaining 2 table-spoons of olive oil over a medium heat for about 25 minutes, until tender. Toward the end of the cooking period, add the asparagus.

5 Meanwhile, bring a pan of water to the boil, uncovered, on a high heat. Add a small splash of olive oil to prevent the strands of spaghetti from sticking together. Add the spaghetti and cook for about 12 minutes, or according to package instructions.

6 Drain the spaghetti in a colander, making sure that no liquid remains in the pan.

7 Add the walnut-basil sauce to the spaghetti and toss to coat.

8 Distribute the spaghetti in warmed pasta bowls and top with the sautéed vegetables.

Per serving: *Calories 691; Fat 47g (Saturated 6g); Cholesterol 0mg; Sodium 35mg; Carbohydrate 59g; Dietary Fibre 10g; Protein 18g.*

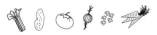

Part VI
Serving Up Sweet Finishes

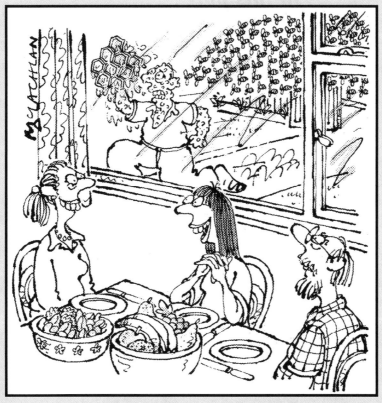

'To go with our nuts and fruit, we need a
<u>natural</u> sweetner – Quentin's just
gone to get that now.'

In this part . . .

This part contains recipes for luxurious, yet 'legal', desserts. Chapter 21 gives you ways to assemble healthy fruit desserts to finish a meal, and explains which fruits are the highest in soluble fibre and colourful, antioxidant nutrients. For those watching their weight and glucose balance, this chapter also points out which fruits raise blood sugar only minimally. We also discuss how you can mix wholegrains with natural sweeteners to bake biscuits and cakes healthy enough to serve for breakfast. Finally, we show you how to use substitute ingredients such as tofu and fromage frais to make some delicious quick-and-easy, lower-cholesterol desserts.

Noble motives aside, these recipes are so yummy that you can easily forget that they're healthy foods.

Chapter 21

Dishing Up Fruit for Dessert

'An apple a day keeps the doctor away' takes on greater meaning when you consider all the ways in which apples and other fruits control cholesterol. Fruit is not only naturally low in fat, but also a source of soluble fibre, just like oatmeal. Colourful melons, citrus, and berries also provide a wealth of antioxidants and phytonutrients that all do their part in preventing heart disease.

Despite all the nutritional benefits of fruit, however, and the drive to get people to eat five-a-day of fruit and veg, the average intake for adults is only 2½ servings a day.

Take a fresh look at fruit and increase your intake the easiest way possible, in the form of fruit desserts. Read on for information and inspiration, and top off your meals with fruit. Try the recipes, and chop, spice, and freeze fruit, or add something low-fat, yet creamy. You can't go wrong!

Picking Fruit Enhances Heart Health

Whole fruit – flesh, skin, core, and all – provides fibre and an array of nutrients that are associated with the prevention of heart disease. Research shows that eating three or more servings of fruit and vegetables a day significantly reduces the risk of dying from heart attack and stroke. Imagine the benefits of eating five or more servings a day, as the Department of Health currently recommends.

Soaking up cholesterol with soluble fibre

Many fruits contain a significant amount of soluble fibre, especially *pectin*, which is the fibre that allows cooked fruits to gel when making jam and marmalade. Soluble fibre in the intestinal tract also has a gelling effect, acting like a sponge to absorb fats and cholesterol. And because the body can't digest fibre, it passes on through, taking the cholesterol with it.

The following list shows you how many grams of soluble fibre are present in 100 grams of the fruits that are the best sources. Considering that 100 grams of oatmeal, long promoted as an excellent source of soluble fibre, provides 0.7 grams, the amounts in these fruits are close behind:

- Oranges: 0.6
- Apricots: 0.5
- Bananas: 0.5
- Nectarines: 0.4
- Pears: 0.4
- Plums: 0.4
- Strawberries: 0.4
- Tangerines: 0.4
- Granny Smith apples: 0.3
- Blueberries: 0.3

Figures for soluble fibre content in foods vary depending upon what method of analysis researchers use. The above data are based on research conducted at the University of Wisconsin and published in the *Journal of the American Dietetic Association*.

Choosing a variety of fruit

If you eat a variety of fruit, you have cause for celebration. This is the only way you are certain to consume all the different vitamins and minerals that various fruits contain. Some are great sources of antioxidants, while others are tops for certain minerals. You need the whole range.

Enjoy different kinds of fruit individually or prepare a luscious bowlful of cut-up mixed fruit, such as in a classic fruit salad. This dish always feels like a luxury, especially if you buy it ready-made, with the fruit trimmed and cut and all the work done for you.

Take a look at the following list of nutrients, all good for the heart, and the fruits that contain them. The first fruit in each list is the richest source of that nutrient with the others arranged in descending order. (Chapter 2 gives you specifics about how these vitamins and minerals help control cholesterol.)

- **Betacarotene:** Cantaloupe melon, mangoes, apricots, persimmons (also known as Sharon fruit), and papayas.

- **Vitamin B6:** Mangoes, watermelon, bananas, plantains, and melons.

- **Vitamin C:** Papayas, guava, kiwis, lychees, oranges, grapefruit, mangoes, cantaloupe melon, watermelon, strawberries, and blackcurrants.

- **Calcium:** Figs, papayas, oranges, tangerines, and boysenberries.

- **Folate:** Boysenberries, cantaloupe melon, oranges, loganberries, strawberries, and papayas.

- **Magnesium:** Figs, raisins, passion fruit, apricots, and bananas.

- **Potassium:** Raisins, papayas, figs, blackcurrants, cantaloupe melon, apricots, and bananas.

Exploring and trying out new fruits is always fun, and you can also explore new ways to enjoy old standbys. Melons, in particular, are very versatile. Figure 21-1 shows ways in which you can cut and serve them.

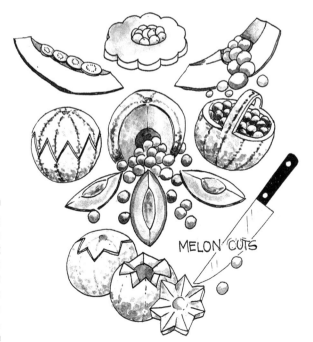

Figure 21-1:
Various ways to cut and serve melons, by themselves or with other fruits.

Don't make a habit of eating tinned fruit because the heating process used in tinning destroys some of the vitamins and some phytonutrients. In addition, manufacturers often pack the fruit in heavy syrup that contains loads of refined sugar. Fresh fruit is best, but tinned fruit is better than none at all. If selecting tinned fruit, choose those preserved in juice rather than heavy syrup.

Nothing is wrong with supplementing your fresh fruit intake with fruit in other forms. Dried fruit retains its minerals, although it's lower in vitamins, and is very handy to snack on when you're out and about. Just remember that eating a handful of raisins, a condensed food, is equivalent to consuming a large bunch of grapes and delivers as many calories.

Frozen fruit is another good option. After harvesting, ripe fruit is flash-frozen within 24 hours and is likely to contain at least as many nutrients as fruit picked before it has ripened and then transported long distances to market. Try supplementing the limited variety of fresh fruit available in winter months with frozen mango, blueberries, mixed berries, or apples. Also keep some fruit spreads on hand that are made without added sugar. The Crepes with Brandied Apricot Conserve (the recipe is later in this chapter) are filled with a thick spread of flavoured apricot, for example.

Feeling fruity controls cholesterol

Fruit is an abundant source of phytonutrients, a huge range of plant compounds that are as important to good health as vitamins and minerals. (Chapter 2 introduces these in detail.) The various phytonutrients perform an array of functions, including controlling cholesterol.

Doing double-duty as pigments

Many phytonutrients are also pigments – the red in cherries, the blue in blueberries, and the orange in oranges – and so they're easy to spot at the supermarket. The two main classes are *carotenoids*, which are the yellow-orange-red hues, and *anthocyanins*, which range from crimson and magenta to violet and indigo. You get the picture. Buy fruit in an assortment of colours, and you bring home a variety of phytonutrients.

In terms of cholesterol, some of these pigments function as antioxidants. They help to prevent oxidation of LDL cholesterol, prevent unwanted blood clots, and reduce chronic inflammation, now considered a factor in heart disease.

The antioxidant potential of various fruits is measured in ORAC (Oxygen Radical Absorbance Capacity) units. Scientists calculate that ideally you need to consume at least 7000 ORAC units per day. Those eating the most fruit and veg obtain at least 20,000 ORAC units per day – the more the better. The figures in Table 21-1 show the ORAC units you can obtain from servings of various fruits, with the most beneficial at the top.

Table 21-1	Antioxidant Score of Various Fruits	
Fruit	Weight of Average Serving (Grams)	ORAC Score per Average Serving
Blueberries	145	13,427
Pomegranates	100	10,500
Cranberries	95	8,983
Blackberries	144	7,701
Prunes	85	7,291
Raspberries	123	6,058
Strawberries	166	5,938
Red Delicious apples	138	5,900
Cherries	145	4,873
Plums (black)	66	4,844
Plums (red)	66	4,118
Gala apples	138	3,903
Golden Delicious apples	138	3,685
Dates	89	3,467
Lemons/Limes	140	3,378
Pears (green varieties)	166	3,172
Pears (Red Anjou)	166	2,943
Oranges (navel)	140	2,540
Figs	75	2,537
Raisins	82	2,490
Red grapes	160	2,016
Red grapefruits	123	1,904
Peaches	98	1,826
Green grapes	160	1,789
Mangoes	165	1,653

ORAC scores show how well the antioxidants in fruit and vegetables prevent the breakdown of a chemical called *fluorescein* after mixing it with a strong oxidating agent. Fluorescein is luminescent, and the intensity of light it emits decreases as it breaks down. This provides an easy way of measuring how much fluorescein remains intact at set intervals after adding the fruit extract and the oxidant. Fruit with low ORAC values provides little protection and the mixture's luminosity rapidly decreases. Foods with high ORAC values protect the fluorescein from degradation and the sample remains luminescent for longer.

Discovering other fruity nutrients

All sorts of other compounds in fruit help control cholesterol in intriguing ways. The following list tells you about some of these:

✔ Betasitosterol competes with cholesterol for absorption into the bloodstream and comes in first place, lowering the level of circulating cholesterol. You get betasitosterol in oranges, cherries, bananas, and apples.

✔ D-glucaric acid is a cholesterol-lowering compound found abundantly in grapefruit and Granny Smith apples, and in cherries, apricots, and oranges, too.

If you take calcium-channel blocker medication or statin drugs, check the data sheet provided to see if you're advised to avoid grapefruit and grapefruit juice. These medications are partly deactivated before they reach your blood stream by a certain enzyme. Prescription dosages compensate for this. However, compounds in grapefruit deactivate this enzyme. A drug overdose can result.

✔ Inulin is a fibre-like carbohydrate in raisins (but not in grapes) that signals the liver to make less cholesterol.

✔ Hesperetin in oranges and other citrus fruits reduces the liver's production of certain compounds that are essential for the formation of 'bad' LDL cholesterol.

Picking top fruits for dessert

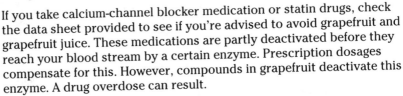

You can hardly go wrong no matter what fruit you decide to slice and serve at the end of a meal. Raw, baked, or stewed, fruit makes a great finish. The tartness of citrus balances the taste of fat in an oily dinner. That's one reason why a wedge of lemon is often provided alongside your grilled salmon, and why duck goes so well with orange. The juiciness of melon also makes a refreshing end to lunch in hot weather.

Fruits are perfect desserts – low in both calories and hassle. Therefore, include the following fruits on your shopping lists so that you always have dessert on hand:

✔ **The usual suspects:** Apples, pears, bananas, melon, red grapes, oranges, and apricots

✔ **Berries:** Blueberries, strawberries, raspberries, blackberries, and cranberries

✔ **Special treats:** Cherries, mango, papaya, pineapple, and kiwi

✔ **Seasonal fruits:** Berries in summer and apples in autumn

You're best off eating bluish-red, purple, and blue fruits (such as cherries, strawberries, black grapes, and plums) raw because tinning and baking them damages the anthocyanin pigments that give them their colour. Raw fruit itself is very colourful and versatile. Figure 21-2 shows examples of how you can arrange raw fruit as attractive desserts.

SINGLE SERVING FRUIT ARRANGEMENTS FOR DESSERT

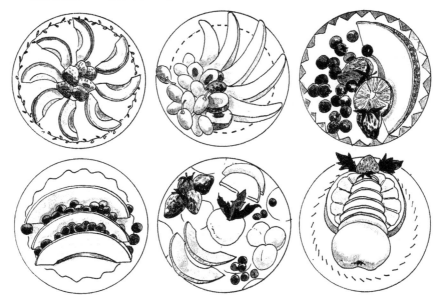

Figure 21-2:
Attractive
ways to
serve raw
fruit.

Selecting fruits for low-glycaemic diets

Cutting back on sugar intake is important to help control your weight and your blood sugar levels. For this reason, *low-glycaemic index (GI) diets* that reduce your intake of sugar and refined carbohydrates are a good idea. Low GI essentially means that you select foods that do not cause a spike in blood sugar levels, followed by an energy slump a few hours later as the sugar levels fall.

Many people mistakenly assume that, because fruit contains sugar, and tastes sweet, it causes a rapid spike in blood levels of the sugar, *glucose*, after you eat some. But fruit doesn't just contain glucose. It also contains other sugars – *fructose* and *sucrose* – that take time to digest and process. As a result, most fruit actually has a low to medium glycaemic index. Whole fruit also contains fibre that slows its effect on blood glucose levels, and eating fruit with some protein and fat slows its absorption even further. For instance, when you make baked apples, stuff the hollowed out core with walnuts, for a satisfyingly low-GI dessert.

Like all foods, each fruit has a *glycaemic index*, or a number that tells you how fast it causes blood sugar (glucose) levels to rise. The higher the index number for a fruit, the faster it raises sugar in the bloodstream. The fruits in the following lists are those that researchers have studied so far. Each list begins with the fruit with the highest glycaemic index in each category.

- **Over 70:** Watermelon.
- **60–69:** Pineapple, cantaloupe, honeydew melon, raisins, and tinned apricots in syrup.
- **50–59:** Fresh apricots, mangoes, tinned fruit cocktail, bananas, kiwis, papayas, and orange juice.
- **40–49:** Grapefruit juice, tinned peaches, pineapple juice, grapes, tinned pears, oranges, peaches, and apple juice.
- **30–39:** Plums, apples, pears, dried apricots, grapefruit, cherries, strawberries, and raspberries.

When you want a sweet snack, choose fruit over cakes and cookies made with white sugar. The types of sugars in fruit have a more gentle effect on blood sugar than the sugars in most baked goods.

Having Fun with Fruity Recipes

Now for the sweet stuff. The following recipes include gourmet desserts such as elegant French crepes, homemade sorbet, and poached pears, as well as a homely apple crumble. With its colour, flavour, and natural sweetness, fruit is the perfect food to start with when inventing desserts. What an easy way to add a serving of fruit to your daily intake.

☙ Crepes with Brandied Apricot Conserve

This elegant dessert gives you just enough fat and protein to balance the carbohydrate it contains. Fill the crepes with the fruit of your choice or with fruit conserves, which are all-fruit spreads; but not with fruit preserves or jam, which contain fruit plus sugar.

Preparation time: 15 minutes

Cooking time: 30 minutes

Serves: 4 (2 crepes per serving)

80 grams plus 2 tablespoons all-fruit apricot spread

1 tablespoon brandy

60 grams spelt flour (see Chapter 22)

60 grams wholemeal flour

Pinch of salt

1 egg white

160 millilitres buttermilk

180 millilitres water

Safflower oil for cooking the crepes

About 60 millilitres non-fat sour cream, for garnish

About 3 tablespoons toasted almonds, for garnish

1 Preheat the oven to 165 degrees. In a small bowl, mix the apricot spread and brandy. Set aside.

2 Sift the spelt flour, wholemeal flour, and salt into a medium-sized bowl. Make a well in the centre of the flour and add the egg white. Slowly add the buttermilk and water, while beating hard with a whisk to incorporate all the liquid and create a smooth, frothy batter.

3 Wipe a nonstick crepe pan or frying pan with shallow sides with an oiled paper towel and heat until very hot. The pan has reached a sufficiently high temperature when a drop of water you flick into the pan skitters across the surface before evaporating. Pour in enough batter to cover the bottom of the pan (around 60 millilitres), swirling the batter around to distribute it evenly. Cook the crepe on a medium heat for about 1 minute, until it is set and golden.

4 Turn the crepe over to cook the other side for an additional 15 to 20 seconds. The crepe is finished when the edges are just beginning to brown and it is not at all crisp. Transfer to a platter and place in the oven to keep warm. Place waxed paper between the layers of crepe so they don't stick together as they cool. Proceed to make all the crepes. Keep the crepes thin and delicate by adding a few teaspoons of water if the batter thickens.

5 To serve, lay a crepe on a work surface and spread 1¹/₂ teaspoons of the apricot mixture in a stripe across the middle. Roll the crepe into a log and place on an individual desert plate. Garnish the crepe with non-fat sour cream and scatter the almonds over the sour cream and crepes. Serve immediately.

Per serving: Calories 233; Fat 4g (Saturated 1g); Cholesterol 2mg; Sodium 99mg; Carbohydrate 41g; Dietary Fibre 2g; Protein 6g.

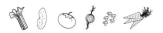

☞ Blueberry and Lemon Mousse

This fruit and yogurt mixture, which becomes a mousse, is a good candidate for using berries because you use the fruit raw and so don't damage the antioxidants in berries by heating. The blueberries in this dish contain a phytonutrient, *pterostilbene*, which appears to lower 'bad' LDL cholesterol, according to preliminary research. The recipe also gives you a simple technique for making yogurt cheese, which involves draining off the watery liquid, known as whey, leaving the solid parts or curds. (Of course, you don't want to do this if you happen to be Little Miss Muffet, sitting on a tuffet, and you want to eat both the curds and whey.)

Special tools required: *Cheesecloth, food processor fitted with a metal blade, whisk*

Preparation time: *45 minutes, plus 6 hours or longer for the yogurt to drain and 1 hour to refrigerate the finished dessert*

Cooking time: *2 minutes*

Serves: *4*

240 millilitres low-fat plain bio yogurt

240 millilitres low-fat lemon yogurt

240 millilitres water

1 sachet unflavoured gelatine (or a vegetarian alternative such as agar-agar, carrageen, or Vege-gel)

150 grams fresh blueberries, rinsed and patted dry

Blueberries, for garnish

1 Line a strainer with several layers of cheesecloth and set the strainer over a large bowl. To drain the yogurt, turning it into 'cheese', spoon the plain and lemon yogurts into the strainer. Cover with a spare saucepan lid to press down on the yogurt and remove more liquid. Place in the refrigerator to drain for at least 6 hours, preferably longer.

2 When the yogurt is drained, put the water in a small saucepan and sprinkle the gelatine over the top. Set aside for 5 minutes while the gelatine softens. Bring to the boil over a medium-high heat, stirring for around 2 minutes to dissolve the gelatine. Remove the pan from the heat and pour the gelatine into a bowl. Place the bowl in the refrigerator for 10 minutes to cool the gelatine sufficiently so that you can comfortably touch it.

3 Purée the blueberries in the bowl of a food processor fitted with a metal blade. Add the cooled gelatine mixture and process to blend.

4 Put the drained yogurt cheese in a large bowl. Slowly add the blueberry mixture, using a whisk to combine thoroughly. Pour into individual dessert dishes or long-stemmed glass-ware. Refrigerate for about 1 hour until firm. Serve topped with fresh whole blueberries.

Tip: *You can use non-fat yogurt cheese to add that needed touch of creaminess, but not the calories, to all sorts of fruit desserts, including baked apples and fruit tarts. Yogurt cheese is also a satisfying substitute for cream cheese smeared on a bagel.*

Per serving: *Calories 109; Fat 0g (Saturated 0g); Cholesterol 2mg; Sodium 83mg; Carbohydrate 21g; Dietary Fibre 1g; Protein 8g.*

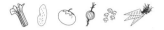

ᴥ Poached Pears with Frozen Yogurt

You can make a whole range of fancy flavoured ice creams if you start off with plain vanilla ice cream or yogurt and mix in your own ingredients. This recipe uses firm pears of whichever type is available fresh locally.

Special tools required: *Food processor fitted with a metal blade*

Preparation time: *30 minutes, plus several hours or overnight refrigeration*

Cooking time: *20 minutes*

Serves: *4*

25 grams crystallised ginger, chopped	*360 millilitres white wine*
600 millilitres low-fat, frozen vanilla yogurt, slightly softened	*4 firm pears, ripe but not mushy, peeled, cored, and sliced (see the tip at the end of this recipe)*
½ teaspoon cardamom, ground	*1 lemon, sliced*
360 millilitres water	*2 tablespoons chopped pistachios, for garnish*

1 Put the chopped crystallised ginger into the bowl of a food processor fitted with a metal blade and process until the ginger is in very small pieces. Spoon the frozen yogurt into the processor and add the cardamom. Pulse briefly, taking care that the frozen yogurt stays as chilled as possible. Immediately return the frozen yogurt mixture to its container and place in the freezer for at least 30 minutes.

2 In a medium saucepan, bring the water and wine to the boil. Lower the heat to medium-low and add the pears and lemon. Cover the pan and simmer for at least 20 minutes until the pears are very tender. Remove the cooked lemon slices.

3 Transfer the cooked pears to a bowl, leaving the pear juice to cook over a medium-high heat until reduced by half. Strain the juice over the pears and refrigerate for several hours or overnight.

4 Place a scoop of the frozen yogurt in each of four shallow dessert bowls and top with slices of poached pear. Sprinkle with the pistachios and serve immediately.

Tip: *To core a pear without ruining the shape of the slices, first peel the pear with a vegetable peeler. Then cut the pear in half lengthwise. Next, using a melon baller, dig out the core in each half. Now slice the pear if you like.*

Per serving: *Calories 217; Fat 4g (Saturated 1g); Cholesterol 7mg; Sodium 96mg; Carbohydrate 42g; Dietary Fibre 3g; Protein 7g.*

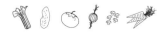

⊙ Creamy Apple Crumble

A *crumble* is pie the easy way, with a fruit mixture on the bottom and a flour mixture on top, but no pie crust to make. This version uses apples, oats, and walnuts, which are all foods that help control cholesterol. The soluble fibre in apples reduces the amount of 'bad' LDL cholesterol produced in the liver, while the apples' insoluble fibre latches on to LDL in the digestive tract and removes it from the body. In a study appearing in 2003 in the *European Journal of Clinical Nutrition* researchers combining the results of seven studies involving over 100,000 men and women, singled out apples as one of a small number of fruits that contribute to low rates of heart disease. So make this crumble and tuck in! An apple a day really does keep the doctor away.

Preparation time: *20 minutes*

Cooking time: *35 minutes*

Serves: *8*

60 grams raw rolled oats

60 grams plus 2 tablespoons wholegrain flour

60 grams chopped walnuts

½ teaspoon cinnamon

Pinch of salt

60 millilitres unrefined safflower oil

60 millilitres pure maple syrup

900 grams Golden Delicious or Bramley apples, peeled, cored, and sliced

Rind and juice of ½ lemon

½ teaspoon allspice

¼ teaspoon nutmeg

1 egg

120 millilitres non-fat sour cream

1 Preheat the oven to 180 degrees. In a large bowl, mix together the rolled oats, 60 grams of the flour, the walnuts, cinnamon, and salt. Add the safflower oil and 30 millilitres of the maple syrup. Stir to combine thoroughly. Set the crumble aside.

2 Place the apples, the remaining 30 millilitres of the maple syrup, the lemon rind, and lemon juice in a large bowl. Toss gently with a wooden spoon to coat the apples.

3 Put the remaining 2 tablespoons of flour, the allspice, and nutmeg in a small sieve and shake the sieve over the apple mixture, occasionally stirring the apples to make sure that the dry ingredients are evenly distributed.

4 In a small bowl, whisk together the egg and sour cream. Pour over the apple mixture and toss to combine.

5 Fill the bottom of a 20-centimetre-square baking pan with the apple mixture. Distribute spoonfuls of the oatmeal crumble evenly over the apples. Bake in the centre of the oven for about 35 minutes until the crumble is golden.

Per serving: Calories 283; Fat 14g (Saturated 1g); Cholesterol 27mg; Sodium 48mg; Carbohydrate 39g; Dietary Fibre 5g; Protein 5g.

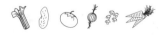

⌕ Mango Sorbet with Minted Strawberry Sauce

Making this dessert earns you high marks for content – zero fat – and presentation, thanks to all the colourful and heart-healthy phytonutrients that make up the palette of this elegant summer dessert. This dish is convenient to serve when you're entertaining and want time with your guests, because you can partially assemble it in advance.

Special tools required: *Food processor*

Preparation time: *15 minutes*

Serves: *4*

200 grams frozen mango chunks, prepared from fresh at home or commercial frozen chunks

15 medium-sized strawberries

2 large sprigs of mint (about 1 heaped tablespoon)

1 tablespoon pure maple syrup

3 tablespoons water or sparkling white wine, or as needed

¼ honeydew melon, cut into 4 slices, rind removed

1 Have on hand a small bowl and a plate pre-chilled in the freezer. Put the mango in the bowl of a food processor and chop the fruit, pulsing until the mango is puréed. Immediately transfer the fruit to the chilled bowl and chill in the freezer section of your refrigerator for 40 minutes, so that a scoop of purée holds its shape.

2 Using a small ice cream scoop that's 5 centimetres in diameter, scoop out some mango and somewhat flatten the top of the sorbet in the scoop. Squeeze the handle of the ice cream scoop to release the sorbet onto the chilled plate, flat side down. Repeat to make 3 more scoops. Reserve the mango sorbet in the freezer.

3 Meanwhile, put 7 strawberries, the mint, and maple syrup into the processor and blend. Add the water or wine to thin the strawberry purée to the consistency of a sauce, to make about 240 millilitres of sauce.

4 To assemble the fruit, place an arc of melon on each of 4 individual dessert plates. In the curve of the melon, put one of the reserved scoops of mango. Next to the mango, place 2 strawberries.

5 With a large soup spoon, drizzle 60 millilitres (4 tablespoons) of the strawberry sauce over each plate of fruit and mango sorbet, making 3 stripes that cross the melon at right angles. Garnish with a sprig of mint and serve immediately.

Per serving: Calories 90; Fat 0g (Saturated 0g); Cholesterol 0mg; Sodium 7mg; Carbohydrate 23 g; Dietary Fibre 3g; Protein 1g.

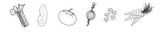

Chapter 22

Baking Up a Storm

In This Chapter

▶ Finding reasons to do your own baking

▶ Switching to healthy substitutes when baking

▶ Enjoying heart-healthy recipes

*B*elieve it or not, you can enjoy cakes and biscuits even though you're watching your cholesterol. The pleasure of that first bite into the tawny, rich flavours of warm muffins fresh from the oven, is quite permissible! An afternoon cup of tea with a slice of Banana and Date Tea Loaf is yours! Baked goods such as these are possible on a cholesterol-controlling diet. It's all a matter of substituting ingredients.

In this chapter's recipes, wholegrain flour replaces refined. Sweeteners with redeeming qualities stand in for white sugar. The addition of nuts brings a good dose of minerals and healthy fats and, at the same time, replaces butter with its saturated fat. Admittedly, the flavour of wholegrain, unrefined flour is quite robust and distinctive when you're accustomed to the blandness of white flour and white sugar. With this in mind, these recipes take advantage of the complex flavours of natural ingredients to enrich the final product. As you find out, they taste surprisingly good, and as they're so nutritious, having them for breakfast is absolutely fine!

Finding Reasons to Bake

Home-made baked goods protect the heart as much for what they don't contain as for what they do. In comparison, manufacturers design their store-bought baked products with ingredients that have a long shelf life, and the products are well-priced and good for the bottom line. However, these ingredients aren't necessarily good for your heart.

Turning out baked goods made with quality oils

One of the great health advantages of doing your own baking is that you control the quality of oil you use. The recipes in this chapter use unrefined safflower oil, available in health food shops, to add richness, small amounts of various nutrients, and healthy polyunsaturated fats. (For more on this subject, see the section 'Including healthy fats' later in this chapter.) A good alternative is rapeseed oil. In contrast, so many commercial breads, cakes, biscuits, and crackers are made with partially hydrogenated vegetable oils. Unfortunately, the process of hydrogenation produces trans fatty acids that increase total cholesterol including the 'bad' LDL cholesterol.

Avoiding white flour and sugar

Commercially baked products are virtually synonymous with white flour and sugar. White flour, as used commercially to make white bread, is low on many vitamins and minerals that keep the heart humming. Refined white sugar has no vitamins or minerals at all. If you check the label on many products, you're likely to see that the first ingredient (the most abundant substance in the product) is white sugar.

Typical commercial baked goods, particularly low-fat versions, consist mostly of carbohydrates, thanks to the flour and sweeteners. Eating such foods, which have a high glycaemic index, is associated with low levels of the 'good' HDL cholesterol. Researchers examining the eating habits of over 1,400 British men and women found that levels of HDL are inversely associated with the glycaemic index of carbohydrates consumed: the lower the glycaemic index, the higher the HDL. Perhaps even more interesting, the intake of total fat, the type of fat, cholesterol, fibre, and alcohol show no such relationship to HDL levels. (For more about the effect of high glycaemic foods on heart health, see Chapter 1.)

So here's another good reason to bake your own: you get to choose the flour! Of course you're going to use wholegrain flours, which, because of their fibre, are absorbed more slowly than white flour. Hence, wholegrain flours have a lower glycaemic index than their refined versions. They also retain all their original nutrients just like the wholegrains we describe in Chapter 20. And you don't miss the blandness of white flour because you discover the authentic flavour of wholegrain flour.

Upgrading Your Ingredients

Baking without refined wheat and sugar is not a hardship because many alternative kinds of flour and sweeteners are available. In fact, the refining of flour and sugar only began around 150 years ago – before then, using wholegrains and natural sugars was the norm.

The following sections tell you about some of the most useful and popular healthy baking ingredients, such as flour made from whole grain, natural sweeteners, and unrefined cooking oils.

Baking with wholegrain flours

You can always find wholewheat flour in supermarkets, but you may need to visit a health food store to find the full array of wholegrain flours that are available, such as:

- **Spelt flour:** This wholegrain substitute for wheat flour has a mellow flavour. Spelt is an ancient grain that has a slightly higher protein content than wheat. As with wheat flour, avoid this if you have a gluten intolerance.

- **Oat flour:** Made from hulled oats that are ground into powder, oat flour still contains most of the original nutrients. Combine it with other flours that contain gluten for baked goods that need to rise, because oats contain no gluten. You can also add oat bran to baked goods, as in the Chewy Oatmeal and Raisin Bites recipe later in this chapter, for extra cholesterol-lowering, soluble fibre.

- **Rye flour:** This tasty flour is heavier and darker than most other flours and contains less gluten than wheat. It adds depth of flavour to the Home-made Crackers with Garlic and Herbs recipe later in this chapter.

Flour spoils, like any other food, but the change is not always obvious. Check for an off odour or flavour, a sign that fats in the flour are rancid. Table 22-1 shows flour storage times to ensure that you bake with fresh flour. Remember, also, to check for weevils – small, brown insects scurrying around in the powder.

As soon as you bring flour home, take it out of the bag and store it in an air-tight canister, or store the bag or box inside an air-tight plastic bag. Keep flour cool, dry, and in the dark.

Wheat germ is the heart of the wheat kernal and is packed with nutrients such as vitamin E. After opening, store the wheat germ in a fridge.

Table 22-1	Storage Times for Flour	
Types of Flour	*Months at Room Temperature*	*Months in Fridge or Freezer*
White flour and other refined flours	6 to 12	12
Wholewheat flour	1	12
Other wholegrain flour	1	2 to 3
Wheat germ	0	2 to 3

Sweetening with natural sugars

The whole point of cakes and biscuits is that they are pleasantly sweet, and so the goal is not to eliminate all sugars completely. You can improve the nutritional value of these goodies by using smaller amounts of sweetener and including those that also provide some vitamins, minerals, or fibre. You can use maple syrup, honey, and blackstrap molasses, as well as fruits such as apples and bananas to replace the white sugar, adding nutrients and a distinctive flavour. For some other examples of substitutions you can try, see the section 'Converting recipes to healthier ingredients' later in this chapter.

Unrefined sugar cane in its natural state contains several minerals – calcium, iron, and phosphorous – as well as B vitamins, which the body needs to metabolise sugar. When the cane is refined, the juice is squeezed from the plants and boiled, producing a syrupy mixture from which sugar crystals are extracted. The brownish-black liquid that remains is molasses. The first boiling of the sugar syrup produces light molasses, the second dark molasses, and the third boiling produces blackstrap molasses. Blackstrap molasses is slightly richer in nutrients.

Brown sugar isn't a health food just because it's brown. Brown sugar is just white sugar combined with molasses.

Treat yourself to unsulphured molasses, which health food shops sell. Other names for this are Barbados or West Indies molasses. Unsulphured molasses is a better option for baked goods because the flavour is more mellow than standard supermarket molasses, and it doesn't overwhelm the flavour of other ingredients. Try the recipe for Ginger and Apple Muffins later in this chapter to experience this.

Including healthy fats

Some recipes, such as butter shortbread, just aren't themselves without you know what. But many baked goods are just as tasty and light made without the butter, using oils that contain less saturated fat and no cholesterol.

In this chapter, the cake and cracker recipes call for unrefined safflower oil, a minimally processed, quality oil. The results are rich and moist. An alternative is rapeseed oil. Olive oil is also nutritious but you probably don't want its olive flavour in most baked goods.

Oil produces a softer, more tender biscuit than butter.

Another option is to bake with one of the butter alternatives you find in the dairy section of supermarkets. (See Chapter 5 for a full description of these products.) These alternatives are made with vegetable oils to create products with no cholesterol and less fat than butter. But not all are good for baking. You need a product in 'stick' form rather than the spreadable kind, which contains ingredients that can make baking too soggy, or worse. You also want to avoid products made with partially hydrogenated oils, which contain trans fatty acids. These fats can raise both total and LDL cholesterol.

Read the labels of products that call themselves 'natural oil blend', 'buttery spread', and 'vegetable oil spread'. The fine print tells you if the product is not suitable for baking.

Using nuts and seeds

Adding some nuts to baked goods is an easy way to increase the amount you eat for their healthy monounsaturated and omega-3 fatty acid content:

- ✔ Whole and chopped nuts give a needed crunch to cakes and biscuits.

- ✔ Garnish baked goods with nuts roasted in an oven set at 220 degrees. Toss 60 grams of nuts with 1 tablespoon of oil and roast them on a baking sheet, shaking this occasionally. Roast the nuts for 10 minutes, until lightly browned. Alternatively, toast them in a dry frying pan on a medium-high heat, stirring frequently, for about 3 to 5 minutes, until they begin to brown.

- ✔ Use ground almonds to augment or substitute for a portion of the flour. The delicate flavour of almonds is welcome in all sorts of cakes. Their heart-healthy monounsaturated oils replace the saturated fat of butter. Ground almonds are one of the ingredients used in the Banana and Date Tea Loaf later in this chapter.

Almonds also contain betasitosterol, a phytonutrient that has a structure similar to cholesterol. Because of this, betasitosterol competes with cholesterol for absorption into the body and comes in first place! Consequently, less cholesterol enters the system, lowering your blood cholesterol levels.

 Nuts and seeds make special additions to all sorts of dishes. Sprinkle chopped pistachios on basmati rice pilaf and toasted flaked almonds over mixed fruit. Scatter sesame seeds on a Chinese vegetable stir-fry and add poppy seeds to baked goods, as in the later recipe for Home-made Crackers with Garlic and Herbs.

 Peanuts can cause an acute and dangerous allergic reaction in people who are sensitive to the proteins these nuts contain. People who are allergic to peanuts often react to tree nuts, such as Brazil nuts and hazelnuts, too. Seek medical advice for proper allergy testing.

 When you get them home, store nuts in airtight containers in cool, dry conditions away from light. Buy little and often, or store in a fridge or freezer, because their oil content is susceptible to oxidation.

Converting recipes to healthier ingredients

Cooks over the years have worked out many types of substitutions, such as how much honey you need to replace the sugar in a recipe. This information is handy to have when you want to convert an old recipe to fit into your current way of healthy eating, or when you discover a new recipe that sounds yummy but forbidden. The trick is to improve the nutrition without ruining the flavour and texture. Who hasn't sampled one of those wholewheat, no anything, super sweet cookies you can use as a doorstop?

Saving your eggs for baked goods

Even when watching your cholesterol, you still need eggs in your diet, especially omega-3 enriched eggs, as we describe in Chapter 1. For many people, a heart-healthy eating plan includes four eggs a week – but you decide when you eat them! If you like, save an egg or two for baked goods such as those in the recipes in this chapter. They're loaded with nutrient and fibre-rich ingredients but require egg to hold all this together. Remember, when it comes to baked goods, you're eating only part of the recipe and a small fraction of the egg the recipe asks for.

Going crackers over crackers

When preparing your own home-made crackers, you control the amount of added salt and the quality of the flour and oil. The basic formula for making crackers – just flour, a source of fat, and some liquid – is very forgiving, and so you can experiment with all sorts of ingredients. Try adding fresh and dried herbs, spices, crushed garlic, a sprinkling of Parmesan cheese, or just freshly ground black pepper. Tailor your cracker invention to what you're serving it with – such as a garlic crackers with minestrone soup, or herby crackers with salad.

If you have a child who wants to find out about baking, start with cracker making, a quick and easy process just one step beyond playing with dough.

To create your own recipes, start with the following formulas, fiddling a bit with the amounts, depending upon how the dough handles and the final baked good tastes:

✔ **125 grams of white flour:** Substitute 125 grams minus 2 tablespoons of wholewheat flour. Then, per 125 grams of flour replaced, reduce the oil by 1 tablespoon and increase the liquid (such as buttermilk or apple juice) by 1 to 2 teaspoons.

✔ **200 grams of granulated sugar:** Substitute 250 grams (175 millilitres) of honey or 240 grams (175 millilitres) of maple syrup. Then, per 200 grams of sugar replaced, decrease the liquid ingredients in the recipe by 60 millilitres, or add 30 grams of flour.

✔ **225 grams of butter, lard, or other solid shortening:** Substitute 240 millilitres of vegetable or nut oil minus 2 tablespoons.

✔ **100 millilitres of melted butter:** Use 100 millilitres of vegetable oil.

Baking with Guilt-Free Recipes

Do you feel inspired to bake? Even if you haven't turned out a batch of home-made biscuits for years or have never used an oven, give it a try, starting with the easy recipes that follow.

☞ Home-made Crackers with Garlic and Herbs

Making crackers is as much fun as baking biscuits, and definitely worth the time. You prepare a dough mixture, moisten it, and roll it out. The process is quick and easy, and with this recipe you have crackers made with the healthiest of ingredients.

Special tools required: *Baking paper*

Preparation time: *15 minutes*

Cooking time: *15 minutes*

Yield: *About 18 crackers*

70 grams oat flour	*¼ teaspoon salt*
70 grams rye flour	*60 millilitres warm water*
35 grams cornmeal	*3 tablespoons unrefined safflower oil, plus oil to brush the cracker dough*
1 clove garlic, crushed and chopped	
1 teaspoon dried mixed Italian herbs	*1 tablespoon cider vinegar*
¼ teaspoon baking soda	*½ teaspoon poppy seeds*

1 Preheat the oven to 200 degrees. Put the oat flour, rye flour, cornmeal, garlic, Italian herbs, baking soda, and salt in a large bowl. Mix together with a fork.

2 To the flour mixture, add the water, oil, and vinegar and mix thoroughly.

3 Place the dough on a work surface. Knead until the dough is stiff, around 1 to 2 minutes.

4 Cut a length of baking paper about 45 centimetres in length. Place the paper on a work surface and transfer the dough to the paper. With a floured rolling pin, roll the dough into a flat sheet about 2 to 3 millimetre thick and 30 centimetres in diameter. Toward the end of the process, sprinkle with the poppy seeds and press these into the dough as you continue to roll out the crackers.

5 Score the dough, by cutting almost all the way through with a knife, to mark out square or rectangular crackers. These allow you to break the cooked dough easily into cracker shapes. Brush with oil.

6 Place the baking paper with the dough on a baking sheet and bake for about 15 minutes, until the crackers begin to crisp and turn golden. Transfer the crackers to a cake rack to cool. Break the scored cracker dough into pieces and serve immediately, or when cooled, store in an airtight container. The crackers stay fresh for 2 to 3 days.

Vary It! *This recipe also tastes great if you add sesame seeds on top.*

Per serving: *Calories 58; Fat 3g (Saturated 0g); Cholesterol 0mg; Sodium 38mg; Carbohydrate 7g; Dietary Fibre 1g; Protein 1g.*

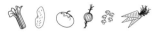

🖐 *Ginger and Apple Muffins*

These satisfying muffins provide soluble fibre, an array of heart-healthy vitamins and minerals, and healing spices. They dress up nicely, too! Top them with a dollop of reduced-fat sour cream or yogurt and more crystallised ginger. Serve with baked apples or poached pears. (You can find a recipe for poached pears in Chapter 21.) Or just spread with marmalade, for breakfast. Yummm.

Preparation time: *20 minutes*

Cooking time: *20 minutes*

Yield: *12 muffins*

240 grams wholegrain wheat flour	*¼ teaspoon salt*
1½ teaspoons baking soda	*80 grams raisins*
1 teaspoon ground ginger (more for a stronger flavour)	*30 grams chopped, crystallised ginger*
1 teaspoon cinnamon	*80 grams molasses*
½ teaspoon allspice	*125 grams unsweetened apple purée*
¼ teaspoon ground cardamom or nutmeg	*120 millilitres cultured, reduced-fat buttermilk*
	6 tablespoons unrefined safflower oil

1 Preheat the oven to 180 degrees. Using a muffin tin designed to make 12 muffins, place a paper cupcake liner in each muffin cup.

2 In a medium-sized bowl, put the wholegrain flour, baking soda, ground ginger, cinnamon, allspice, cardamom, and salt. Whisk together to blend. Briefly mix the raisins and crystallised ginger into the flour mixture.

3 Put the molasses, apple purée, buttermilk, and safflower oil in a bowl and whisk to combine.

4 Slowly pour the molasses mixture into the flour mixture, combining with a spoon. Make sure that all the flour is incorporated, but don't over-mix.

5 Spoon the batter into the muffin tin, distributing it evenly among the cups. The muffins are done when the top surface is springy to the touch, or when a toothpick inserted into the centre comes out clean, after about 20 minutes.

Vary It! *You can also bake this apple and ginger dough in a 20-centimetre-square tin. The baking time is 30 to 35 minutes.*

Tip: *Serve with a little honey to bring out the flavour.*

Per serving: *Calories 184; Fat 8g (Saturated 1g); Cholesterol 0mg; Sodium 113mg; Carbohydrate 29g; Dietary Fibre 3g; Protein 3g.*

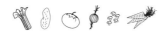

○ Banana and Date Tea Loaf

This moist, rich cake is full of nutritious ingredients, and yet tastes like a treat. The ample sweetness comes from the ripe bananas, which are a source of potassium, and from the smooth-textured dates, a source of fibre and vitamin B6. Instead of using butter to supply fat, the recipe calls for ground almonds and safflower oil, sources of healthy oils that don't clog your arteries. This recipe also gives you a chance to bake with spelt flour, which you can buy in health food stores.

Special tools required: *Food processor fitted with a metal blade*

Preparation time: *20 minutes*

Cooking time: *45 minutes*

Yield: *12 slices*

3 very ripe bananas

60 millilitres lemon juice (juice of 1 lemon)

60 millilitres unrefined safflower oil, plus extra for oiling the loaf pan

200 grams spelt flour

50 grams ground almonds

½ teaspoon baking soda

½ teaspoon baking powder

¼ teaspoon nutmeg

½ teaspoon salt

4 dates, pitted and chopped

1 Preheat the oven to 180 degrees. In a food processor fitted with a metal blade, pulse the bananas for 15 seconds, until they're smooth (or mash with a fork or potato masher). Add the lemon juice and safflower oil and process briefly to combine.

2 In a medium-sized bowl, put the spelt flour, ground almonds, baking soda, baking powder, nutmeg, and salt. Whisk together.

3 Add the banana mixture and the dates to the flour mixture. Using a spoon, mix until the ingredients are thoroughly combined.

4 Grease a 23-x-10-centimetre loaf tin with safflower oil. Turn the dough into the tin and bake for 45 minutes. The cake is done when a knife inserted into the loaf comes out clean. Serve with afternoon tea or with sliced oranges for dessert after dinner, or start your day with a piece of it rather than cereal.

Per serving: *Calories 161; Fat 7g (Saturated 1g); Cholesterol 0mg; Sodium 166mg; Carbohydrate 23g; Dietary Fibre 1g; Protein 3g.*

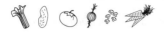

☺ Chewy Oatmeal and Raisin Bites

If you're curious about substituting ingredients, play with this recipe, packed full of all sorts of ingredients to lower cholesterol and protect the heart. Instead of unrefined safflower oil, try walnut, almond, or macadamia nut oils. You can also use currants rather than raisins and make the cookies even more chewy by using thick-cut, rolled oats rather than regular oats. Have fun.

Special tools required: *Baking paper*

Preparation time: *15 minutes*

Cooking time: *15 minutes*

Yield: *30 cookies*

120 millilitres unrefined safflower oil	*130 grams rolled oats*
120 millilitres maple syrup	*120 grams wholewheat flour*
1 egg, slightly beaten	*50 grams oat bran*
1½ teaspoons vanilla	*1 teaspoon baking powder*
½ teaspoon cinnamon	*80 grams raisins*
½ teaspoon salt	*60 grams chopped walnuts*

1 Preheat the oven to 190 degrees. In a medium bowl, use an electric mixer to cream together the oil, maple syrup, egg, vanilla, cinnamon, and salt and mix until well blended.

2 Put the rolled oats, wholewheat flour, oat bran, and baking powder in a bowl and stir together with a fork. Mix in the raisins and walnuts.

3 Slowly add the maple syrup mixture to the oat mixture, combining until all the dry ingredients are moistened. If necessary, add a tablespoon or two of water to hold the dough together.

4 Cover 2 baking sheets with baking paper. On the paper, place the dough using tablespoons to form little mounds. Flatten the dough slightly. Bake for 15 minutes, until the biscuits are lightly browned. Cool for 2 minutes on the baking sheet before using a spatula to transfer them to a wire rack to finish cooling. Store in an airtight container to preserve freshness.

Per serving: Calories 105; Fat 6g (Saturated 1g); Cholesterol 7mg; Sodium 55mg; Carbohydrate 13g; Dietary Fibre 2g; Protein 2g.

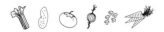

Chapter 23

Cheating with Quick Fix Desserts

In This Chapter

▶ Preparing instant desserts

▶ Creating creamy yet cholesterol-friendly puddings

▶ Enjoying sweet stuffings

Many hard-to-resist popular desserts are full of fat – especially saturated fat – which usually comes hand-in-hand with some dietary cholesterol. This chapter shows you a great, easy-to-prepare array of lower-cholesterol puddings that taste so good you're likely to forget all about the 'bad' concoctions you may be used to!

Considering Alternatives to Cream

You may think that going onto a cholesterol-balancing diet means that you can't enjoy some of your favourite 'naughty-but-nice' desserts any more. For example, you may think that cream is right out. Well, it is really. But although you can enjoy an occasional dollop of the real stuff, you can use other options that taste just as good – if not better – and aren't so full of, er, cream.

Examples of good cream substitutes are silken (or soft) tofu (no, not toffee, but *tofu* – made from soya protein), yogurt, and fromage frais. You can also use crème fraîche, which is a cross between yogurt and cream. This may sound healthier, but crème fraîche typically contains more fat and cholesterol than single cream alone. If you select the reduced-fat version, however, you get a similar taste and texture but make a significant saving in fat.

Table 23-1 shows you how these creamy products compare nutritionally.

Table 23-1	Cholesterol, Total Fat, and Saturated Fat Content in Creamy Foods per 100 grams		
Food Item	*Cholesterol*	*Total Fat*	*Saturated Fat*
Single cream	55 milligrams	19 grams	12 grams
Double cream	137 milligrams	54 grams	33 grams
Clotted cream	170 milligrams	64 grams	40 grams
Crème fraîche	113 milligrams	40 grams	27 grams
Reduced-fat crème fraîche	57 milligrams	15 grams	10 grams
Fromage frais	9 milligrams	8 grams	6 grams
Fat-free fromage frais	1 milligram	0	0
Greek yogurt (sheep's milk)	14 milligrams	6 grams	4 grams
Full-fat yogurt	11 milligrams	3 grams	2 grams
Low-fat yogurt	1 milligram	1 gram	0.7 grams
Tofu	0	4 grams	0.5 grams

Derived from: McCance and Widdowson's The Composition of Foods, 6th Summary Edition. Food Standards Agency.

As you can see, fat-free fromage frais, low-fat yogurt, and tofu are by far the best options for a quick and easy dessert. Just swirl in some chopped fruit or squished berries and you have an instant quick-fix pudding.

Toying with Tofu

Tofu is a Chinese soya bean product made by curdling soya milk with a calcium or magnesium salt, pressing together the curds, and draining away some of the whey. The resulting tofu varies from firm to soft depending on how much whey remains.

A Japanese version, known as kinugoshi, uses a seaweed extract to thicken soya milk without curdling it or draining off any whey. This produces a 'silken' tofu that has a similar texture to yogurt.

You can cut firm tofu into cubes and use it for marinating and stir-frying, whereas soft and silken tofu makes great, creamy desserts.

Because tofu is made from soya beans it contains good amounts of protein but very little fat and no cholesterol. Tofu is also a rich source of *isoflavones*, which are plant substances that help to dilate coronary arteries, reduce blood stickiness, and lower LDL cholesterol levels. Isoflavones also have an antioxidant and anti-inflammatory action that reduces the risk of your arteries hardening and furring up.

Here's a recipe for a quick, creamy tofu dessert that works as well for dinner parties as for the nursery.

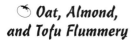

⟲ Oat, Almond, and Tofu Flummery

Flummery is an Old English term for a soft, sweet pudding that usually contains a grain such as rice or oats. This flummery contains four ingredients with a cholesterol-lowering action: tofu, oats, almonds, and bananas. Serve with fresh berries and a drizzle of honey.

Preparation time: *3 minutes plus 1 hour chilling time*

Serves: *6*

300 grams silken tofu (soft)

1 ripe banana

Dash of pure vanilla extract

100 grams rolled oats

50 grams flaked almonds

1 Puree together the tofu, banana, and vanilla extract in a food processor.

2 Add the oats and flaked almonds and mix together. Chill for one hour before serving.

Vary it: *You can top this flummery with some berries if serving it at a dinner party.*

Per serving: *Calories 158; Fat 7g (Saturated 1g); Cholesterol 0mg; Sodium 3mg; Carbohydrate 19g; Dietary Fibre 3g; Protein 7g.*

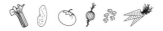

Fooling Around with Fromage Frais

Fromage frais is a white soft curd originating from France and is an excellent alternative to cream in a low-cholesterol diet. The name literally means 'fresh cheese'. Like harder cheeses, manufacturers make fromage frais by adding a mixture of enzymes, called *rennet*, to milk. They then stir the mixture so that it doesn't divide into curds and whey, but thickens into a yogurt-like texture. In contrast, yogurt is made by fermenting milk with bacterial cultures.

Fruit fools are traditional English desserts made simply by whipping up some sweetened puréed fruit with thick custard or cream. People usually make fools with tart, acidic fruits such as gooseberries, lemon, blackcurrants, and rhubarb to balance the added sugar. (Okay, so rhubarb isn't technically a fruit, but a leaf stalk or, strictly speaking, a fleshy petiole!)

If you use a naturally sweet fruit such as raspberries, however, you can make a great fool that doesn't need additional sugar and is healthier than versions made with cream. Here's a recipe for Raspberry Fool that's so simple to make, it's literally fool proof!

🍑 Raspberry Fool

This delicious fool is really easy to make and extremely tasty, yet delightfully low in saturated fat and cholesterol. Use fresh or frozen raspberries – whichever you can find, depending on the season. Just avoid the tinned ones that come in thick, sweetened syrup.

Special tools required: *Food processor fitted with a metal blade*

Preparation time: *2 minutes*

Serves: *4*

225 grams raspberries, fresh or frozen	*4 sprigs mint*
300 millilitres plain very low-fat fromage frais	*Handful of raspberries for garnish*

1 Place the raspberries and fromage frais in a food processor fitted with a metal blade. Process to form a smooth purée.

2 Pile the fool mixture into 4 martini or wine glasses.

3 Decorate with a mint and raspberry garnish.

Vary it: *You can vary this fool as much as you want by substituting other berries or puréed fruit for the raspberries, or adding a handful of flaked almonds as garnish. You can produce a raspberry-ripple effect by puréeing the raspberries separately and folding them into the fromage frais. Low-fat Greek yogurt makes a good substitute for the fromage frais, too.*

Per serving: *Calories 99; Fat 0g (Saturated 0g); Cholesterol 12mg; Sodium 94mg; Carbohydrate 18g; Dietary Fibre 4g; Protein 3g.*

Going Bananas

Bananas are among the most popular fruits and, when mashed, they add an extra creaminess to deserts. Bananas are also nutritious and a good source of potassium, which helps to lower blood pressure. In fact, a single banana provides one tenth of your daily potassium needs.

Bananas also contain a soluble fibre called *pectin*, which lowers LDL cholesterol by reducing its absorption from your intestines, and are a good source of vitamin B6, which helps to control your homocysteine levels (for more on homocysteine, see Chapter 1).

Substances known as *biogenic amines* (serotonin and dopamine) that influence mood are also present in bananas, as is an amino acid, *tryptophan*, which your body converts into serotonin for a potentially calming effect. All this, and bananas are fat-free and cholesterol-free, too!

Bananas taste even sweeter when you bake them, as in the following recipe for baked bananas with pumpkin seeds and lime.

☺ Baked Bananas with Pumpkin Seeds and Lime

Pumpkin seeds contain a type of antioxidant called lignan, which can lower cholesterol levels and improve glucose control. Pumpkin seeds also provide a nice crunch in this otherwise soft and delicious dessert.

Tip: When using lime or lemon zest in a recipe, use only unwaxed lemons, which are usually organic. That way you don't get the wax (with all the dust and dirt it picks up) in your food.

Preparation time: *17 minutes*

Serves: *4*

4 ripe bananas	*4 teaspoons runny honey*
40 grams pumpkin seeds	*Juice and zest of 2 limes*

1 Preheat the oven to 180 degrees.

2 Cut the bananas in half lengthways and arrange them in an oven-proof dish.

3 Sprinkle with the pumpkin seeds, honey, lime juice and zest.

4 Bake for 15 minutes.

Per serving: Calories 189; Fat 5g (Saturated 1g); Cholesterol 0mg; Sodium 4mg; Carbohydrate 37g; Dietary Fibre 3g; Protein 4g.

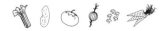

Fooling around with bananas

Bananas are one of the few foods with real potential as an aphrodisiac. They contain an alkaloid called bufotenine that acts on the brain to improve mood, self-confidence, and increase sex drive. You find bufotenine in the greatest quantity just beneath the skin, and you can obtain it by baking the banana and scraping away the soft flesh from inside the skin. Consider yourself warned!

Stuffing Yourself Silly

You can make a quick dessert by stuffing fruit with a creamy concoction of fat-free fromage frais, silken tofu, or reduced-fat crème fraîche. Fruits that contain a stone that leaves a natural hollow when you remove it are the easiest to stuff in this way. Try dates, apricots, lychees, rambutan (a sort of hairy lychee), large plums, peaches, and nectarines. Use very ripe fruits and serve them raw for maximum health benefits.

Even if a fruit doesn't have a natural hollow left when you remove the stone or core, you can make a suitable concave. Try the later Turkish Delight Fresh Figs recipe that opens out succulent, juicy fresh figs to create a tulip-shaped cup ready for a creamy spoonful of something delectable.

You can also core and stuff apples with a sweet mix of raisins, nuts, and honey and bake them in the oven for a quick, nutritious dessert, as in the following recipe for Baked Apples Stuffed with Raisins. Or for something really different, try a savoury stuffing such as the breakfast recipe for Baked Apples with Turkey Sausage and Mango Chutney in Chapter 6.

☺ Baked Apples Stuffed with Raisins

Apples and raisins are both good sources of soluble fibre, which helps to lower cholesterol. The honey in this recipe appears in place of the more usual brown sugar for a lesser effect on blood glucose levels. These apples are delicious served with a dollop of reduced-fat crème fraîche.

Special tools required: *Apple corer*

Preparation time: *45 minutes*

Serves: *4*

4 medium Bramley cooking apples, washed	*4 tablespoons raisins*
200 millilitres water	*4 teaspoons runny honey*
Juice and zest of one lemon	*½ teaspoon cinnamon*

1 Preheat the oven to 180 degrees.

2 Core the apples, cut 1 centimetre off the end of the core, and replug the bottom of the hole. Run a knife around the outside middle of each apple, scoring the peel to help stop the apples splitting as they bake. Place the apples upright in a small baking tray

3 Mix the water and lemon juice together. Fill each apple with 1 tablespoon of the water and pour the rest into the baking dish, around the apples.

4 Mix the raisins, lemon zest, honey, and cinnamon together. Stuff each apple with a quarter of the raisin mix.

5 Bake for 35 to 45 minutes, or until the apples are soft. Baste with pan juices twice during cooking. Serve with the juices from the pan.

Per serving: Calories 181; Fat 0g (Saturated 0g); Cholesterol 0mg; Sodium 8mg; Carbohydrate 48g; Dietary Fibre 6g; Protein 1g.

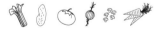

☺ Turkish Delight Fresh Figs

If you're a fan of Turkish delight you're going to love this dish, made from fresh figs. Figs are full of fibre, which has a cholesterol-lowering action. Rose water smells and tastes divine and is available from health food stores and pharmacies. Only buy 100 per cent pure distilled rose water, and not the cheaper versions made with synthetic flavourings and preservatives. If you have fresh rose petals in the garden, use them as an additional garnish on the plate!

Special tools required: *Blender or food processor fitted with a metal blade*

Preparation time: *5 minutes*

Serves: *4*

12 ripe fresh figs	*Juice and zest of 1 lemon*
250 grams silken tofu (soft)	*3 tablespoons pure distilled rose water*
4 teaspoons runny honey	*4 tablespoons chopped pistachios*

1 Cut a deep cross in the top of each fig, without cutting all the way through the fruit. Gently open out the figs quarters to form a tulip shape.

2 Place the tofu, honey, lemon juice and zest, rose water, and pistachios in a blender or food processor fitted with a metal blade, and process until smooth.

3 Spoon the creamy rose-scented tofu mix into the centre of each fig.

4 Serve three to a plate, garnished with pistachios. Drizzle with additional rose water if you like.

Per serving: *Calories 215; Fat 6g (Saturated 1g); Cholesterol 0mg; Sodium 5mg; Carbohydrate 40g; Dietary Fibre 6g; Protein 6g.*

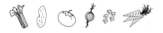

Part VII
The Part of Tens

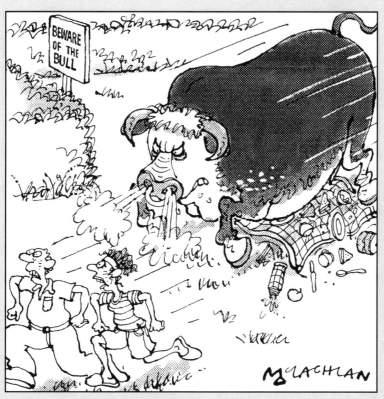

'You and your healthy picnic in the countryside with plenty of exercise.'

In this part . . .

This part gives you lots of useful advice, such as explaining why certain beverages protect the heart from disease, and why waving goodbye to high-sugar drinks – which can trigger chemical effects in the body that affect cholesterol balance – makes sense. We also give you a recipe for a tasty drink to sip while you read.

The other chapter in this part offers advice on buying healthy ingredients that aren't necessarily expensive if you know how and where to shop. This helps to ensure that your kitchen is filled with quality foods for evermore!

Chapter 24

Ten Beverages That Say, 'Here's to Your Health!'

You hear about the importance of drinking water over and over again, and now you're going to hear it one more time. No substitute for the plain stuff, which flushes your system and refreshes your body, exists. Water is essential for nutrient absorption, chemical reactions, and proper circulation in the body. In these many ways, drinking sufficient water supports the health of your heart.

But what about the other liquids you drink from morn till night? This chapter gives you an overview of some of the most common beverages and takes a look at the health benefits of these drinks, as well as some of the drawbacks. Why not sit with a glass of your favourite drink right now as you read about some of the healthier ways to quench your thirst?

Benefiting from Black Tea

If you don't already drink tea, give it a try. Yes, it has less of a kick than coffee, but your body does adjust. You'll soon hum along on tea just as you did on the high-octane stuff. To make the transition from coffee to tea easier, start with a complex, richly flavoured tea, such as Earl Grey, which is perfumed with bergamot oranges.

But these pleasures aside, tea benefits the heart in many ways. Here are some reasons, based on the results of many large studies, to brew a pot full of tea (it's a great British institution, don't you know!):

✔ Antioxidants in tea help prevent LDL cholesterol from *oxidising* – a harmful chemical change that hastens the development of atherosclerosis. In fact, tea contains even higher levels of antioxidants than many fruits and vegetables.

✔ Experts now consider heart disease to be an inflammatory process, and phytonutrients in tea have an anti-inflammatory effect.

✔ Tea helps keep blood vessels functioning normally.

If this section has inspired you to try some tea, don't start with the pack of tea lurking in the cupboard forever. When you buy tea in the supermarket, it's probably already a year old, and so keep tea no longer than six months to a year. Black tea stays fresh longer than green or white tea.

Enjoying Green Tea

The delicate flavour of green tea, suggestive of twigs and herbs, is a refreshing change from the richer flavour of black tea. Sip it slowly, to savour its subtle flavour, as is the practice in the traditional Japanese tea ceremony. The flavour of green tea is also a perfect complement to Japanese specialities such as sushi, sashimi, and tempura.

Green tea contains more beneficial nutrients than black tea, which is fermented, a process that converts some of these compounds into weaker versions. The nutrients in green tea that are most important for heart health are the polyphenols, some of which are antioxidants and others anti-inflammatory substances (see Chapter 1). Many studies, although not all, have shown that green tea helps to mildly lower total cholesterol, increasing the 'good' HDL cholesterol while lowering the 'bad' LDL, and protecting LDL from oxidation. Green tea may also help prevent the formation of blood clots that can cause heart attack and stroke. Research published in the *Journal of the American Medical Association* in 2006 also suggests that green tea consumption is associated with reduced mortality from cardiovascular disease.

One of the polyphenols in green tea, epigallocatechin gallate (EGCG), is a mouthful and an antioxidant 20 times stronger than vitamin E.

Considering Chamomile Tea

Chamomile tea earns its place in a heart-healthy diet because of its anti-inflammatory properties. Very mild but chronic (long-term) inflammation of body tissues such as those lining the arteries can set the stage for heart disease. Chamomile tea bags are now for sale in just about every supermarket: steep in a cup of hot water for five to ten minutes.

Curbing coffee to cut cholesterol

The latest word on whether coffee raises cholesterol is that it does, when you drink too much. Aim to drink no more than one or two cups a day.

Earlier research suggests that the brewing method is the deciding factor. Boiled coffee, the kind favoured in Scandinavia, raises cholesterol levels, but filtered coffee does not. However, conclusions from a more recent Norwegian study, published in 2001 in the *American Journal of Clinical Nutrition,* question the safety of drinking even filtered coffee. When participants who drank an average of 4 cups of filtered coffee daily for one year abstained for the test period of six weeks, they experienced a drop in total cholesterol and homocysteine levels, both risk factors for heart disease (see

Chapter 1). Controversy surrounds this issue, but drinking excessive amounts of coffee isn't a good idea.

Experiment with coffee alternatives, which are healthier drinks than actual coffee because of what they don't contain, specifically, caffeine and alkaloid compounds. These compounds are cardiac stimulants that can stress the heart muscle and lead to heart palpitations. Coffee substitutes consist of clever mixes of ingredients such as roast barley, chicory, figs, orange peel, oats, rye, roast soy, roast acorns, and even dandelions! The results are surprisingly satisfying, often pleasantly bitter, and usually rich-tasting. Gourmet versions are scented with nuts and carob, which is an alternative to chocolate.

Chamomile also has a mild relaxing effect, and so it's the right drink when you're feeling stressed. It also helps you sleep.

Winning with Red Wine

The civilised habit of having a couple of glasses of wine with lunch and dinner, an established part of meals in Europe, is considered one of the main reasons that the French have a low incidence of heart disease, despite having high cholesterol and eating a diet that includes fatty duck, cream sauces, cheese, and pâté.

Flavonoids, also known as polyphenols, in red wine are mainly responsible for these benefits. One important flavonoid, quercetin, has antioxidant and anti-inflammatory properties. Tannins, which are found in the skin and seed of grapes and give red wine its colour, protect the body from harmful cholesterol. Red wine raises 'good' HDL cholesterol levels and promotes the break-up of 'bad' LDL cholesterol. It may also help keep arteries open.

Choose red wine over white and rosé, both of which contain only relatively small amounts of heart-protective tannins.

Alcohol may reduce the risk of coronary heart disease, but of course, abusing alcohol increases the chance of life-threatening liver disease as well as heart disease. The Department of Health advises that men should not regularly drink more than 3 to 4 units per day, and women should not have more than 2 or 3 units per day. 1 unit of alcohol (10 grams) is equivalent to:

- ✔ 300 millilitres (½ pint) normal strength beer, lager, or cider that is 3.5 per cent alcohol in strength. But remember that many lagers now contain 5 per cent and some versions supply as much as 9 per cent alcohol.

  or

- ✔ 100 millilitres wine (10 per cent alcohol by volume). But be aware that most wines are now much stronger (12 to 15 per cent alcohol) and many pubs sell wine in 250- millilitre glasses. Depending on the alcohol percentage, a bottle of wine typically contains between 8 and 11 units of alcohol.

  or

- ✔ 50 millilitres sherry.

  or

- ✔ 25 millilitres of 40 per cent spirits. Many pubs now serve 35-millilitre measures as standard, and often serve a double unless you specifically say you want a single.

A bottle (275 millilitres) of 5 per cent alcopop contains around 1.5 units of alcohol.

Working out exactly how many units you've had is often difficult. To help, take a look at the www.drinkaware.co.uk website and use their handy unit calculator. You may get a surprise when you add up what you drink – it's often more than you think.

Aim to have two or more alcohol-free days per week.

Enjoying a Drop of the Grape

Drinking purple grape juice, just like red wine, benefits the heart in many ways such as inhibiting the formation of blood clots. A study published in the medical journal, *Circulation*, in 1999, showed that grape juice also prevents LDL cholesterol from oxidising and helps keep arteries elastic. The 15 adults with coronary artery disease who participated in this study consumed 350 to 455 millilitres of purple grape juice daily for two weeks. Admittedly this quantity of juice adds calories but it's certainly a better choice than a sugary cola.

If you decide to start drinking lots of grape juice, have only about 125 millilitres at a time. Sip it slowly, preferably with food, to avoid quickly swallowing a lot of sugar, which can rapidly elevate blood glucose levels (see Chapter 1)

Like red wine, purple grape juice protects your heart in the following ways:

✔ Reduces the stickiness of blood to help prevent blood clots.

✔ Protects LDL cholesterol from oxidation, which promotes the accumulation of plaque on artery walls.

✔ Triggers the arteries to dilate when necessary to respond to an increased flow in blood.

Read the label and make sure that you buy juice made with Concord grapes, the dark purple-blue grape with the highest levels of antioxidants. White and red grape juices have far less. The juice is very sweet while the tannin-rich skins are super tart.

For a non-alcoholic treat, look for gourmet brands of grape juice that are designed to taste like wine.

Going for Orange

Buy some juicy oranges, such as smooth, thin-skinned Valencias, and give them a squeeze. Oranges are full of nutrients, especially when juice is freshly-made. Although the mineral content remains the same, the amount of the more fragile vitamin C and B vitamins in orange juice rapidly declines over time. For instance, vitamin C is destroyed when exposed to air, and folate and thiamin are lost to heat. So it's best to squeeze and quickly drink your OJ for the greatest benefits. Here is a list of nutrients in orange juice that are good for the heart:

✔ All sorts of antioxidants, including vitamin C.

✔ Vitamin B6 and folate, both associated with lower levels of homocysteine (see Chapters 1 and 2 for more on homocysteine).

✔ Potassium in good amounts, an important mineral for preventing high blood pressure.

Including Other Fruit Juices (but Not Too Much!)

Besides grape and orange juice, how about other good-for-you juices such as apple, apricot, pear, pineapple, papaya, and watermelon – great mixed with orange juice. And don't forget such exotics as pomegranate and cherry juice. (See Chapter 8 to find out their benefits.) Just as eating a variety of fruit lets you take in an assortment of nutrients, drinking their juice does the same thing.

However, juice also has its downside. You can quickly add a surprising amount of calories to your daily intake as you guzzle glassfuls of juice to quench your thirst. Take a look at Table 24-1.

Table 24-1	Calories in 240 millilitres of Fruit Juice
Type of Juice	*Calories (Kilocalories)*
Apple juice (unsweetened)	91
Cranberry juice	146
Grape juice (unsweetened)	110
Orange juice (unsweetened)	110
Pineapple juice (unsweetened)	98

Drinking 240 millilitres of orange juice is equivalent to eating two oranges. Although the bulk of actual oranges prevent you from quickly taking in all the sugar in this amount of fruit, you can gulp a glass of juice in 5 seconds and cause your blood sugar to rise rapidly. Making this a habit can contribute to weight gain and even lead to insulin resistance, and consequently high cholesterol (see Chapter 1.)

To reduce calories and concentrated sugars, dilute fruit juice with plain water, soda water, or herbal tea. Try these combinations:

- Orange juice and ginger tea
- Grapefruit juice and mint tea
- Grape juice and sparkling water

Most commercial fruit juice is missing the soluble fibre that is in the whole fruit. But you can remedy this by making your own juice. Use a blender that liquefies the entire peeled fruit, rather than a juice extractor, which removes all the pulp and fibre. Then, what you have is a really healthy smoothie. When making your own smoothies from whole fruit, each serving you put in can count towards your 5-a-day goal. Shop-bought smoothies are often made with fruit juice plus yogurt, however, so the same doesn't necessarily apply.

Lifting a Stein

Imagine! A beer a day keeps the doctor away. Some research suggests that drinking the equivalent of one beer a day can reduce the level of fatty deposits in artery walls. Like red wine, which is accepted as good for the heart in moderation, beer is full of flavonoid antioxidants that can slow ageing and may help to prevent heart disease. Dark beers contain more flavonoids than light.

The prescription for beer is one a day. Drinking more than this does not produce additional benefits, and you may end up with a genuine beer belly, which can stress the heart.

Sipping Healthy Sparkling Beverages

Instead of regular commercial soft drinks, enjoy some of the sparkling alternatives now available. Try some carbonated apple juice, a little sparkling cider, or even sparkling grapefruit juice (just add soda or sparkling mineral water). Ginger beer is also worth discovering.

But always read the labels. Manufacturers have a habit of adding sugar and artificial sweeteners to all sorts of speciality fruit juices, sparkling drinks, and herbal tea mixtures. Although these drinks are healthier than heavily sweetened, acidic colas, they aren't necessarily health foods because they often contain non-nutritive sweeteners.

Lassi Come Home

In India, a *lassi* is a popular chilled yogurt drink. The yogurt is mixed with water and/or crushed ice and is flavoured with salt, or served sweet by mixing it with sugar, fruit, and fruit juices. Mint and cumin are also common additions. All Indian restaurants serve lassi, but making it in your own kitchen is easy. For a delightful treat, put 250 millilitres plain, low-fat yogurt and the flesh of one mango in a blender. Add a pinch of cumin and blend until light and frothy. Enjoy this drink at room temperature, chill in the fridge, or simply pour over ice. Serve with Indian food such as the Chicken Tandoori with Yogurt-Mint Sauce in Chapter 13.

Chapter 25

Ten Ways to Trim Your Food Bill

Saving money on food is easy, because prices for meals vary so much depending on whether you eat at home or out, which restaurants you go to, and how cleverly you shop for groceries. Here are ten ways to cut food expenditures that are just a matter of thinking ahead and trying new places to shop and eat. If you save just £1 a day, that comes to £365 a year – and that's not peanuts!

Shopping More Often but Buying Less

When you shop for perishable items, buy only as much as you think you're going to eat before it goes off. Follow Noah's example, and allow items into the kitchen, two by two. You can always finish two avocados before they go rotten, but not three or four.

Freezing a loaf of sliced bread means you can take slices out, as and when you need them, without letting the whole loaf go stale.

Showing Up at Farmers Markets

Buy seasonal; buy local. Why pay an apple's travel expenses from Central Europe, or even farther afield, when you can purchase one that's grown closer to home? At farmers' markets you also find reasonably priced speciality items such as baby lettuce, heirloom tomatoes, fresh herbs, and speciality cheeses produced on a small scale. Produce at farmer's markets often costs about the same as fruit and vegetables at the supermarket, but those bought in the farmers market are almost certainly fresher and of higher quality. To find farm shops, pick-your-own farms, and farmers' markets in your area, visit www.farmersmarkets.net.

Buying Produce in Season

Take advantage of fruit and vegetables in season, because when the supply is plentiful, prices drop, and flavour is at its peak. In-season produce is also likely to contain more of the antioxidants and phytonutrients that help control cholesterol. Of course, you're probably used to seeing strawberries for sale at Christmas, but despite their holiday colours, these berries are not a winter fruit.

The website of the Women's Food and Farming Union contains a handy table showing the seasonal availability of fruit and vegetables in the UK – very useful for the more exotic produced available. Check it out at www.wfu.org.uk/seasonalveg.htm.

Going Shopping with a Plan

Experts advise you to have a written shopping list and stick to it when you head out to do your Christmas shopping. The same advice applies when you're on your way to the supermarket. This way, you aren't as likely to pick up gourmet and exotic foods that you don't really need. Alternatively, you can plan to have no plan at all. Wander the aisles and look for special bargains on offer, such 'buy one, get one free'. If you see that pork loin, new potatoes, apples, and cabbage are on sale, that's nearly a complete dinner menu. Take care not to select less healthy offers that encourage you to eat foods that are high in fat, sugar, or salt, however.

Scouting Out Neighbourhood Food Shops

You can shop at a snazzy supermarket and buy a few Medjool dates for £5, or you can go to a little speciality ethnic store and buy another type of date that's equally tasty for half the price. The same goes for other delicatessen items such as feta and marinated olives. Taking the time to find new places to shop can save you money.

Wising Up On How To Keep Food Fresh

Storing your food properly prevents it from spoiling before you can use it. If you have to throw away food that you didn't store or freeze properly, it's like throwing out your hard-earned cash. Know the special storage requirements of all sorts of foods, from flour and nuts to basil and filet of sole. Here are some suggestions:

✔ Collect storage containers of various sizes and with airtight lids, and keep plastic freezer bags on hand.

✔ Make room in your refrigerator or freezer for wholegrain flour and nuts. Store them in tightly lidded containers or seal them in airtight plastic bags. Wholegrain flour stays fresh for 2 to 3 months in the refrigerator and most nuts keep at least 6 months.

✔ Put perishables such as avocados and mangoes on display in your kitchen where you can see them every day and so are more likely to eat them.

✔ Resist the temptation to keep cooking oils in clear glass bottles in a kitchen window. Light causes oil to go rancid even faster than exposure to air.

Stocking Up on Stock

Always have some sort of stock on hand – vegetable, meat, or poultry-based – frozen in 1-litre portions. Use these to create a quick soup (see Chapter 9 for some ideas) made with trimmings and leftovers, a thrifty way to use up all sorts of foods in your fridge. At last, a free lunch!

Travelling with Snacks

Don't leave home without something to munch on, whether on a cross-country trip with your family or just an outing for the day in your home town. You're sure to eat healthier and far cheaper than if you rely on fast food outlets and coffee shops when you feel peckish. If you're looking for snacks that are low in cholesterol and high in healthy fats and fibre, try these:

✔ Peanuts and a banana, which is great for travelling because the banana comes with its own handy package and doesn't drip juice.

✔ Cut, raw veg in a plastic bag and yogurt dip stored in the yogurt container.

Keep perishable snacks such as yogurt dip in a small cooler.

✔ Ready-made hummus, sold as party food in small containers, and wholemeal pittas.

✔ Cracker sandwiches made with a nut butter such as almond butter, which is readily available in health food stores. Use crackers that don't contain partially-hydrogenated oil, and add a nice juicy apple.

Bring along something to drink. Whether in the car or at work, make sure that you have fresh, bottled water handy. Then, when you feel tired and thirsty, reach for what you really need – a refreshing glass of water – instead of making a pit stop for an expensive sugary, fizzy drink or frozen latte.

Finding Cheap Restaurant Eats

Often, the best restaurant meals, and the best deals, are in those modest ethnic restaurants that feature the cooking of various cultures, such as Italian fish restaurants and Spanish tapas bars. As long as you remain willing to make some mistakes, you can find new favourites that you can frequent regularly without breaking your dining-out budget.

If you want only a smallish meal, try ordering one or two appetisers rather than a pricy main course. Ordering this way also lets you put together a creative vegetarian meal; for instance, a salad with bean soup.

Cooking at Home More Often

Preparing food at home usually amounts to a fraction of the cost of eating out. Even when you spend the same amount, the pounds that give you wild salmon and fresh pineapple in a supermarket buy only fish and chips in a restaurant. And if you have leftovers when you cook for yourself, you have two meals for the price of one – you've guessed it, make some all-in soup! Cooking at home also gives you control over the quality and nature of your ingredients. You can fashion meals with all those foodstuffs that help to bring down a raised cholesterol level.

Index

• *C* •

• N •

• *Q* •

• *R* •

• *S* •

• Z •

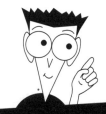

FOR DUMMIES®

Do Anything. Just Add Dummies

UK editions

BUSINESS

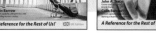

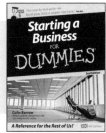

Starting a Business For Dummies
978-0-470-51806-9

Understanding Business Accounting For Dummies
978-0-470-99245-6

Lean Six Sigma For Dummies
978-0-470-75626-3

FINANCE

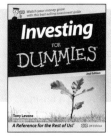

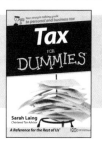

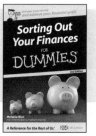

Investing For Dummies
978-0-470-99280-7

Tax For Dummies
978-0-470-99811-3

Sorting Out Your Finances For Dummies
978-0-470-69515-9

PROPERTY

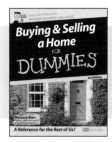

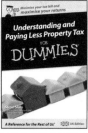

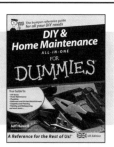

Buying & Selling a Home For Dummies
978-0-470-99448-1

Understanding and Paying Less Property Tax For Dummies
978-0-470-75872-4

DIY & Home Maintenance All-In-One For Dummies
978-0-7645-7054-4

Backgammon For Dummies
978-0-470-77085-6

Body Language For Dummies
978-0-470-51291-3

British Sign Language For Dummies
978-0-470-69477-0

Children's Health For Dummies
978-0-470-02735-6

Cognitive Behavioural Coaching For Dummies
978-0-470-71379-2

Counselling Skills For Dummies
978-0-470-51190-9

Digital Marketing For Dummies
978-0-470-05793-3

Divorce for Dummies
978-0-7645-7030-8

eBay.co.uk For Dummies, 2nd Edition
978-0-470-51807-6

English Grammar For Dummies
978-0-470-05752-0

Fertility & Infertility For Dummies
978-0-470-05750-6

Genealogy Online For Dummies
978-0-7645-7061-2

Golf For Dummies
978-0-470-01811-8

Green Living For Dummies
978-0-470-06038-4

Hypnotherapy For Dummies
978-0-470-01930-6

Available wherever books are sold. For more information or to order direct go to www.wiley.com or call +44 (0) 1243 843291

13902_p1

FOR DUMMIES®

A world of resources to help you grow

UK editions

SELF-HELP

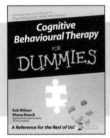

Cognitive Behavioural Therapy For Dummies

978-0-470-01838-5

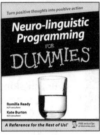

Neuro-linguistic Programming For Dummies

978-0-7645-7028-5

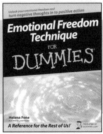

Emotional Freedom Technique For Dummies

978-0-470-75876-2

HEALTH

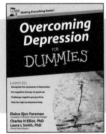

Overcoming Depression For Dummies

978-0-470-69430-5

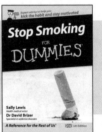

IBS For Dummies

978-0-470-51737-6

Stop Smoking For Dummies

978-0-470-99456-6

HISTORY

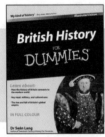

British History For Dummies

978-0-470-99468-9

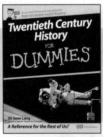

Twentieth Century History For Dummies

978-0-470-51015-5

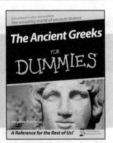

The Ancient Greeks For Dummies

978-0-470-98787-2

Inventing For Dummies
978-0-470-51996-7

Job Hunting and Career Change All-In-One For Dummies
978-0-470-51611-9

Motivation For Dummies
978-0-470-76035-2

Origami Kit For Dummies
978-0-470-75857-1

Personal Development All-In-One For Dummies
978-0-470-51501-3

PRINCE2 For Dummies
978-0-470-51919-6

Psychometric Tests For Dummies
978-0-470-75366-8

Raising Happy Children For Dummies
978-0-470-05978-4

Starting and Running a Business All-in-One For Dummies
978-0-470-51648-5

Sudoku for Dummies
978-0-470-01892-7

The British Citizenship Test For Dummies, 2nd Edition
978-0-470-72339-5

Time Management For Dummies
978-0-470-77765-7

Wills, Probate, & Inheritance Tax For Dummies, 2nd Edition
978-0-470-75629-4

Winning on Betfair For Dummies, 2nd Edition
978-0-470-72336-4

Available wherever books are sold. For more information or to order direct go to www.wiley.com or call +44 (0) 1243 843291

13902_p2

FOR DUMMIES®

The easy way to get more done and have more fun

LANGUAGES

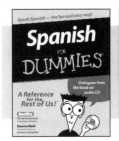
978-0-7645-5194-9

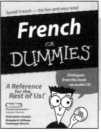
978-0-7645-5193-2

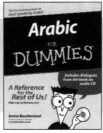
978-0-471-77270-5

MUSIC

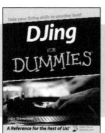
978-0-7645-9904-0

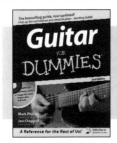
978-0-470-03275-6
UK Edition

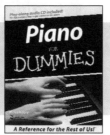
978-0-7645-5105-5

SCIENCE & MATHS

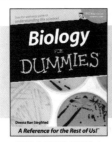
978-0-7645-5326-4

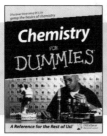
978-0-7645-5430-8

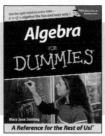
978-0-7645-5325-7

Art For Dummies
978-0-7645-5104-8

Baby & Toddler Sleep Solutions For Dummies
978-0-470-11794-1

Bass Guitar For Dummies
978-0-7645-2487-5

Brain Games For Dummies
978-0-470-37378-1

Christianity For Dummies
978-0-7645-4482-8

Filmmaking For Dummies, 2nd Edition
978-0-470-38694-1

Forensics For Dummies
978-0-7645-5580-0

German For Dummies
978-0-7645-5195-6

Hobby Farming For Dummies
978-0-470-28172-7

Jewelry Making & Beading For Dummies
978-0-7645-2571-1

Knitting for Dummies, 2nd Edition
978-0-470-28747-7

Music Composition For Dummies
978-0-470-22421-2

Physics For Dummies
978-0-7645-5433-9

Sex For Dummies, 3rd Edition
978-0-470-04523-7

Solar Power Your Home For Dummies
978-0-470-17569-9

Tennis For Dummies
978-0-7645-5087-4

The Koran For Dummies
978-0-7645-5581-7

U.S. History For Dummies
978-0-7645-5249-6

Wine For Dummies, 4th Edition
978-0-470-04579-4

Available wherever books are sold. For more information or to order direct go to www.wiley.com or call +44 (0) 1243 843291

13902_p3

FOR DUMMIES®

Helping you expand your horizons and achieve your potential

COMPUTER BASICS

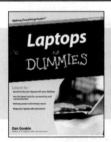

978-0-470-27759-1

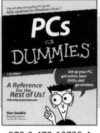

978-0-470-13728-4

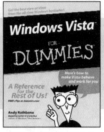

978-0-471-75421-3

DIGITAL LIFESTYLE

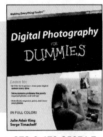

978-0-470-25074-7

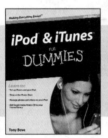

978-0-470-39062-7

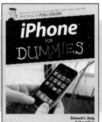

978-0-470-17469-2

WEB & DESIGN

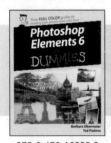

978-0-470-19238-2

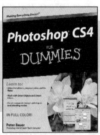

978-0-470-32725-8

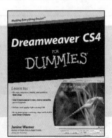

978-0-470-34502-3

Access 2007 For Dummies
978-0-470-04612-8

Adobe Creative Suite 3 Design Premium
All-in-One Desk Reference For Dummies
978-0-470-11724-8

AutoCAD 2009 For Dummies
978-0-470-22977-4

C++ For Dummies, 5th Edition
978-0-7645-6852-7

Computers For Seniors For Dummies
978-0-470-24055-7

Excel 2007 All-In-One Desk Reference F
or Dummies
978-0-470-03738-6

Flash CS3 For Dummies
978-0-470-12100-9

Mac OS X Leopard For Dummies
978-0-470-05433-8

Macs For Dummies, 10th Edition
978-0-470-27817-8

Networking All-in-One Desk Reference
For Dummies, 3rd Edition
978-0-470-17915-4

Office 2007 All-in-One Desk Reference
For Dummies
978-0-471-78279-7

Search Engine Optimization For
Dummies, 2nd Edition
978-0-471-97998-2

Second Life For Dummies
978-0-470-18025-9

The Internet For Dummies, 11th Edition
978-0-470-12174-0

Visual Studio 2008 All-In-One Desk
Reference For Dummies
978-0-470-19108-8

Web Analytics For Dummies
978-0-470-09824-0

Windows XP For Dummies, 2nd Edition
978-0-7645-7326-2

Available wherever books are sold. For more information or to order direct go to www.wiley.com or call +44 (0) 1243 843291

13902_p4